YOUR PREGNANCY & BIRTH

FOURTH EDITION

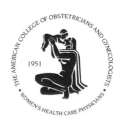

The American College of
Obstetricians and Gynecologists
Women's Health Care Physicians

Your Pregnancy & Birth, Fourth Edition, was developed by a panel of experts working in consultation with staff of the American College of Obstetricians and Gynecologists (ACOG):

Editorial Task Force
Members
Bonnie J. Dattel, MD
Nancy Chescheir, MD
Charles Lockwood, MD
Susan F. Meade, RNC, FPNP
Lynnae K. Millar, MD
Laura E. Riley, MD
Catherine Y. Spong, MD
Paul G. Tomich, MD

ACOG staff
Sterling B. Williams, MD, MS, FACOG
Rebecca D. Rinehart, Director of Publications
Tatum Birdsall, Senior Editor
Thomas P. Dineen, Associate Director of Publications
Barbara Gasque, Design

The assistance of the following people is greatly appreciated:
Chris Briscoe/Index Stock, *Cover photograph*
Marian Wiseman, *Editorial assistance*
John Yanson, *Illustration*

Library of Congress Cataloging-in-Publication Data

ACOG guide to planning for pregnancy, birth, and beyond.
   Your pregnancy and birth / American College of Obstetricians and Gynecologists.-- 4th ed.
        p. cm.
   Previously published in 1990 under the title: ACOG guide to planning for pregnancy, birth, and beyond.
   Includes index.
   ISBN 0-696-22591-3 (alk. paper)
   1. Pregnancy--Popular works. 2. Childbirth--Popular works. I. American College of Obstetricians and Gynecologists. II. Title.

   RG525.A26 2005
   618.2--dc22
                                    2005000052

Designed as an aid to patients, *Your Pregnancy & Birth* sets forth current information and opinions on subjects related to women's health and reproduction. The information does not dictate an exclusive course of treatment or procedure to be followed and should not be construed as excluding other medical opinions or acceptable methods of practice. Variations taking into account the needs of the individual patient, resources, and limitations unique to the institution or type of practice may be appropriate.

6/9

Contents

Preface

Your Pregnancy & Birth is designed for pregnant women who want authoritative advice from experts they can trust. The American College of Obstetricians and Gynecologists (ACOG)—America's preeminent authority on women's health—has published *Your Pregnancy & Birth* to be the most reliable source of information on childbirth.

ACOG represents the nation's leading group of professionals that provide health care for women. Throughout its 50-year history, ACOG has strived to maintain the highest standards of women's health care. *Your Pregnancy & Birth* is a culmination of those efforts and the knowledge of 47,000 ACOG members, developed under the direction of a committee of experts in the field.

Today, women may feel overwhelmed by all the information and advice about pregnancy and birth that is available. *Your Pregnancy & Birth* is a unique resource that a woman can use alone or to complement other sources of information to lead her through prenatal care, labor, delivery, and the postpartum period. It answers the common questions patients ask ob-gyns before, during, and after pregnancy in a factual, straightforward style. *Your Pregnancy & Birth* encourages a woman to become informed about her pregnancy and empowers her to work with her doctor to become an active participant in one of the most fulfilling times of her life.

Now in its fourth edition, *Your Pregnancy & Birth* has undergone extensive revision and reorganization to reflect the latest scientific advances and practice guidelines. The chapter on genetic disorders covers advances in identifying women who may be at risk and describes how some disorders can be detected and in some cases prevented. New tests—both routine and optional—and approaches to monitoring the health of mother and baby are described to help parents understand the screening techniques they may encounter. Women who need special care will appreciate the expanded information on how certain medical conditions are affected by pregnancy and what steps they can take to stay healthy. This edition also includes the latest recommendations on what foods a pregnant woman can safely enjoy, as well as things to avoid to maintain a healthy pregnancy. Because a woman needs to maintain her health not only during pregnancy, but also throughout her life, an all-new chapter on how to stay healthy has been added. It includes information on nutrition, exercise, family planning, and the routine tests and exams that are recommended for women at certain ages.

In addition to medical information, *Your Pregnancy & Birth* provides advice to help ease a woman and her family through the childbirth process. Tips are offered on how to find a doctor that meets a woman's specific needs and locate a facility that can best accommodate her. Options are described to help a woman plan her birth experience. Advice on how to cope with the many changes—physical and emotional—that occur during pregnancy and ease discomforts also are included. What to expect after birth and how to care for the newborn at home, including breastfeeding, are covered in detail.

Although the content has been completely updated in this edition into an attractive new format, many popular features of earlier editions have been retained. These features include a complete subject index, a personal pregnancy diary that can be used to chart the progress and note key events of the pregnancy, and an extensive glossary that defines terms marked in *boldface italic* type at first mention in the text.

Your Pregnancy & Birth is intended to be a complete guide to childbirth. Its goal—and that of ACOG—is to help women and their families have a safe pregnancy and healthy baby and to get the most from this special time of their lives.

YOUR PREGNANCY & BIRTH

FOURTH EDITION

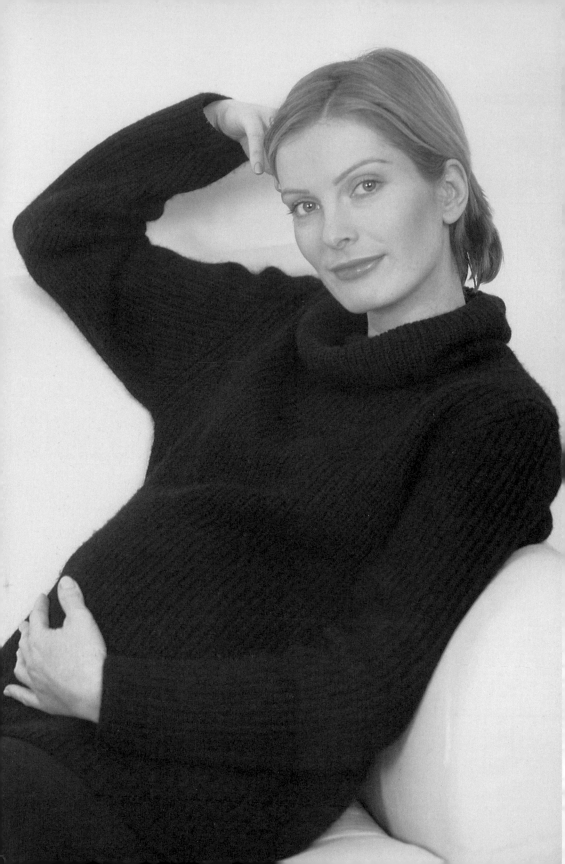

PREGNANCY

Congratulations! You're pregnant. Pregnancy is an exciting time of major change. From the very start, your baby-to-be alters your body and the way you live your daily life. For the entire pregnancy, the baby depends on you for all the things it needs to grow and thrive.

Learning about what to expect during pregnancy—what is normal and why it happens—is an important step toward a healthy and happy pregnancy. You can take an active role in your pregnancy. See your doctor as soon as you suspect you are pregnant, get regular prenatal care, make well-informed decisions, and stick to a healthy lifestyle. You will be helping your baby to have a healthy start in life, and helping yourself to feel your best.

CHAPTER 1

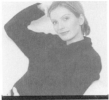

A New Life Begins

A finely tuned series of events must take place for pregnancy to occur. Knowing how reproduction works will help you understand the rapid changes that will take place in your body during early pregnancy to nurture the new life inside you. Knowing how your body will support the growing baby will help you understand the changes in your body that will continue to occur throughout pregnancy.

Your Growing Baby

The first step in a new life begins with *fertilization*, the fusion of a woman's *egg* and a man's *sperm*. Together the sperm and egg join to form cells that will develop over time into a baby. As the baby grows, the mother's body adapts to create a support system for it during the 9 months of pregnancy.

Reproduction

A woman's fertility depends on her menstrual cycle. Changes that occur during each cycle are caused by hormones—substances made by a woman's body to control certain functions. Each month, hormones direct the uterus to build up a lining of blood-rich tissue (endometrium). These hormones also send a signal for an egg to ripen in a follicle—tiny, fluid-filled clusters of cells in the *ovaries*. When the egg is ripe, it's released from an ovary and moves into a *fallopian tube*,

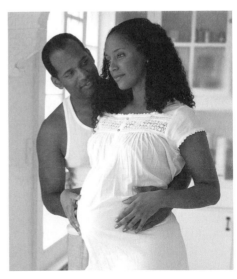

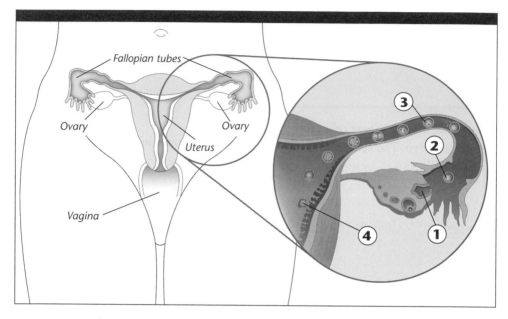

Each month during ovulation an egg is released (1) and moves into one of the fallopian tubes (2). If a woman has sex around this time, an egg may meet a sperm in the fallopian tube and the two will join (3). The fertilized egg then moves through the fallopian tube into the uterus and becomes attached there (4) to grow during pregnancy.

one of a pair of ducts that connects the ovaries to the **uterus**. This process is called ovulation. Ovulation most often occurs halfway through the cycle—on day 14 of 28, for instance.

During sex, when a man climaxes, semen spurts (ejaculates) from his penis through a tube called the urethra. This deposits millions of sperm in a woman's **vagina**. After ejaculation, the sperm "swim" up through the **cervix**, into the uterus, and out into the fallopian tubes. Although sperm can live inside a woman's body for up to 6 days, once an egg is released it must be fertilized within 12–24 hours.

After an egg is fertilized, it splits into identical cells, which then split again and again—two cells become four, four cells become eight, and so on. Within about a week after fertilization, this tiny ball of cells, called a **blastocyst**, moves through the fallopian tube to the uterus. There it implants and starts to grow. This fertilized egg is called an **embryo** for the first 8 weeks. Then it is called a **fetus**.

The lining of a woman's uterus thickens and grows a rich blood supply to nourish the fetus. As pregnancy progresses, the uterus will expand to make room for the growing baby. By the time the baby is born, the uterus may be 60 times its normal size.

Built-in codes in the cells of the blastocyst signal the cells to change as they multiply. Some cells grow into an organ called the **placenta**, which connects the baby to the mother. Some cells grow into the embryo. The cells in the embryo soon start to become different parts of the baby. Some cells become

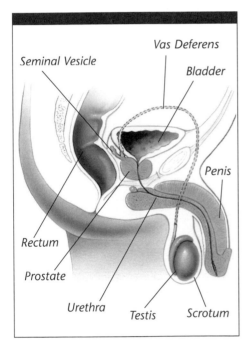

Sperm are tiny cells made by a man's testes in the sac (scrotum) below his penis. When sperm cells mature, they leave the testes through small tubes called the vas deferens. The vas deferens transports the sperm to the seminal vesicles and the prostate gland, which are small organs located near the bladder. There, the sperm mix with seminal fluid to create semen.

the brain, for instance, and others become other organs, such as the stomach. The figures on the following pages show how a baby grows during the 40 weeks of pregnancy.

Hormones

The hormones in your body play a leading role in reproduction, pregnancy, and birth. Each step in the creation of new life is led by these hormones:

➤ *Estrogen* and *progesterone.* Initially produced by the ovaries, these hormones trigger the lining of the uterus to thicken during each menstrual cycle and to be shed if pregnancy doesn't occur. After an egg is fertilized, a sharp increase in estrogen and progesterone levels prevents further ovulation.

➤ *Follicle-stimulating hormone (FSH)* and *luteinizing hormone (LH).* These hormones are made by the *pituitary gland*, a small organ at the base of the brain. FSH causes an egg to ripen each month in one of the ovaries. LH triggers the egg's release.

➤ *Gonadotropin-releasing hormone (GnRH).* This hormone, also made in the brain, signals the pituitary gland when to produce FSH and LH.

➤ *Human chorionic gonadotropin (hCG).* Made by certain cells from the fertilized and quickly dividing egg, hCG spurs increased estrogen and progesterone production during pregnancy. It's the hormone that pregnancy tests detect.

Growth and Changes of the Fetus

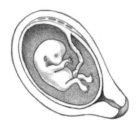

Week 8: 1½–2 inches, less than 1 ounce

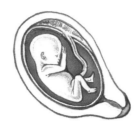

Week 12: 2½ inches, less than 1 ounce

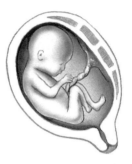

Week 16: 6–7 inches, 5 ounces

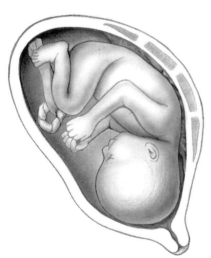

Week 28: 14 inches, 2–2½ pounds

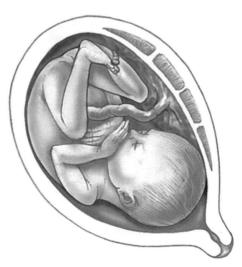

Week 32: 15 inches, 3 pounds

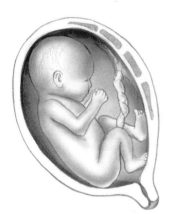

Week 20: 10 inches,
½–1 pound

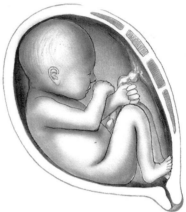

Week 24: 12 inches,
1–1½ pounds

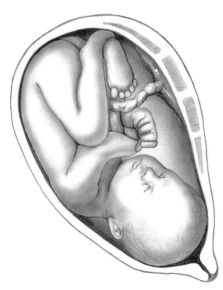

Week 36: 18 inches,
5 pounds

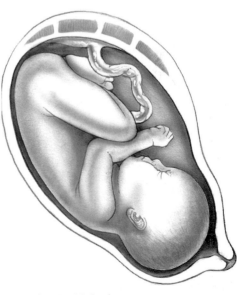

Week 40: 20 inches,
6–9 pounds

The Placenta

The placenta is the life-support system for the fetus. It has small finger-like growths that tuck into the wall of the uterus. On one side of the placenta, the **umbilical cord** connects the placenta with the fetus. Inside the cord are three blood vessels. One delivers blood enriched with oxygen and nutrients from the placenta to the fetus. Harmful agents, such as drugs or viruses, also can be transferred to the fetus this way. The other two blood vessels carry blood filled with waste products from the baby back to the placenta. The placenta filters waste products from the baby's blood and deposits them in the woman's blood. The woman's body then disposes of them. Blood itself is not exchanged between the mother and fetus. After the baby is born, the placenta is expelled, which is why it is sometimes called the "afterbirth."

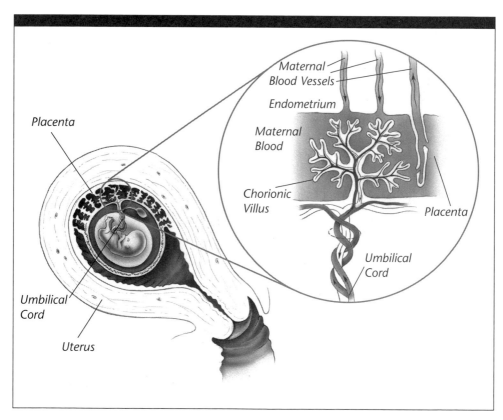

The placenta is composed of many lobes of chorionic villi. Chorionic villi contain fetal cells. One of these lobes is shown above on a larger scale (*right*).

Amniotic Fluid

The baby grows safely inside the *amniotic sac*. This sac is formed by two membranes: the amnion and the chorion. Inside the sac, a liquid called *amniotic fluid* collects to support and protect the fetus.

Amniotic fluid starts forming around the tiny embryo a few weeks after conception. At first, it's made up mostly of fluid from your body. Because the fetus swallows some of this fluid, new fluid is needed all the time.

As early as 11 weeks of pregnancy, the baby's kidneys start to put out urine. After 20 weeks of pregnancy, this urine makes up most of the amniotic fluid.

Amniotic fluid helps your growing baby in many ways:

➤ It cushions the fetus if you fall or have an accident.

➤ It creates pressure to push out on the walls of your uterus. This gives the fetus room to grow.

➤ It provides a safe, warm place for the fetus to exercise muscles and practice the movements he or she will need after birth.

➤ The fetus breathes in and swallows amniotic fluid. This helps develop the baby's ability to breathe and swallow.

➤ This fluid stops the growth of some kinds of bacteria. This protects the fetus from infection.

The fluid also has cells that have been shed from the skin of the fetus. These cells have all of the baby's genetic material. That's why amniotic fluid is sometimes used for prenatal testing.

Signs of Pregnancy

Your first sign of pregnancy probably was missing your menstrual period. Along with a late period, you may have had one or more of these other early signs of pregnancy:

➤ Spotting or having a very light menstrual period

➤ Feeling nauseated or queasy

➤ Having tender or swollen breasts

➤ Feeling very tired

➤ Urinating frequently

➤ Being moody

➤ Feeling bloated

These signs are normal in pregnancy. You may not have all of them, but you will most likely have at least one. Some signs are not normal, though. Call the doctor right away if you have any of the symptoms listed in the box. These could be signs of early pregnancy loss or *ectopic pregnancy*. An ectopic pregnancy occurs outside the uterus and could be a medical emergency.

The Length of Pregnancy

A "typical" pregnancy lasts for 280 days, or 40 weeks, counting from the first day of the last menstrual period. A normal pregnancy can last anywhere from 37–42 weeks. Since most women *ovulate* 2 weeks after their period begins, the actual pregnancy is 2 weeks less.

It is useful to talk about the length of pregnancy using the number of weeks rather than the number of months. The average pregnancy of 40 weeks is divided into three *trimesters*. Each trimester lasts about 13–14 weeks (or about 3 months):

➤ 1st trimester: 0–13 weeks

➤ 2nd trimester: 14–28 weeks

➤ 3rd trimester: 29–40 weeks

Planning Your Pregnancy Care

In most cases, you should schedule an appointment with your doctor to start prenatal care as soon as possible, preferably by the 8th or 10th week of your pregnancy. If you have any factors that might make your pregnancy high risk, let the doctor's office know right away.

Choosing Your Doctor or Midwife

Choosing the right person to care for you during pregnancy is an important decision. That person will play a major role in your pregnancy. Some women are happy to stick with the doctor they have been seeing for routine gynecologic care. Other women ask friends or relatives who are new mothers for recommendations. Still others first pick the hospital or birthing center where they'd like to have their babies and ask the staff there to refer them to someone. Your health insurance may limit your choices.

Four types of practitioners offer medical care for pregnancy and birth: obstetrician–gynecologists (ob–gyns), maternal–fetal medicine specialists (high-risk ob), family physicians, and certified nurse–midwives.

1. *Obstetrician–gynecologists.* Ob-gyns are doctors who specialize in the health care of women. After completing medical school, ob-gyns complete 4 years of special-

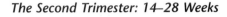

The First Trimester: 0–13 Weeks

➤ The placenta develops.

➤ The major organs and nervous system form.

➤ The heart starts beating.

➤ The lungs begin to develop.

➤ Bones appear.

➤ The head, face, eyes, ears, arms, fingers, legs, and toes form.

➤ Hair starts to grow.

➤ Buds for 20 temporary teeth develop.

The Second Trimester: 14–28 Weeks

➤ The organs develop further and begin to function.

➤ Eyebrows, eyelashes, and fingernails form.

➤ The skin is wrinkled and covered with a waxy coating (*vernix*).

➤ The genitals develop.

➤ Fine hair (*lanugo*) covers its body.

➤ The fetus moves, kicks, sleeps, and wakes.

➤ The fetus can swallow, hear, pass urine, and suck its thumb.

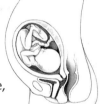

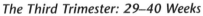

The Third Trimester: 29–40 Weeks

➤ The fetus kicks and stretches. (This activity may slow down as the fetus grows and space in the uterus decreases.)

➤ Lanugo disappears.

➤ With its major development finished, the fetus gains most of its weight—about half a pound each week until the 37th week.

➤ Bones harden, but the skull remains soft and flexible for delivery.

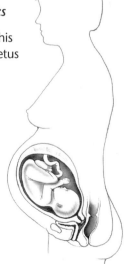

ized training in obstetrics and gynecology. To be certified, an ob-gyn must pass written and oral tests to show that he or she has obtained the knowledge and skills required for the medical and surgical care of women. A certified ob-gyn can then become a Fellow of the American College of Obstetricians and Gynecologists. This group helps doctors stay up-to-date on the latest medical advances.

2. *Maternal–fetal medicine specialists.* These doctors have completed 4 years of training in obstetrics and gynecology and then received fur-ther training and certification in high-risk obstetrics for 2–3 years. Women who have high-risk pregnancies may be referred to a maternal–fetal medicine specialist for care.

3. *Family physicians.* Doctors in family practice provide general care for most conditions, including pregnancy. After completing medical school, family physicians complete 3 years of advanced training in family medicine (including obstetrics) and become certified by passing an exam. They are able to care for normal pregnancies and deliveries.

Risk Factors That May Need Special Care in Pregnancy

Medical

➤ High blood pressure

➤ Heart, kidney, lung, thyroid, connective tissue, or liver disease

➤ Sexually transmitted diseases (such as HIV or hepatitis), urinary tract infections, or other infections caused by a virus or bacteria

➤ Diabetes

➤ Asthma

➤ Severe anemia

➤ Epilepsy or other seizure disorders

➤ Mental health problems

➤ Obesity

Obstetric

➤ Problems in past pregnancies

➤ Being younger than 15 years or older than 35 years during pregnancy

➤ Previous birth defects

➤ Multiple pregnancy (carrying more than one baby)

➤ Bleeding, especially during the second or third trimester

➤ Pregnancy-induced high blood pressure (**preeclampsia**)

➤ Abnormal fetal heartbeat

➤ Intrauterine growth restriction (the fetus doesn't grow at the rate it should)

4. *Certified nurse–midwives.* Certified nurse–midwives are registered nurses who have been specially trained to care for women and their babies from early pregnancy through labor, delivery, and the weeks after birth. They have completed an accredited nursing program and have a graduate degree in midwifery. To be certified, they must pass a national exam and maintain an active nursing license. They also must work with a qualified doctor who will provide backup support. Certified nurse–midwives are trained to care for healthy women with normal pregnancies. They consult with a doctor if medical problems arise or refer patients to a doctor for special care.

Another factor to think about is whether a provider is in a solo, group, or collaborative practice. In a solo practice, one doctor works alone, but may have help from other physicians to cover deliveries. In a group practice, two or more doctors share duties for constant coverage of their patients' health care. A collaborative practice is led by an ob–gyn and brings together a team of health care professionals, such as nurses, nurse–midwives, nurse practitioners, physician assistants, and childbirth educators, with different knowledge and skills. The contributions of each member are key to the care of the patient.

No matter what type of practitioner you are considering for your prenatal care, getting answers to the following questions may help you make your decision:

➤ *Office visits:* When is the office open? What is the usual length of a visit?

➤ *Personnel:* Will you always be seen by the same doctor? What other caregivers might be scheduled to see you? Who covers for the doctor when he or she is sick or on vacation?

➤ *Phone calls:* Who will answer questions over the phone during office hours? Does the doctor charge for phone calls? How are calls and emergencies handled after regular office hours?

➤ *Hospitals:* Where does the doctor have privileges to treat patients? Is the hospital fully equipped and close to you?

Choosing Where Your Baby Will Be Born

The setting can have a major impact on your birth experience. Depending on where you live, the following options may be available:

➤ *L&D (labor and delivery).* A woman labors in one room and gives birth in another room. She will then be transferred to a recovery room and then to a hospital room for the rest of her stay.

➤ *LDR (labor/delivery/recovery).* A woman will be in the same room throughout her labor and delivery and recovery and is then transferred to a hospital room for the rest of her stay.

➤ *LDRP (labor/delivery/recovery/post-partum).* A woman is in the same room throughout her stay at the hospital.

There also are freestanding birthing centers that are not in a hospital. These centers may not offer all the services you may need if an emergency arises. Because of this, the safest places to give birth are thought to be a hospital or a birthing center within the hospital complex.

When choosing a birth setting, you may wish to ask about its policy on the presence of others in the delivery room. Most hospitals permit support people in both labor and delivery rooms. It is wise to know the hospital's policy in advance so you can plan.

Your choice will depend on what your area offers, where your caregiver performs deliveries, and what your health insurance will cover. Your caregiver will let you know about the choices available. You can tour the hospitals in your area to see which settings appeal to you.

Money Matters

You should consider in advance how you will pay for your pregnancy care. If you have insurance, check to see if your health plan covers complete pregnancy care or only the most routine medical tests and procedures. That could become an issue if problems arise during pregnancy or birth or if the baby has health problems. Check your plan to see how much of the cost it will pay for the following items:

➤ Obstetric care

➤ Prenatal tests

➤ Hospital charges

➤ Well-baby care

➤ Postpartum birth control

Also make sure that the provider and the hospital where you want to give birth are part of the plan. In many

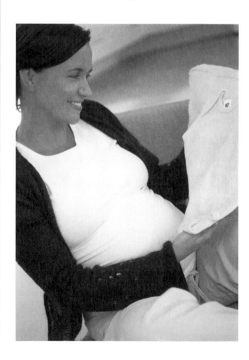

cases, seeing a provider or going to a hospital that is "out of network" — meaning not part of the insurance health plan—means that you'll have to pay for some or all expenses yourself.

The Health Insurance Portability and Accountability Act (HIPAA) protects most women who switch health insurance plans during pregnancy or enroll in a plan after they become pregnant. This means that if you change jobs and insurance plans during your pregnancy, you cannot be denied insurance coverage for care related to your pregnancy. It does not matter how long you were with your insurance plan before you switched. Also, your newborn cannot be denied coverage as long as you sign him or her up for health insurance within 30 days of birth.

The Countdown Begins

The basics of having a baby are the same for almost every woman, but each pregnancy is unique. Being well-informed and taking the time to plan for prenatal care can help ensure a healthy start for your pregnancy. Knowing what is taking place in your body and with your developing baby will help you prepare for the exciting weeks ahead.

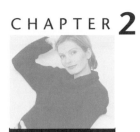

CHAPTER 2

Prenatal Care

Prenatal visits allow your doctor to keep close tabs on your health and your baby's progress. Pregnancy and birth are a natural part of life, but problems can arise. That's why it's important to get prenatal care as soon as you know you are pregnant.

During prenatal visits, you'll learn about what's going on in your body. You can ask for advice on coping with common changes during pregnancy and gather the information you need to make important choices.

During your pregnancy, each member of your health care team—your doctor, midwife, and others—will keep an eye on your health and well-being. Tests will be done to check on the health of the baby.

Prenatal care isn't just medical care. It helps you learn good health habits, get counseling or support if needed, find out about local family services, and prepare for childbirth and being a parent.

Informed Care

The more you know about your health care, the better equipped you are to make choices. During prenatal visits, your doctor will explain what's happening and why. Before you give your OK for a test or a treatment, be sure you know what it is and why it's needed. You also should be told about the risks, benefits, and options. This is called "informed consent."

If you don't understand something you have heard, ask for a more clear explanation. In some cases, you may be asked to sign a form saying that you have been informed of something or stating your decision on whether to have a certain procedure or test done.

Trust and good communication between you and your health care team are important. The box on the following page spells out the ways each of you can help build that trust and have open communication.

Partners in Health Care

Both you and your health care providers have rights and responsibilities. You have the right to:

➤ Get quality care without discrimination

➤ Be given privacy

➤ Know the professional status of your health care providers and their fees

➤ Know your diagnosis, treatment options, and expected outcome

➤ Be involved in decisions about your care

➤ Refuse treatment

➤ Agree or decline to be involved in research that affects your care

➤ Read your chart and get a copy of it if you wish

➤ Ask your caregiver to keep letters and calls about your health care private by calling or writing to you only at a certain place

You have the responsibility to:

➤ Provide correct and complete health information

➤ Let your providers know that you understand what's being done to you and what you are expected to do

➤ Accept responsibility if you refuse treatment or don't follow the doctor's plan

Your health care provider has the responsibility to:

➤ Give you quality medical treatment while you are in his or her care

➤ Notify you of your privacy rights and the privacy practices used in his or her office

➤ Charge a reasonable fee for copying your medical records if you ask for a copy

➤ Not release your health information to a nonhealth insurance company, bank, or marketing firm unless you grant permission by signing a document

➤ Comply with your request for special private handling of calls and letters if he or she can reasonably do so

Your health care provider has the right to:

➤ Ask you to sign a notice that you were told about your privacy rights

➤ Stop treating you as long as you have time to find other care

Prenatal Visits

One of your early prenatal checkups may be longer and more involved than later visits. This visit will include a detailed health history, a physical exam, lab tests, calculation of your due date, and a schedule for your prenatal care. Throughout your pregnancy you will see your doctor on a regular basis. These visits provide a good chance to discuss any questions or concerns and learn more about your pregnancy.

History

A review of your health history and previous pregnancies can help your doctor provide any special care you may need during your pregnancy. Each pregnancy is different and problems often arise without warning. The more information you can provide, the better equipped your doctor will be to plan your care. The checklist "Your Health History" can help you organize this information. You may want to complete it and take it with you to your doctor's visit.

Physical Exam

After your health history is obtained, your height, weight, and blood pressure will be measured. You will then have a general physical exam. The doctor will listen to your heart and lungs and check your body for any health problems.

Next, a *pelvic exam* may be done to check your reproductive organs: cervix,

vagina, ovaries, fallopian tubes, and uterus. Using a device called a *speculum,* the doctor can look at your vagina and cervix and may collect cells for testing.

The doctor may insert one or two gloved fingers into your vagina to check the size of your uterus. He or she also may feel the ovaries and check their size, shape, and position.

Many women have a light spotting of blood after the pelvic exam. This spotting is not related to the pregnancy. However, if the spotting does not stop, becomes heavy bleeding, or is accompanied by pain, call the doctor.

Your doctor also may check your cervix during the last weeks of pregnancy to look for changes that can sig-

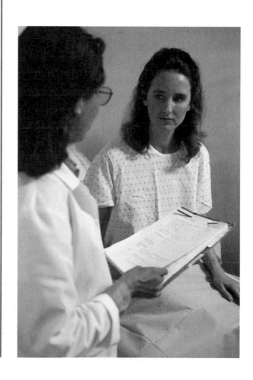

Your Health History

Fill out this list and take it with you to your first doctor's visit.

Medications you are taking_____

_____

Allergies you have (including latex)_____

_____

Medical conditions you have_____

_____

Surgical procedures you have had_____

_____

Immunizations you have had, and when you had them_____

_____

Childhood diseases you have had_____

_____

Your age when you got your first period_____

Usual number of days between your periods_____

When your last period started_____

What birth control you have used_____

Whether you smoke, drink alcohol, or use drugs_____

Whether you are exposed to anything that could put your baby at risk

_____

If you have been pregnant before, the doctor will ask the following questions:

Have you had a *miscarriage*, induced abortion, ectopic pregnancy, *still-birth*, or *multiple pregnancy*?_____

Did you have problems such as preterm labor or high blood pressure during pregnancy?_____

How long did your labor last?_____

Did you give birth vaginally or by cesarean birth?_____

Did you or the baby have any problems before, during, or after delivery?

_____

How much did your children weigh at birth?_____

Have you had a child with a birth defect?_____

What kind of pain relief, if any, did you use?_____

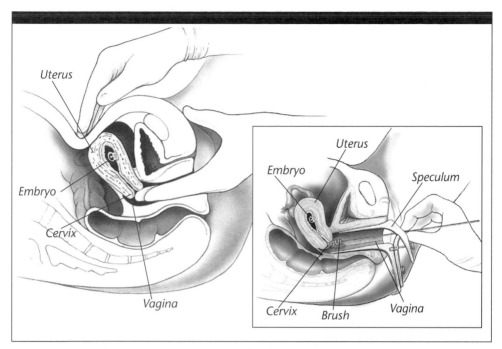

During your visit, your caregiver may check your pelvic organs for any changes (*left*). A Pap test also may be done (*right*). For the Pap test, a speculum is inserted into the vagina. A sample of some cells is collected with a small brush or swab and scraper. The brush or swab is inserted into the cervical canal to reach cells from deeper inside.

nal the onset of labor. Before delivery, the cervix often begins to move forward in the vagina, thin out, soften, and open slightly as it gets ready for delivery. All of these things may happen weeks before labor begins. However, many women have none of these signs before going into labor.

Due Date

The day your baby is due is called the "estimated date of delivery," or EDD (also known as estimated date of confinement or EDC). Although only about 1 in 20 women deliver on their exact

due date, the EDD is useful for a number of reasons. It is used as a guide for checking the baby's growth and your pregnancy's progress. Your due date also affects the timing of prenatal tests. In some cases, the test results depend on the stage of pregnancy. Finally, the EDD gives a rough idea of when your baby will be born. Most women go into labor within about 2 weeks of their due dates—either before or after.

There are a number of methods to figure your due date. They often are used together to help predict when your baby will be born.

Date of Ovulation

The best way to figure the age of a fetus (and thus your due date) is to know the date you ovulated. However, a woman rarely knows her exact date of ovulation unless she uses an ovulation prediction kit. Women may use these kits when they are trying to get pregnant.

Date of Menstruation

Your due date is most often figured out by counting from the first day of your last period. This method isn't exact, though. The length of your menstrual cycle affects your due date. These cycles differ from one woman to another and from one month to the next. Also, unless you made a note of it, it's easy to forget when your last period started. This is why it is a good idea to make a note of your period on the calendar. To get an idea of your due date, take the date that your last normal period started. Add 7 days. Then count back 3 months. Say the first day of your last period was January 1. Add 7 days to get January 8. Then count back 3 months. Your due date is October 8. The chart on the following pages can help you use this method. This technique is based on a 28-day cycle, with conception occurring 2 weeks afterward, which does not apply to all women.

Size of Your Uterus

At about 12 weeks of pregnancy, the top of the uterus (**fundus**) has grown up and out of the pelvic cavity and can be

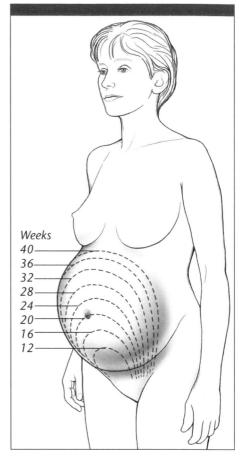

Weeks
40
36
32
28
24
20
16
12

Even early in pregnancy, the size of your uterus can help show how long you have been pregnant.

felt just above the pubic bone. At 20 weeks, it reaches the navel. At term, when the baby is fully grown, it will be under the rib cage.

Ultrasound

Ultrasound uses sound waves to create a picture of the uterus and the fetus growing inside it. The size of the fetus can be measured to figure its age. During the first half of pregnancy, ultrasound can be used to set the age of the fetus within a week or so. Later on, this method is less reliable.

Fetal Heartbeat

The doctor also may be able to tell how far along you are in your pregnancy by hearing the fetal heartbeat. By about 12 weeks, your doctor may be able to hear your baby's heart by using a Doppler ultrasound device. This device uses a form of ultrasound to convert sound waves into signals that can be heard.

Future Visits

The timing of prenatal visits depends on your health and any special needs you may have during pregnancy. Healthy women with no known risk factors often need fewer visits than women with medical or obstetric problems. If a problem develops, you'll need to see the doctor more often.

As long as mother and baby are both doing well, checkups often follow a basic schedule. From your first prenatal visit to 28 weeks of pregnancy, you most likely will have a checkup every 4 weeks. From 28 to 36 weeks of pregnancy, you will have a checkup every 2–3 weeks. After 36 weeks of pregnancy until you give birth, you will have a weekly checkup. The following items are checked at each visit:

➤ Weight

➤ Blood pressure

➤ Urine to detect protein and sugar

➤ Height of uterus to gauge the baby's growth

➤ Face, ankles, hands, and feet for signs of swelling

➤ Fetal heartbeat (after about the 12th week)

➤ Position of the fetus (later in the pregnancy)

If you have any questions or concerns, it's a good idea to jot them down ahead of time and bring them with you. Also make a note of any symptoms you have between visits and mention them to the doctor. The "Pregnancy Diary" at the back of this book is a handy way to chart the course of your pregnancy.

If your questions are pressing or your symptoms alarm you, don't wait until your next visit. Talk to your doctor or nurse right away.

Prenatal Tests

Lab Tests

To confirm the findings of a home pregnancy test, your blood or urine may be tested for the hormone human chorionic gonadotropin (hCG). Also, the doctor can order lab tests to check for any diseases or infections. These tests may include:

➤ *Urine tests.* Urine is collected to look for sugar, protein, and bacteria. Their presence can signal diabetes or a bladder or kidney problem.

What's Your Due Date?

There's no way to know for sure your delivery date. Here's how to get an idea: simply find the first day of your last menstrual period (LMP) on this chart. Then look at the estimated date of delivery (EDD) directly below it.

LMP: Jan.	1	2	3	4	5	6	7	8	9	10	11	12	13	14	15	16	17	18	19	20	21	22	23	24	25	26	27	28	29	30	31
EDD: Oct./Nov.	8	9	10	11	12	13	14	15	16	17	18	19	20	21	22	23	24	25	26	27	28	29	30	31	1	2	3	4	5	6	7

LMP: Feb.	1	2	3	4	5	6	7	8	9	10	11	12	13	14	15	16	17	18	19	20	21	22	23	24	25	26	27	28
EDD: Nov./Dec.	8	9	10	11	12	13	14	15	16	17	18	19	20	21	22	23	24	25	26	27	28	29	30	1	2	3	4	5

LMP: Mar.	1	2	3	4	5	6	7	8	9	10	11	12	13	14	15	16	17	18	19	20	21	22	23	24	25	26	27	28	29	30	31
EDD: Dec./Jan.	8	9	10	11	12	13	14	15	16	17	18	19	20	21	22	23	24	25	26	27	28	29	30	31	1	2	3	4	5	6	7

LMP: April	1	2	3	4	5	6	7	8	9	10	11	12	13	14	15	16	17	18	19	20	21	22	23	24	25	26	27	28	29	30
EDD: Jan./Feb.	8	9	10	11	12	13	14	15	16	17	18	19	20	21	22	23	24	25	26	27	28	29	30	31	1	2	3	4	5	6

LMP: May	1	2	3	4	5	6	7	8	9	10	11	12	13	14	15	16	17	18	19	20	21	22	23	24	25	26	27	28	29	30	31
EDD: Feb./Mar.	8	9	10	11	12	13	14	15	16	17	18	19	20	21	22	23	24	25	26	27	28	1	2	3	4	5	6	7	8	9	10

LMP: June	1	2	3	4	5	6	7	8	9	10	11	12	13	14	15	16	17	18	19	20	21	22	23	24	25	26	27	28	29	30
EDD: Mar./April	8	9	10	11	12	13	14	15	16	17	18	19	20	21	22	23	24	25	26	27	28	29	30	31	1	2	3	4	5	6

	1	2	3	4	5	6	7	8	9	10	11	12	13	14	15	16	17	18	19	20	21	22	23	24	25	26	27	28	29	30	31
LMP: July	1	2	3	4	5	6	7	8	9	10	11	12	13	14	15	16	17	18	19	20	21	22	23	24	25	26	27	28	29	30	31
EDD: April/May	8	9	10	11	12	13	14	15	16	17	18	19	20	21	22	23	24	25	26	27	28	29	30	1	2	3	4	5	6	7	8
LMP: Aug.	1	2	3	4	5	6	7	8	9	10	11	12	13	14	15	16	17	18	19	20	21	22	23	24	25	26	27	28	29	30	31
EDD: May/June	8	9	10	11	12	13	14	15	16	17	18	19	20	21	22	23	24	25	26	27	28	29	30	31	1	2	3	4	5	6	7
LMP: Sept.	1	2	3	4	5	6	7	8	9	10	11	12	13	14	15	16	17	18	19	20	21	22	23	24	25	26	27	28	29	30	
EDD: June/July	8	9	10	11	12	13	14	15	16	17	18	19	20	21	22	23	24	25	26	27	28	29	30	1	2	3	4	5	6	7	
LMP: Oct.	1	2	3	4	5	6	7	8	9	10	11	12	13	14	15	16	17	18	19	20	21	22	23	24	25	26	27	28	29	30	31
EDD: July/Aug.	8	9	10	11	12	13	14	15	16	17	18	19	20	21	22	23	24	25	26	27	28	29	30	31	1	2	3	4	5	6	7
LMP: Nov.	1	2	3	4	5	6	7	8	9	10	11	12	13	14	15	16	17	18	19	20	21	22	23	24	25	26	27	28	29	30	
EDD: Aug./Sept.	8	9	10	11	12	13	14	15	16	17	18	19	20	21	22	23	24	25	26	27	28	29	30	31	1	2	3	4	5	6	
LMP: Dec.	1	2	3	4	5	6	7	8	9	10	11	12	13	14	15	16	17	18	19	20	21	22	23	24	25	26	27	28	29	30	31
EDD: Sept./Oct.	8	9	10	11	12	13	14	15	16	17	18	19	20	21	22	23	24	25	26	27	28	29	30	1	2	3	4	5	6	7	8

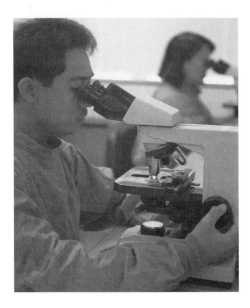

➤ *Blood tests.* Blood is drawn and checked for **anemia** and infection. All women are offered testing for **human immunodeficiency virus (HIV)** infection. Most women also are tested for **syphilis** and **hepatitis B virus** surface **antigen.** Your blood also may be studied to look for other sexually transmitted diseases (STDs) and signs that you are immune to rubella (German measles) and chickenpox (varicella). Your blood type and **Rh factor** also are noted.

➤ **Pap test.** The cells from the cervix collected during a pelvic exam may be examined for signs of infection, cancer, or conditions that could lead to cancer. Samples also may be collected to check for infections, such as chlamydia or gonorrhea.

➤ *Glucose screening test.* This test measures the **glucose** level in the mother's blood to test for **gestational diabetes.**

➤ *Group B streptococci (GBS) testing.* The cells from the mother's vagina and rectum are tested for GBS infection, which can be passed to the baby during delivery.

➤ *Human immunodeficiency virus testing.* There are several types of HIV tests. The most common test—called ELISA—searches for HIV **antibodies** in your blood. If this test result is positive, another test called the Western blot is used to confirm the results.

Tests can be done to help your doctor spot possible health problems. They also will give clues to how your baby is growing and developing. The results of these tests will be noted on your chart. The specific tests you have depend on your medical history, family background, racial and ethnic background, and exam results. Other tests may be needed later in pregnancy. (Chapter 13 has more information about tests that can be done to detect genetic disorders and birth defects.)

Fetal Movements

In mid-pregnancy, you will have a new sensation: a gentle flutter that is your baby moving inside you. The first time you feel the baby move is called **quickening**, and it's likely to be one of the most thrilling moments of your pregnancy.

Quickening usually occurs between 16 and 20 weeks of pregnancy. With first-time mothers, it often occurs toward the end of that range—around 20 weeks. It can be felt sooner by thin women and in women who have been pregnant before. The feeling varies from woman to woman. Many compare it to a fluttering sensation.

During the second half of pregnancy, your baby's soft movements will become stronger and more lively. Such movement is a sign of fetal well-being. If you notice any change in the way your baby moves, be sure to mention it to your doctor. He or she also may ask you to perform daily **kick counts** to gauge the baby's movements. (Chapter 3 gives details on how to perform kick counts.)

Childbirth Options

If you haven't done so yet, now is the time to make choices about your baby's birth and care after delivery. It is best to think about your options and resolve as much as you can well before delivery. You can ask your doctor about what to expect during labor and delivery and get answers to your questions about childbirth options. The box lists some of the options that you may want to discuss with your doctor. You can express your preferences and get answers to any questions you and your partner may have.

Choices To Consider

Now is the time to make choices about your baby's birth and after-delivery care. Even the best-laid plans may not work out, but think about your options and resolve as much as you can well before the delivery day.

Among the issues to think about ahead of time:

➤ What kind of childbirth preparation do you want, and what classes are offered nearby?

➤ Do you want pain relief during labor, or will you try for a natural childbirth? (For more information, see Chapter 8)

➤ Who will be at your side during labor and delivery? (For more information, see Chapter 8)

➤ If you have a boy, do you want him circumcised? (For more information, see Chapter 11)

➤ Will you breastfeed your baby? (For more information, see Chapter 10)

Work and travel plans, which also may need advance planning, are covered in Chapter 4.

Choosing Your Baby's Doctor

Pediatricians are doctors who care for children. The best time to choose a doctor for your baby is before the baby is born. If you have children who use a doctor you like, check to be sure he or she will take new patients. You may need to choose a new doctor for the baby. Find out if he or she also will care for your older children.

If you have health insurance, look for a doctor who is part of your insurance plan. You can choose a pediatrician or a family physician to take care of your baby. Look for a doctor who is board certified.

It's a good idea to have a get-acquainted office visit while you are pregnant. This will let you get a feel for how the office is run and what the staff is like. You also can ask the doctor questions you have about the baby.

These are some topics you may want to cover with the doctor:

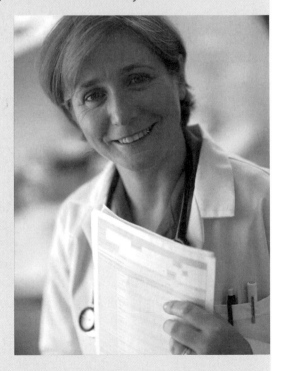

➤ Office visits: When is the office open? What is the usual length of a visit? Is there a separate waiting room for children who are sick?

➤ Personnel: Will your baby always be seen by the doctor? What other caregivers might be scheduled to see your baby? Who covers for the doctor when he or she is sick or on vacation?

➤ Phone calls: Who will answer questions over the phone during office hours? Does the doctor charge for phone calls? How are calls and emergencies handled after regular office hours?

➤ Hospitals: To what hospital does the doctor admit patients? What emergency room does the doctor recommend?

Now is also the time to choose a doctor for your baby (see box). It's a good idea to talk to the baby's doctor ahead of time so you can ask questions and be sure you are comfortable with your choice.

Childbirth Education Classes

Childbirth education classes are a good way to learn what happens during labor and birth and how to prepare for it. Your doctor can direct you to a childbirth education class that's a good match for you and the kind of birth you expect.

These classes often meet over the course of a few weeks or months, so start looking into them as soon as you can. The class will inform you about the labor and delivery process and teach you how to help it go smoothly. Childbirth preparation will help ease your fears, teach you methods for coping with labor pain, and help you feel more in control.

The most common methods of preparation—Lamaze, Bradley, and Read—vary greatly, but each is based on the idea that pain is made worse by fear and tension. Classes aim to relieve labor pain through education, emotional support, relaxation techniques, and touch.

Some childbirth education classes will help you draft a birth plan. This is a written outline of what you would like to happen during labor and delivery. It might include the setting you want to deliver in, the people you want to have

with you, and the pain medications you want, if any. A birth plan is useful to make sure your doctor is aware of your wishes and agrees with them.

Once you have drawn up your plan, go over it with your doctor. He or she will help you tailor the plan to your needs and wishes. The doctor also will let you know if there is any conflict with hospital policies. It is best to keep your birth plan both realistic and flexible so changes can be made based on events that can arise during labor and delivery.

Your Childbirth Partner

A childbirth partner can be a spouse, partner, relative, or friend who provides support during pregnancy. Such support helps ease the many stresses of pregnancy and provides comfort during labor and delivery.

If possible, your partner should come with you to prenatal visits and tests. Your partner also needs to attend childbirth classes with you. Your childbirth partner has almost as much to learn as you do. This person will help you practice breathing or relaxation exercises. On delivery day, your partner will coach you through contractions and help you carry out what you learned in class.

A growing number of mothers-to-be also hire a professional labor assistant, or doula. Although the childbirth partner still plays a vital role, a doula can take some of the pressure off of the partner during a long or intense labor. The doula provides support for both the mother and the partner.

Teamwork

In the coming months, you and your prenatal caregivers will work as a team to ensure the health of you and your baby. Early and regular prenatal care allows your doctor to monitor your progress and detect any problems and allows you the chance to ask questions. Your doctor and the other members of the health care team can give you advice, explain options, and be your partners in this exciting time in your life.

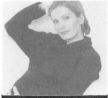

CHAPTER **3**

Testing for Fetal Well-Being

Many techniques are used to check the well-being of your fetus throughout pregnancy. The methods described in this chapter often are used in the second half of pregnancy, although some also can be done earlier. These tests may be done to confirm other test results or to provide further information. The results of these tests may assure you and your doctor all is going well.

These tests cannot cure a problem, nor can they ensure a healthy baby. What they can do is alert your doctor that you may need special care.

Kick Counts

You may be asked to keep track of your baby's movements. Kick counts is a test that you can do at home to help check on your baby's health. Sometimes it is called fetal movement counts.

If you have been asked to note your baby's kick counts, your doctor will tell you how often to do it and when to call him or her. One method is to write down how long it takes the fetus to make 10 movements. Choose a time when the fetus usually is active. Often, a good time is after a meal. Each baby has its own level of activity, and most have a sleep cycle of 20–40 minutes. Alert your doctor if there is a change in the normal pattern or number of movements.

Ultrasound

Ultrasound is energy in the form of sound waves. The sound waves move at a frequency too high to be heard by the human ear. Ultrasound creates pictures or sounds of the baby from sound waves. It is used today in all major hospitals and in many doctors' offices. No harmful effects to either the mother or the baby have been found in more than 30 years of using ultrasound.

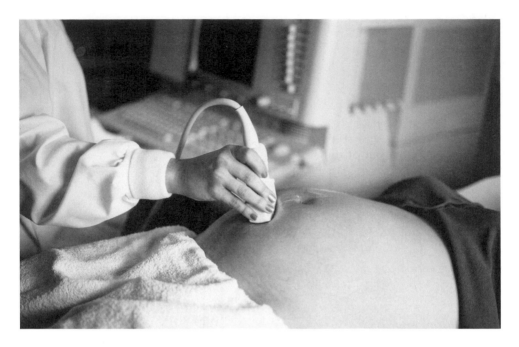

When It Is Used

Ultrasound can provide useful information about the fetus's health and well-being, such as the following:

➤ Age of the fetus

➤ Growth of the fetus

➤ Location of the placenta

➤ Fetal position, movement, breathing, and heart rate

➤ Amount of amniotic fluid in the uterus

➤ Number of fetuses

➤ Some birth defects

➤ Length of the cervix

In the first trimester, ultrasound also may be used to help find out the reason for bleeding or pelvic pain (see "Vaginal Bleeding" in Chapter 15). It also is used to confirm the dates of pregnancy.

Sometimes ultrasound is used if the doctor wants to check on possible problems. For instance, if you are at risk for the baby not growing well, the doctor may do an ultrasound exam every 2–4 weeks to check the rate of growth.

How It Is Done

To prepare for an ultrasound exam, wear clothes that allow your abdomen to be exposed easily. You may be asked to wear a hospital gown.

The doctor or a technician will perform the ultrasound exam by using a device called a ***transducer.*** It directs the sound waves into the body. There are two types of transducers: one that is moved around by hand on the outside of the abdomen and one that is placed in the vagina.

For an ultrasound exam using the transducer on the outside of your abdomen, you will lie on the table with your abdomen exposed from the lower part of the ribs to the hips. The doctor or technician will put a gel on your abdomen. This improves the contact between the transducer and the skin surface. The transducer then is moved around on the outside of your abdomen. The sound waves sent out from the transducer enter the body and reflect back when they make contact with your internal organs and the baby. They are changed into pictures that appear on a screen that looks like a TV.

The vaginal transducer is inserted in the vagina to help view the pelvic organs and the baby. Ultrasound with a vaginal probe may feel like the exam you have for a Pap test. This exam is done to detect certain disorders, such as ***placenta previa.***

Special Cases

A detailed ultrasound exam can be done to look at specific areas of concern, such as the baby's heart or spinal cord. This is called a detailed or comprehensive ultrasound exam. This exam

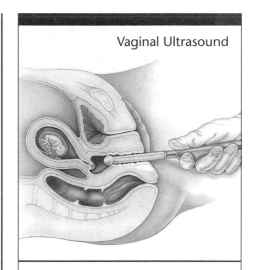

Vaginal Ultrasound

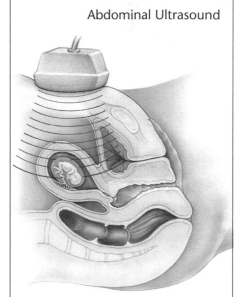

Abdominal Ultrasound

With ultrasound, energy in the form of sound waves is reflected off the fetus. The reflected sound waves are changed into pictures of the fetus that you and your doctor can see on a TV-type screen.

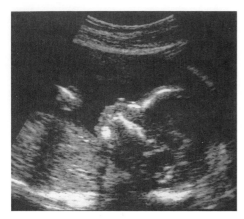

Ultrasound of a fetus in the mother's uterus.

may be done if the fetus is at increased risk for birth defects based on family history or other test results (see "Diagnostic Tests" in Chapter 12). Ultrasound also can be used along with other tests to screen for birth defects in early pregnancy.

Sometimes a special ultrasound test called Doppler flow is used to check the blood flow in the umbilical cord. This test also is called Doppler velocimetry. It uses a special kind of ultrasound that allows the doctor to both see and hear the wave form produced by ultrasound.

Fetal Heart Rate Monitoring

There are three methods of fetal heart rate monitoring. One method—called auscultation—involves listening to your baby's heartbeat at certain times. The other method—electronic fetal monitoring—uses equipment to record the heart rate on an ongoing basis. Finally, the *biophysical profile* uses a combination of values to assess the fetus.

Auscultation

The baby's heartbeat can be heard with auscultation. Auscultation is done with Doppler ultrasound.

Doppler ultrasound changes sound waves into signals that can be heard. With Doppler ultrasound, a small, handheld device is pressed against your abdomen to detect your baby's heart beat.

Electronic Fetal Monitoring

There are two kinds of tests that use the fetal heart rate to assess a baby's well-being before labor starts: 1) the *non-stress test* and 2) the *contraction stress test.* Both of these tests measure the fetal heart rate in response to some form of stimulus. These tests can reassure you if the results are normal. If the results are not normal, further testing is needed.

For both tests, the Doppler ultra-sound device is pressed against your abdomen. Sometimes belts are used to strap it on, just as they may be during labor (see "Monitoring" in Chapter 8). When the fetal heartbeats are reflected, they make sounds you can hear. These signals are shown on a graph.

Nonstress Test

The nonstress test measures the fetal heart rate in response to the fetus's own movements. Often the fetal heart rate beats faster when the baby moves, just as your heart does when you exercise. Such changes in your baby's heart rate are believed to be a sign of good health.

During the nonstress test, you lie on a bed or examining table or a chair with a belt around your abdomen. The belt is attached to ultrasound transducers. The fetal heart rate is measured by Doppler ultrasound. You push a button each time you feel the baby move. This causes a mark to be made on a paper that is recording the fetal heart rate. (The nonstress test also can be done with a device that senses fetal movement.) It takes 10–40 minutes to complete the test.

If the baby does not move for a while during the nonstress test, your baby may be asleep. A device like a buzzer may be used to produce sound and vibration to wake the baby and cause movement. This test is called **vibroacoustic stimulation.** The doctor also may suggest you have something to eat or drink to make the fetus active.

Contraction Stress Test

The contraction stress test measures how the fetal heart rate reacts when the uterus contracts. The fetal heart rate is recorded at the same time the contractions of the uterus are measured. The contraction stress test often is used if the nonstress test shows no change in the fetal heart rate when the fetus moves. To make your uterus contract mildly, you are given a drug called oxytocin. (In rare cases, a woman's uterus may contract on its own, especially if the test is done late in pregnancy.)

During a contraction, the blood flow to the placenta decreases for a brief

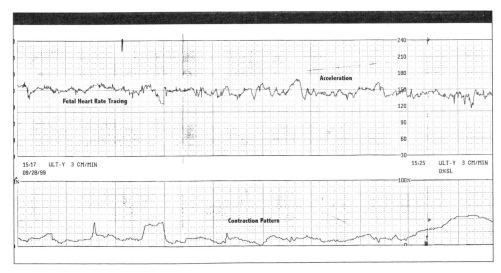

Sample of a nonstress test graph that records the fetal heart rate.

time. Normally, contractions do not affect the fetal heart rate. If there is something wrong with the placenta or the baby is showing signs of having a problem, the contraction can decrease the oxygen flow and cause the fetal heart rate to decrease.

Biophysical Profile

The biophysical profile assesses fetal well-being in these five areas:

➤The nonstress test

➤Breathing movements

➤Body movements

➤Muscle tone

➤Amount of amniotic fluid

For the biophysical profile, in addition to the nonstress test results, the doctor uses ultrasound to measure the amniotic fluid and to see how often the fetus breathes, moves, and flexes muscles during a 30-minute period. Each of the areas is given a score of 0 or 2 points, for a possible total of 10 points. A score of 8 or 10 is normal.

In measuring the amount of amniotic fluid, your doctor may use the term "amniotic fluid index" or AFI. For this test, ultrasound is used to measure the depth of the amniotic fluid in four different areas of your uterus. The sum of these measurements is the AFI.

Sometimes a modified biophysical profile is performed. This includes a nonstress test and AFI.

The biophysical profile does not cause any harm to the fetus. It can be repeated if needed at various times to check the well-being of the fetus. The score will help decide whether you need special care or whether your baby should be born sooner than planned.

Test Results

Testing during the second half of pregnancy can assure you and your doctor that all is going well with you and your baby. If there is a problem, tests may help your doctor find and treat it. Keep in mind tests cannot always find a problem, or the results may say there is a problem when there isn't one. Results of your test may mean that you and your baby will need special care before and during pregnancy. This will help keep you and your baby as healthy as possible.

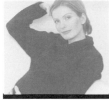

CHAPTER **4**

A Healthy Lifestyle

Many choices you make in your daily life during pregnancy can affect your health as well as the health of your baby. Some women may need to make a few changes in their lifestyle after they become pregnant. They may simply need to get extra rest and eat healthy foods. (Chapter 6 has information about good nutrition during pregnancy.) A healthy lifestyle during pregnancy is the best thing you can do for yourself and for your baby.

Exercise

If you are active now, pregnancy need not cause you to alter your fitness routine. If you have not been active, now is a good time to start. Exercise during pregnancy can benefit your health in the following ways:

➤ Increase your energy

➤ Relieve constipation, leg cramps, bloating, and swelling

➤ Lift your spirits

➤ Help you relax

➤ Improve your posture

➤ Promote muscle tone and stamina

➤ Control gestational diabetes

➤ Improve sleep

Exercise can help prepare your body for labor and delivery. It will give you a head start in getting back in shape after the baby is born.

Some exercise routines can help you relieve pregnancy-related aches and pains. For instance, the extra weight you are carrying affects your posture and can be hard on your back. Exercise may help ease back pain by stretching muscles and making them stronger. (Specific back exercises are described in Chapter 7.)

Some of the changes in your body during pregnancy affect the kinds of activities you can do safely. It is important to choose an exercise program that will be safe for you during this time:

➤ *Joints.* Some pregnancy hormones cause the ligaments that support your joints to stretch. This makes them more prone to injury.

➤ *Balance.* The weight you gain in the front of your body shifts your center of gravity. This puts stress on your joints and muscles—mostly those in the lower back and pelvis. It also can make you less stable and more likely to fall.

➤ *Heart rate.* Extra weight also makes your body work harder than it did before you were pregnant. This is true even if you are working out at a slower pace. Intense exercise boosts oxygen and blood flow to the muscles and away from other parts of your body—such as your uterus. If you can't talk at a normal level during exercise, then you are working too hard.

Before you start your exercise program, talk with your doctor to make sure you do not have any health conditions that may limit your activity. If you have heart disease, are at risk for preterm labor, or have vaginal bleeding, for example, your doctor may advise you not to exercise. Ask about specific exercises or sports that you like to do. Unless your doctor tells you not to, you should do moderate exercise for 30 minutes or more on most days, if not every day. The 30 minutes do not have to be all at one time—it can be a total of different exercise periods. If you have not been active, start with a few minutes each day and build up to 30 minutes or more.

Almost any form of exercise is safe if it is done with caution and if you don't do too much of it. Be aware of signs that may signal a problem (see box).

Warning Signs When to Stop Exercise

➤ Dizziness or faintness

➤ Increased shortness of breath

➤ Uneven or rapid heartbeat

➤ Chest pain

➤ Trouble walking

➤ Calf pain or swelling

➤ Headache

➤ Vaginal bleeding

➤ Uterine contractions that continue after rest

➤ Fluid gushing or leaking from your vagina

➤ Decreased fetal movement

Follow these tips for a safe and healthy exercise program that's geared to the special needs of pregnancy:

DOs

➤ Start your workout routine with slow, low-impact activities such as walking, swimming, or cycling, if you didn't exercise much before getting pregnant. As you become more fit, you can move to higher levels slowly.

➤ Be sure you have all the equipment you need for a safe workout. Wear the right shoes for your sport and be sure the shoes have plenty of padding and give your feet good support. Be sure to wear a sports bra that fits well and gives plenty of support. Your breasts are growing and may be very tender.

➤ Drink enough fluid. Take a bottle of water with you for a drink before, during, and after your workout. If you're getting hot or feeling thirsty, take a break and drink more water or sports drink.

➤ Begin your workout with stretching and warming up for 5 minutes to prevent muscle strain. Slow walking or riding a stationary bike are good warm-ups.

➤ Work out on a wooden floor or a tightly carpeted surface. This gives you better footing.

➤ Get up slowly after lying or sitting on the floor. This will help keep you from feeling dizzy or fainting.

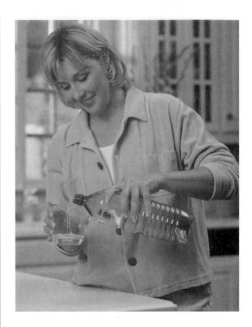

Once you're standing, walk in place briefly.

➤ Follow intense exercise with cooling down for 5–10 minutes. Slow your pace little by little and end your workout by gently stretching. Don't stretch too far, though. This can injure the tissue that connects your joints.

DON'Ts

➤ Don't exercise to shed excess pounds. Instead try to reach or keep a safe fitness level during pregnancy. Spurts of heavy exercise followed by long periods of no activity put strain on your body and offer few benefits.

➤ Don't do brisk exercise when it's hot and humid outside. Wear comfortable clothes that will help you stay cool. Also, don't exercise if you have a fever.

Are Hot Tubs, Baths, and Saunas Safe?

A warm bath can be a safe—and relaxing—treat during pregnancy. But, just as it is not safe to exercise until you are overheated during pregnancy, it also is not a good idea to become overheated in a hot tub, very hot bath, or sauna. During pregnancy, your core body temperature should not increase above 102.2°F (39°C) for more than 10 minutes. You can check the water temperature by dipping a thermometer into the water. One sign of being overheated is that you feel uncomfortable or you stop sweating.

If you soaked in a hot tub before you knew you were pregnant, most likely your baby will be fine. Most women get out of the hot tub before the temperature reaches a harmful level because they start to feel too hot.

➤ Don't do jerky, bouncy, or high-impact motions. Jumping, jarring motions, or quick direction changes can strain your joints and cause pain. Low-impact exercise such as walking or swimming is best.

➤ Don't do deep knee bends, full sit-ups, double leg lifts (raising and lowering both legs at once), and straight-leg toe touches. After the first trimester, you also should avoid exercises in which you lie on your back. This can cut down the blood flow to your baby.

If you are a competitive athlete or engage in strenuous exercise, talk to your doctor about what level of activity is safe for you.

Certain sports are safe even for beginners. Others are acceptable for those who have done them for a while. Still others are off-limits during pregnancy (see box). With any type of exercise you would like to try, be sure to discuss it with your doctor ahead of time. With your doctor's OK, here are some safe options:

➤ *Walking.* If you were not active before getting pregnant, walking is the ideal way to start an exercise program. Try to walk briskly for 30 minutes every day, if possible.

➤ *Swimming.* This sport is great for your body because it works many different muscles. The water supports your weight so you avoid injury and muscle strain.

➤ *Cycling.* This activity provides a good aerobic workout. However, your changing body shape can affect your balance and make you more prone to falls. Later in pregnancy, stationary cycling may be best.

➤ *Jogging.* If you were a runner before you became pregnant, you can keep it up now. Be careful, though. Avoid getting too hot. Stop exercising if you have pain or feel too tired.

➤ *Aerobics.* Low-impact aerobics is a safe and good way to keep your heart and lungs strong. There are aerobics classes designed just for pregnant women. Water aerobics also is a good activity. It combines the benefits of swimming and aerobics.

➤ *Yoga.* Yoga exercises or postures can stretch and strengthen muscles and help develop good breathing techniques.

➤ *Body building or strength training.* Your muscles will become stronger with strength training. The workouts also help prevent some of the aches and pains so common in pregnancy. To avoid harming your muscles and joints, do strength training only under the watchful eye of an expert. Use slow, controlled movements and do short sets (10 or fewer repetitions). Don't hold your breath while bearing down.

Sports to Avoid During Pregnancy

The following activities should be avoided during pregnancy:

➤ *Racquet sports.* Your changing balance affects rapid movements in sports such as badminton, tennis, or racquetball. This can increase your risk of falling.

➤ *Downhill snow skiing.* Downhill skiing also poses a risk of severe injuries and hard falls. In addition, you should not exercise at heights of more than 6,000 feet.

➤ *In-line skating, gymnastics, horseback riding.* Again, your balance is affected and there's a risk of crashes and falls.

➤ *Water skiing, surfing, diving.* Hitting the water with great force can be harmful. Taking a fall at such fast speeds could harm you or your baby.

➤ *Contact sports.* Avoid playing fast-paced team sports such as ice hockey, soccer, basketball, and volleyball. Collisions or falls could result in harm to both you and your baby.

➤ *Scuba diving.* High pressure from the water puts your baby at risk for decompression sickness.

➤ *Pilates.* With its focus on healthy breathing and improving flexibility, a Pilates exercise program is a good way to improve posture and build muscle strength.

➤ *Cross-country skiing.* This activity is safer for pregnant skiers than skiing on downhill slopes. Also, the ski machines at a gym or in your home will give you a safe workout.

➤ *Golf and bowling.* These sports may be fun and usually are safe. But they don't do much to tone your body, heart, and lungs. With either sport, you may have to adjust to your change in balance.

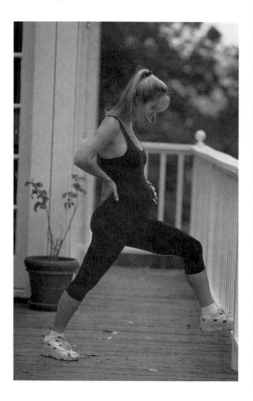

Alternative Medicine

Some women benefit from forms of health care that are different from conventional medicine as practiced in the United States. This type of care is called complementary and alternative medicine (CAM) and includes herbal products and other types of treatments.

You may have already been using some form of CAM before you became pregnant. If you want to continue using it, be sure to tell your doctor about it. This is a way to be sure it will be safe to use during your pregnancy. Also, be sure to tell your CAM provider that you are pregnant.

You also may want to try an approach you have heard about but never tried. Again, talk it over with your doctor. In all cases, it is important to seek CAM treatment from a qualified practitioner.

Herbal Products

Many drugs we use today come from plants. Some drugs that are now manmade first came from plants. Herbal treatments also come from plants and can be given in many forms. Some doctors may suggest herbal treatments in addition to conventional treatments or drugs prescribed.

Some people think of herbal treatments as being more "natural." They may think natural means safer and better. But natural things can hurt you too.

Practitioners of Herbal Treatments

➤ *Herbalists*—People who treat illness with herbs

➤ *Homeopaths*—People who treat conditions by giving small doses of a remedy that would produce symptoms of the condition in a healthy person.

➤ *Acupuncturists*—People who use the Chinese method of placing needles at points on the body to treat disease and pain

Just because something is natural does not mean it is good for you.

It also can be hard to know if a product is safe because herbs are not tested the same way as drugs are tested. There are risks to pregnancy with many herbal supplements, including black or blue cohosh, ephedra, dong quai, feverfew, juniper, pennyroyal, St. John's wort, rosemary, and thuja. You should definitely not take any supplements for weight-loss or weight-gain during pregnancy.

Other Treatments

Besides herbal products, there are many other kinds of CAM approaches to aid health and well-being. These are some of the most common treatments:

➤ *Acupuncture.* Very fine sterile needles are placed under the skin at key points. If done for labor, this may be done over a period of several weeks before labor begins. If you use acupuncture, be sure the practitioner uses a new set of disposable needles in a sealed package every time.

➤ *Aromatherapy.* Extracts or essences from plants such as flowers and herbs are used to promote health and well-being.

➤ *Chiropractic care.* The spine and other joints are manipulated to bring about alignment. Chiropractic care focuses on the way the body (mainly the spine) affects health.

➤ *Herbal and nutritional supplements.* Dietary supplements may include vitamins, minerals, herbs, or other plant or animal products. (See Chapter 6, Nutrition, for more details on supplements.)

➤ *Hypnosis.* Hypnosis is a state of concentration and focus. Some people seem to be more able to let themselves be hypnotized than do others. Some people have used it to help quit smoking or to relieve the pain of childbirth.

➤ *Massage.* Massage therapists manipulate and apply pressure to muscles and soft tissue. This can help muscles relax and promote oxygen flow.

During pregnancy, the best position for a massage is lying on your side.

As with any treatment, CAM methods help some people and not others. If you want to use CAM, ask your doctor to help you find an approach that is best for you and your baby.

Work

Most women of childbearing age in the United States work outside the home. Pregnant women often work right up until delivery and return to their jobs within weeks or months of the baby's birth.

As long as you and your baby are healthy and your job presents no special hazards, you should be able to work as long as you want. There are some jobs that could pose a risk for a pregnant woman. No matter what type of work you do, discuss it with your doctor early in pregnancy.

Jobs That May Cause Concern

Women often can keep doing their normal jobs while they are pregnant. However, some jobs may expose a woman to heavy duties or harmful substances. You may need to cut back on the hours you work, give up certain tasks, transfer to another position, or stop working until after the baby is born.

Heavy Duties

Strenuous jobs—those that involve a lot of heavy lifting, climbing, carrying, or standing—may not be safe during pregnancy. That's because the dizziness, nausea, and fatigue common in early pregnancy can increase the chance of injury. Later on, the change in body shape can throw off your balance and can lead to falls.

Harmful Substances

Being exposed on the job to harmful substances is fairly rare. Still, agents found in some workplaces pose a risk. It makes sense, then, to think about the things you come into contact with during the course of your workday. You also may come in contact with these agents through a hobby.

Pesticides, chemicals, cleaning solvents, and heavy metals such as lead can potentially cause serious problems during pregnancy. Women who work in farming, factories, dry cleaners, electronics, printing, or crafts such as painting or pottery glazing may be exposed to harmful agents.

Health care workers also are at risk. Breathing or absorbing medical gases and toxic drugs is another danger. Radiation is used to take X-rays and treat certain diseases, such as cancer. In high doses, it can harm a fetus. Most women who work around radiation are protected from exposure.

Keep in mind that just because a toxic agent is present doesn't mean you are exposed to harmful levels of it. In some cases, proper clothing and safety measures such as gloves or a mask can greatly reduce or prevent exposure.

Infections

Child care workers, health care workers, teachers, and mothers with young children may be at risk for exposure to certain viruses and childhood diseases. (See Chapter 17 for more information.) Viruses such as German measles (rubella), and chickenpox (varicella) can cause miscarriage or birth defects if a woman is infected during pregnancy. Most women are immune to these diseases or have a **vaccination** against them before they become pregnant.

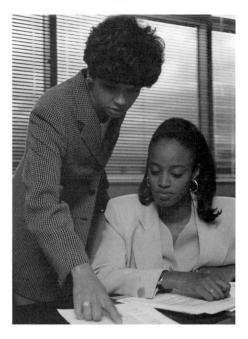

If you think your job may bring you into contact with something harmful, find out for sure by asking your personnel office, employee clinic, or union. Let your doctor know right away if you and your baby are at risk. Workplace safety hazards and tips can be found at the web sites of the Occupational Safety and Health Administration (www.osha.gov) and the National Institute for Occupational Safety and Health (www.cdc.gov/niosh).

Pregnancy-Related Disability

Having a disability means that health problems keep you from doing your normal duties. Most pregnancies are not disabling. For some women, pregnancy could become a disability if problems arise. Your pregnancy may be partly or totally disabling—only you and your doctor can decide. There are two types of pregnancy-related disability:

1. *Disability caused by the pregnancy itself.* Some symptoms of pregnancy may cause short-term or partial disability. Giving birth also causes short-term disability.

2. *Disability due to pregnancy complications.* More severe problems or conditions you had before getting pregnant may worsen during pregnancy and cause longer disability.

If your doctor decides that your pregnancy is disabling, the appropriate forms must be completed. Likewise, if your employer wants you to stop working but your doctor says you can continue, get a letter from the doctor to give to your employer.

The federal Pregnancy Discrimination Act requires employers that have at least 15 workers to treat workers disabled by pregnancy or childbirth the same as workers disabled by illness or accident (see box). If you are partly disabled by pregnancy and your company gives lighter duty to other partly disabled workers, it must do the same for you. However, because many employers don't offer their workers any disability benefits, they don't have to provide paid leave. If you are not covered by a disability plan at work, you may be able to get state unemployment or disability benefits. For details, contact your local unemployment office. Many states also have maternity and family leave laws.

Leave

Policies about maternity leave and disability leave vary from company to company and state to state. Only about 4 in 10 working women in the United States get paid leave after giving birth. Others must use sick leave and vacation time or take time off without pay.

The Family and Medical Leave Act protects your right to leave, with certain limits, for pregnancy-related problems or after giving birth. This federal law says you may be on leave up to 12 weeks without pay during any 12-month period and have your job back afterwards.

To qualify for this family leave protection, you must meet the following conditions:

➤ Work for a company at a location where there are at least 50 employees of the same employer within a 75-mile area (at a branch office, for instance)

➤ Have worked there for at least 12 months

➤ Have worked at least 1,250 hours during the past 12 months

You may have to use vacation or personal or sick leave for some or all of your time off. If an employer provides health care benefits, this coverage must be kept at the same level during the leave period. When you return to work, you must be given the same or an equal job and the same benefits you had when you left. If you use some of the 12 weeks for a difficult pregnancy, it may be counted as part of the 12-week family-leave entitlement.

Changes for Your Partner and Family

Pregnancy is a special time for a couple. It also can strain your relationship. Your old roles are shifting, and you need to adapt to new ones. You'll both spend a lot of time thinking about the baby, but try to make time for your partner, too.

Your Workplace Rights

Three major federal laws protect the health, safety, and employment rights of pregnant working women. If you are denied your rights, contact the agencies listed.

Pregnancy Discrimination Act

The Pregnancy Discrimination Act requires employers to treat pregnancy as they would treat any other medical condition. That means they must offer the same disability leave and pay as they would to workers disabled by illness or injury. This federal act also makes it illegal to hire, fire, or refuse to promote a woman because she's pregnant. If you think you are the victim of pregnancy discrimination, contact the Equal Employment Opportunity Commission 1-800-669-4000 (voice) or 1-800-669-6820 (TDD/TTY). The commission's website (www.eeoc.gov) also gives details on how to file a claim.

Occupational Safety and Health Act

The Occupational Safety and Health Administration (OSHA) requires employers to provide a workplace free from known hazards that cause or are likely to cause death or serious physical harm. It also requires employers to give workers facts about harmful agents. If you think your employer may be breaking these rules, call OSHA at 1-800-321-6742 (voice) or 1-877-889-5627 (TTY) or go to the OSHA website (www.osha.gov) and click on "Contact Us."

The National Institute for Occupational Safety and Health (NIOSH) finds workplace hazards, figures out how to control them, and suggests ways to limit the dangers. If you, your union, or your doctor asks it to, this group will inspect your workplace for hazards. Call NIOSH at 1-800-356-4674.

Certain state and city laws also give workers and unions the right to ask for the names of chemicals and other substances used in the workplace. If you have questions or concerns, ask your employer or call the numbers for OSHA or NIOSH.

Family and Medical Leave Act

The Family and Medical Leave Act (FMLA) requires employers with 50 or more employees to allow up to 12 weeks of unpaid leave during any 12-month period for the following reasons:

1. Upon the birth, adoption, or foster care of a child

2. When needed to care for a spouse, a child, or a parent with a serious health condition

3. When a worker isn't able to do her job because of her own serious health condition, including a pregnancy-related disability or birth-related disability

To find out more about family and medical leave, contact the U.S. Department of Labor at 1-800-827-5335. A few states have better leave laws than the federal FMLA. For details, contact your state's Department of Labor.

Each of you can talk about your feelings and give each other support. Go to your prenatal visits and tests together. Attend childbirth and baby-care classes as a team. Your parents, siblings, and other children also should be involved.

Sex

You may feel more or less desire for sex during pregnancy. During the first and last months, for instance, nausea and fatigue may get in the way of sex. Be open and honest with your partner. Talking can bring you closer and help avoid hurt feelings and loneliness.

You also may worry that having intercourse or having an orgasm will harm your baby. The fetus is safe in the uterus and will not be harmed by sexual relations. The amniotic sac protects the fetus, and the cervix shields the baby from germs.

Unless your doctor has told you not to, you can keep having sex throughout pregnancy. As your belly grows, though, certain positions may be more comfortable for you:

➤ *The side-lying position.* You and your partner can either face each other or your partner can enter you from behind.

➤ *The woman-on-top position.* This takes the pressure off your belly.

➤ *The man-behind position.* This way your growing belly won't come between you.

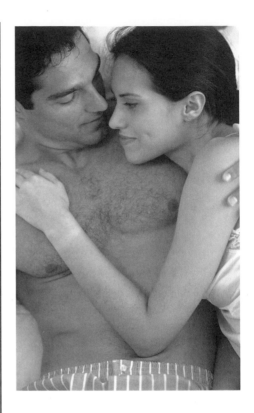

You may be advised to limit or avoid intercourse if these conditions exist:

➤ Preterm labor or birth

➤ Placenta previa

➤ Infection

➤ Vaginal bleeding

➤ Discharge of amniotic fluid

If intercourse is off-limits, there are other ways to express your sexuality. Cuddling, kissing, fondling, mutual masturbation, and oral sex are ways to stay intimate and satisfy desire.

Travel

In most cases travel is not ruled out during pregnancy. If you are planning a trip, it's a good idea to check with your doctor about safety measures to take during travel. Most women can travel safely until close to their due dates. If travel poses a risk, it is wise to change plans.

The best time to travel is mid-pregnancy (14–28 weeks of pregnancy). After 28 weeks, it's often harder to move around or sit for a long time. During mid-pregnancy, your energy has returned, morning sickness is over, and you are still mobile.

Paying heed to the way you feel is the best guide for your activities—whether you are on the road or at home. When choosing your mode of travel, think about how long it will take to get where you are going. The fastest way is often the best. Whether you go by train, plane, car, bus, or boat, take steps to ensure your comfort and safety.

Foreign Travel

If you are planning a trip out of the country, your doctor can help you decide if foreign travel is safe for you. Your doctor also can help you figure out what steps to take before your trip. Allow plenty of time to get any shots you may need. Also be sure to get a copy of your health record to take with you.

When you are planning your trip, call the International Travelers Hotline at the Centers for Disease Control and Prevention (CDC). This service has safety tips and up-to-date vaccination facts for many countries. The number is 1-888-232-3228. The CDC web site (www.cdc.gov) also has world travel health facts and special information for traveling while pregnant.

Even if you are in perfect health before going on a trip, you never know when an emergency will come up. Before leaving home, locate the nearest hospital or medical clinic in the place you are visiting. The International Association for Medical Assistance to Travelers (IAMAT) has a worldwide directory of doctors. To obtain the free directory, call IAMAT at 1-716-754-4883, or check the IAMAT website (www.iamat.org). You must join IAMAT to obtain information, but membership is free (donations are requested).

If you need to see a doctor who doesn't speak English, it's a good idea to have a foreign language dictionary with you. After you arrive, register with an American embassy or consulate. This will help if you need to leave the country because of an emergency.

Here are some tips for healthy travel:

➤ Have a prenatal checkup before you leave.

➤ If you'll be far from home, take a copy of your health record with you.

➤ Ask your doctor for the name and phone number of a doctor where you're visiting, in case of emergency.

➤ Keep your travel plans easy to change. Pregnancy problems can come up at any time and ground you before you leave home. Buy travel insurance to cover tickets and deposits that can't be refunded.

➤ For air travel, book an aisle seat. This will make it easier for you to get up and walk around every hour or so. Try to get a seat near the front of the plane. The ride often is smoother there.

➤ While you are en route, walk around about every hour. Stretching your legs will lessen the risk of blood clots and make you more comfortable. It also will decrease the swelling in your ankles and feet.

➤ Wear comfortable shoes, support stockings, and clothing that doesn't bind. Wear a few layers of light clothing.

➤ Carry some crackers or other light snacks with you to help prevent nausea.

➤ Take time to eat regular meals. A balanced and healthy diet during your trip will boost your energy and keep you feeling good. Be sure to get plenty of fiber to ease constipation, a common travel problem.

➤ Drink extra fluids. Take some juice or a bottle of water with you. In an airplane, the cabin is very dry. Choose water instead of a soft drink.

➤ Traveling can upset your stomach and disrupt your sleep. Don't take any medicine—including motion-sickness pills, laxatives, diarrhea remedies, or sleeping pills—before checking with your doctor.

➤ Rest after a long trip. While away from home, rest often so you won't feel tired. Get plenty of sleep at night.

Car Travel

During a car trip, make each day's drive brief. Spending hours on the road is tiring even when you're not pregnant. Try to limit driving to no more than 5 or 6 hours each day.

Be sure to wear your seat belt every time you ride in a car or truck, even if your car has an air bag (see box). If you get in a crash—even a minor one—see your doctor to make sure you and your baby are not injured.

Many cars have air bags to protect the driver and the passenger riding in the front seat. Air bags are inside the steering wheel, in the dashboard on the passenger side, and sometimes on the sides of the car, inside, near the doors. In a crash, air bags inflate very fast.

Buckling Up During Pregnancy

For the best protection in a vehicle, wear a lap–shoulder belt every time you travel. The safety belt will not hurt your baby. You and your baby are far more likely to survive a car crash if you are buckled in. More damage is caused when they are not used.

Follow these rules when wearing a safety belt:

➤ Always wear both the lap and shoulder belt.

➤ Buckle the lap belt low on your hip bones, below your belly.

➤ Never put the lap belt across your belly.

➤ Place the shoulder belt across the center of the chest (between your breasts)—never under your arm.

➤ Make sure the belts fit snugly.

The upper part of the belt should cross your shoulder without chafing your neck. Never slip the upper part of the belt off your shoulder. Safety belts worn too loosely or too high on the belly can cause broken ribs or injuries to your belly.

The force of an airbag can hurt people who are close to it—especially if they are short. To prevent injury, buckle up with both the lap and shoulder belts on every trip. Keep your seat as far back from the dashboard as you can.

If you plan to travel by bus or train, be sure to have a good hold on railings or seat backs when you are up and about. Don't worry that a bumpy ride could bring on labor—it won't.

Air Travel

Flying in an airplane is almost always safe during pregnancy. Most airlines allow pregnant women to fly until about 36 weeks of pregnancy. For air travel, check with the airline about any rules it may have for pregnant women.

Commercial planes are pressurized. That makes sure there is enough oxygen to breathe even when the plane is at a high altitude where the air outside is low on oxygen. Many private planes are not pressurized. It's best to avoid altitudes higher than about 7,000 feet in unpressurized planes.

Don't worry about walking through the metal detector at the airport security check. These machines give off very low levels of radiation—not nearly enough to harm you or your baby.

Sea Travel

Sea travel can upset your stomach. If you have traveled by sea before and you think your stomach can stand it, check on cruise rules for pregnant women.

Make sure the ship has a doctor or a nurse on board and that it docks in areas with modern medical facilities. Ask your doctor about safe medicines for calming seasickness. You also may want to try a pair of the seasickness bands for sale at many drug stores. These bands use acupressure to help ward off nausea.

Healthy Lifestyle, Healthy Baby

Few things are more vital to your baby's health than your lifestyle choices during pregnancy. If you led an active, healthy lifestyle before pregnancy, keep it up. If you do want to make some changes, make them now to give your baby the best start you can. You'll also make a change for the better in your own life. Years from now, you'll still be reaping the rewards.

CHAPTER 5

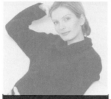

Lifestyle Risks

Almost all women have to make some lifestyle changes during pregnancy. In some cases, this may mean adjusting an exercise routine, resting more, or eating healthier foods. In other cases, it may mean kicking a smoking or drinking habit or ending an abusive relationship. These changes can help you have a healthy pregnancy, as well as a healthy baby.

Harmful Agents

Teratogens are agents that can cause birth defects when a woman is exposed to them during pregnancy. They include certain medications, chemicals, and infections. (Chapter 17 has details about infections during pregnancy.) These agents can prevent the fetus from growing normally and can cause defects of the brain or body. Their effect depends on the level of exposure and when in pregnancy it occurs. Other substances, such as tobacco, alcohol, and illegal drugs, also are harmful during pregnancy.

Some substances once were thought to be harmful but now are considered safe during pregnancy. For instance, many women worry that using hair dye during pregnancy may be harmful to their babies. But hair dyes are believed to be safe to use during pregnancy. Another concern was that caffeine causes problems during pregnancy. However, there's no proof that small amounts of caffeine (for instance, one or two cups of coffee) harm the fetus. Caffeine is a stimulant and a diuretic (it increases urine production). It may be helpful to avoid it in the afternoon and evening if it keeps you from sleeping at night. Caffeine is found in coffee, cola and some other soft drinks, some teas, and chocolate.

If a woman is addicted to harmful substances, it may be hard to stop. It is

Agents to Avoid During Pregnancy

Certain medications (including prescription medications) and drugs are known to be harmful to your baby if you are exposed to them during pregnancy. Some agents may be more harmful than others—it often depends on the amount taken or when in pregnancy the fetus was exposed. If you are prescribed or exposed to any of the following substances, be sure to talk to your doctor:

➤ Alcohol

➤ Androgens and testosterone by-products (for instance, danazol)

➤ Angiotensin-converting enzyme (ACE) inhibitors (for instance, enalapril or captopril)

➤ Coumarin by-products (for instance, warfarin)

➤ Carbamazepine

➤ Anti-folic acid drugs (for instance, methotrexate or aminopterin)

➤ Cocaine

➤ Diethylstilbestrol (DES)

➤ Lead

➤ Lithium

➤ Organic mercury

➤ Phenytoin

➤ Streptomycin and kanamycin

➤ Tetracycline

➤ Thalidomide

➤ Trimethadione and paramethadione

➤ Valproic acid

➤ Vitamin A and its by-products (for instance, isotretinoin, etretinate, or retinoids)

important for a woman to try to quit for her sake and the sake of her baby. A doctor may be able to help a woman get the treatment she needs to make a new start in her life.

Smoking

If a woman smokes when she's pregnant, her baby is exposed to harmful chemicals such as tar, nicotine, and carbon monoxide. Nicotine causes blood vessels to constrict, so less oxygen and nutrients reach the fetus. Carbon monoxide lowers the amount of oxygen the baby receives. Also, women who smoke during pregnancy are more likely to have certain problems:

➤ An ectopic pregnancy

➤ Vaginal bleeding

➤ Problems with the way the placenta attaches to the uterus

➤ A stillbirth

➤ A low-birth-weight baby (weighing less than 5½ pounds)

Smoking is harmful to the baby after birth, too. The baby may breathe in harmful amounts of smoke from cigarettes smoked nearby (secondhand smoke). Breathing secondhand smoke raises the risk of asthma and *sudden infant death syndrome (SIDS).*

The sooner a pregnant smoker quits, the better off both she and her baby will be. If she stops smoking early in her pregnancy, the chance of having a low-birth-weight baby is the same as that of a woman who didn't smoke at all. If a woman kicks the habit while she's pregnant, she may be able to kick it for a lifetime. She and her family will be healthier as a result.

A pregnant smoker may be tempted to cut down on the number of cigarettes she smokes instead of quitting. The less she smokes, the less harm it will do. Cutting down or stopping smoking at any time in pregnancy is better than not stopping at all. However, quitting is the best thing to do for both the mother and baby.

If you are a smoker and have tried to quit on your own but failed, tell your doctor that you need help. If you are a heavy smoker, chewing nicotine gum or wearing a nicotine patch may help. But nicotine replacements also have some risks. They should be used only if the benefits of using them to stop smoking outweigh the risks of using them.

You may want to ask your partner and other family members to quit too. This will help support you in your efforts to give up smoking. Even if you don't smoke yourself, when you are pregnant, secondhand smoke from people around you can be harmful.

Alcohol

Alcohol can harm your baby's health. The degree of harm depends on the amount of alcohol consumed. It's best to stop drinking before you get pregnant because the effect is greatest during early pregnancy, when many of the baby's organs are forming. If you had a drink or two before you knew you were pregnant, most likely it would not harm your baby.

When a pregnant woman drinks alcohol, it quickly reaches her fetus. The same amount of alcohol that's in her blood is in her baby's blood. In an adult, the liver breaks down the alcohol. But a baby's liver is not yet able to do this. Thus, alcohol is much more harmful to a fetus than it is to an adult. The more a pregnant woman drinks, the greater the danger to her baby. Drinking at any time during pregnancy can cause problems. Alcohol may affect the baby in many ways. Alcohol increases the chance of having a miscarriage or a

Do You Have a Drinking Problem?

Do you use alcohol or abuse it? Sometimes it's hard to tell. If you're not sure, ask yourself these questions:

T How many drinks does it take to make you feel high? (TOLERANCE)
A Have people ANNOYED you by criticizing your drinking?
C Have you felt you ought to CUT DOWN on your drinking?
E Have you ever had a drink first thing in the morning to steady your nerves or get rid of a hangover? (EYE OPENER)

Scoring:

➤ 2 points if your answer to the first question is more than two drinks.

➤ 1 point for every "yes" response to the other questions.

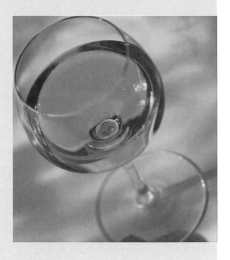

If your total score is 2 or more, you may have an alcohol problem.

Talk to your doctor about your drinking habits. He or she can help you decide if you have a problem. The doctor will refer you for counseling or treatment if needed. You also may want to think about contacting a substance abuse program. These groups can help you find someone to talk to about your problem and give you needed support when you are trying to quit. Check your local yellow-page listings.

Modified from Sokol RJ, Martier SS, Ager JW. The T-ACE questions: practical prenatal detection of risk drinking. Am J Obstet Gynecol 1989;160:865

preterm baby. Alcohol abuse during pregnancy is a leading cause of mental retardation.

One of the worst effects of drinking in pregnancy is *fetal alcohol syndrome.* This is a pattern of major physical,

mental, and behavioral problems in babies exposed to alcohol during pregnancy. Smoking, drug use, poor diet, and stress may play a role in how severely the baby is affected by fetal alcohol syndrome. Babies with fetal alcohol syndrome may have one or more of the following:

➤ Small bodies (even with special care, their growth doesn't catch up)

➤ Problems with joints and limbs (such as *clubfoot*)

➤ Heart defects

➤ Abnormal facial features

➤ Behavioral problems, including hyperactivity, anxiety, and poor attention span

➤ Low IQ

Some babies with fetal alcohol syndrome are born with all of these problems. Some babies may have some of these symptoms, but not to a great extent. Also, severe ear infections and vision and dental problems may appear later in the child's life. There is no cure for fetal alcohol syndrome.

It is not known how much alcohol it takes to harm the fetus. The best course is not to drink at all during pregnancy. Also, there are no types of drinks that are safe. One beer, one shot of liquor, one mixed drink, or one glass of wine all contain approximately the same amount of alcohol. Thus, all forms of alcohol may be harmful.

It may be hard to stop drinking. If this is true for you, you may need help. Talk honestly to your caregiver about your drinking habits.

Drugs

Drug use during pregnancy can lead to long-term problems. Babies may need special care after birth. There's no safe time to use drugs. Severe damage can occur if drugs are used in the first 12 weeks of pregnancy. The baby's organs are forming during this time. Using them in mid to late pregnancy can affect brain growth. During late pregnancy, drug use can stunt fetal growth and bring on preterm labor. After birth, some drugs can be passed to the baby through breast milk.

It's safest to quit taking drugs well before getting pregnant. Still, giving them up or cutting back at any time is better than nothing.

Drug addiction is a chronic illness. Usually, people addicted to drugs cannot quit by themselves. Treatment is needed to end addiction. Ask your doctor for information or a referral. In some states, social services agencies may get involved. You also can check the phone book for support groups and substance abuse treatment centers. The following groups will provide help treating a drug problem:

➤ Narcotics Anonymous. Call 818-772-9999 or go to the web site www.na.org.

➤ Substance Abuse and Mental Health Services Administration. Call 800-662-HELP (4357) or go to the web site findtreatment.samhsa.gov.

Effects of Drugs

Use of illegal drugs during pregnancy can harm your baby. Many are highly addictive and a user's lifestyle can be just as harmful as the drug itself. These are the effects of specific drugs:

➤ *Marijuana.* The active compound in marijuana stays in the body for weeks, leading to higher levels of fetal exposure. Smoking marijuana releases carbon monoxide. This can prevent the baby from getting enough oxygen.

➤ *Methamphetamine.* "Meth" can cause placental abruption or even fetal death. Babies exposed to methamphetamine may grow too slowly in the womb. After birth, they may be very fussy, have trouble bonding with others, and have tremors.

➤ *Heroin and other narcotics.* If heroin is used during pregnancy, it can cause any of these problems:

—Fetal death

—Addiction in the fetus

—Small babies

—Preterm birth

—Low birth weight

—Delays in development

—Behavioral problems

Sudden withdrawal from heroin can harm a woman and her baby. Drug treatment programs often replace heroin with methadone, a prescription drug. Women in methadone treatment programs may be able to stick to a healthier lifestyle than women who are addicted to heroin. Still, the methadone is not good for a growing fetus. It also may be addictive. Because of this, methadone should be used only under a doctor's care.

➤ *"T's and blues."* This is street name for a mix of a prescription drug and an over-the-counter allergy medication. Babies whose mothers use "T's and blues" are more likely to have slow growth before birth. They also may have withdrawal symptoms after birth.

(continued)

Effects of Drugs (continued)

➤ *Cocaine.* During pregnancy, cocaine can cause the placenta to tear away from the uterus—a condition called abruptio placentae (*placental abruption*). This can cause bleeding, preterm birth, or fetal death. These are problems that babies exposed to cocaine may have:

—Withdrawal symptoms

—Slow growth

—Brain injury

—Fussiness

—Long-term behavioral, emotional, and learning problems

➤ *PCP, Ketamine, and LSD.* Users of PCP, or angel dust, may lose touch with what's real. They may become violent. A woman who uses PCP can have flashbacks, seizures, heart attacks, or lung failure. Babies exposed to PCP during pregnancy may have withdrawal symptoms after birth, be smaller than normal, and have poor control of their movements. Ketamine, or Special K, affects the user in much the same way as PCP does. In addition, ketamine can cause a type of amnesia. Babies exposed to ketamine during pregnancy may have behavioral or learning problems. LSD ("acid") can cause someone who has used it to hear and see things that aren't there, have flashbacks, and become violent. LSD use during pregnancy can cause birth defects.

➤ *Glues and Solvents.* Inhalant use makes a user feel light-headed and dizzy. It also can damage the liver, kidneys, bone marrow, and brain. It can even cause sudden death. During pregnancy, glue and solvent abuse can lead to miscarriage, slow growth of the fetus, and preterm birth. The birth defects linked with glue sniffing during pregnancy are much like those caused by alcohol.

➤ *Ecstasy.* Risks from Ecstasy are similar to those found with the use of cocaine or methamphetamines, including mood changes, sleep problems, and loss of appetite. A baby born to a woman who took Ecstasy while pregnant may have long-term learning and memory problems.

Medications

Medications cross the placenta and enter the baby's bloodstream. In some cases, a medication could cause birth defects, addiction, or other problems in the baby. That doesn't mean you need to throw out the contents of your medicine cabinet once you become pregnant. It means that you need to be careful.

Some medicines are safe to take during pregnancy. Also, the risks of some medicines may be outweighed by the effects of not taking them. For instance, certain diseases are more harmful to a fetus than the drugs used to treat them. Don't stop taking a medication prescribed for you. Ask your doctor about it first.

Tell anyone who prescribes medications for you that you are pregnant. That includes any doctors you see for non-pregnancy problems, your dentist, or a mental health provider. Be sure that the doctor who cares for you during pregnancy knows about any medical problems you may have. Tell him or her about all the medications you take and if you have any drug allergies. If a medication you are taking poses a risk, your doctor may recommend switching to a safer drug while you are pregnant.

Prescription medications also can be harmful if they are abused. A woman who abuses prescription drugs risks overdose and addiction.

Medicines sold over-the-counter can cause problems during pregnancy, too. Pain relievers such as aspirin and ibuprofen may be harmful to a fetus. Check with your doctor before taking any over-the-counter drug. This includes pain relievers, laxatives, cold or allergy remedies, and skin treatments. You don't have to have the discomfort of headaches or colds without relief. Your doctor can give you advice about medicines that are safe for pregnant women.

Domestic Violence

Physical, sexual, and emotional abuse of women is one of America's worst health problems. Millions of women are abused each year. Injuries inflicted by a partner are the cause for 1 in 5 visits to an emergency room by a woman. More than 1 in 3 female murder victims is killed by her husband or boyfriend. Domestic abuse crosses all racial, class, economic, and religious lines.

Pregnancy often offers no break from the abuse. In fact, nearly 1 in 6

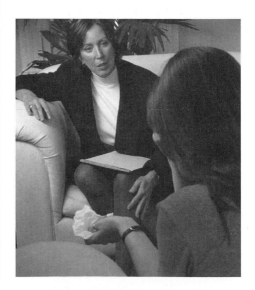

Is Your Relationship Abusive?

Fights, even heated ones, are a normal part of relationships. Physical violence and other abuse are not. How do you know if your relationship has crossed the line? Ask yourself these questions:

➤Does your partner make jokes at your expense or put you down?

➤Has he forced or pressured you to perform a sexual act?

➤Does he threaten you or throw things when he's angry?

➤Has he physically hurt you in the past year?

➤Does he say it's your fault if he hits you?

➤Does he promise it won't happen again, but it does?

If your answer to any of these is "yes," your relationship is not healthy. Get help right away.

pregnant women is abused by her partner. Abuse often starts or gets worse during pregnancy. It puts both the mother and her baby at risk. An abuser is likely to aim his blows at a pregnant woman's breasts and belly. The dangers of this violence include miscarriage, vaginal bleeding, low birth weight, and fetal injury.

Sometimes abuse lessens during pregnancy. A woman may feel safe from her partner only when she's carrying a child. As a result, she may get pregnant to escape her partner's rage. All too often, though, his rage returns and may worsen after the baby is born. Then, there are two victims.

If you are in a violent relationship, it's vital to take steps to protect yourself and your baby. It's important to know that you are not at fault for your part-

ner's actions. Abusers often blame their wives or girlfriends for their own actions. No matter what your partner says, it is not your fault. You do not make it happen. Women also may think they can stop the abuse by trying to please the abuser or avoid getting him or her angry. He or she alone is to blame for his or her actions.

The first step to breaking the pattern of violence is to tell someone about it. Tell someone you trust—a close friend, a family member, your doctor, a counselor, or a clergy member. Talking about a problem can be a huge relief. The person you confide in may be able to put you in touch with crisis hotlines, domestic violence programs, legal-aid services, and shelters for abused women. These services offer counseling that can help you get out of a bad situation.

For your safety, have a plan for a fast exit:

➤ *Pack a suitcase.* Include toiletry items, a change of clothes for you and your children, and an extra set of car and house keys. Store the bag with a friend or neighbor you trust.

➤ *Hide some cash.* Each week, put aside as much money as you can spare.

➤ *Keep needed items in a safe place.* Have these items handy so you can take them with you on short notice:

—Prescription medicines

—Birth certificates

—Social Security cards

—Health insurance cards

—Driver's license

—Extra cash and change for phone calls

—Checkbook

—Savings account book

—Credit cards

—Medical and financial records

—A special toy for each child

➤ *Have a safe place.* Know a friend or relative's home or shelter where you can go, no matter what time of day or night. Keep the address and phone number in your purse.

➤ *Know where to go if you are hurt.* Call your doctor or head to an emergency room if your partner harms you. Tell the doctor how you were hurt. Be sure to ask for a copy of your medical record in case you want to file charges.

➤ *Call the police.* Physical abuse is a crime, even if you are living with or married to your abuser. Tell the police what happened to you. Get the officer's badge number and a copy of the report in case you want to press charges at any time.

It's hard to break the cycle of violence. If you do nothing, though, chances are the abuse will happen more often and become more severe. No one deserves to be abused: not you, not your baby, and not your children. Leaving your partner or having him or her arrested during your pregnancy takes great courage. But you owe your baby a safe and loving home, and you owe yourself an end to the violence.

For more information or to get help, check the section of your phone book for domestic violence services or hotlines. You also can call the National Domestic Violence Hotline at 800-799-SAFE (7233) (voice) or 800-787-3224 (TDD).

Healthy Choices

Taking good care of yourself during pregnancy helps ensure you are taking good care of your baby. Stay healthy by ending harmful habits such as smoking or drinking alcohol, and taking steps to end an abusive relationship. Making healthy choices now will help give your baby a healthy beginning.

CHAPTER 6

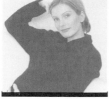

Nutrition

A well-balanced diet is crucial to good health. It is even more important during pregnancy, when there are added demands on your body to meet the needs of the growing fetus. A good diet can help ensure the health of your body and the growth of your baby.

Healthy eating during pregnancy may take a little effort, but it will be a major benefit for you and your baby. If you already have a balanced diet, all you have to do is add a few extra well-chosen *calories.* (Breastfeeding mothers need to pay careful attention to their diets as well. See Chapter 10 for details.)

A variety of foods can be used to create a healthy diet for you and your baby. Women all over the world with vastly varied diets have healthy babies. To nourish your growing baby, make sure you are getting the nutrients both of you need.

A Healthy Diet

The Food Guide Pyramid

One way to be sure you're eating a balanced diet is to follow the Food Guide Pyramid (see box). This pyramid was

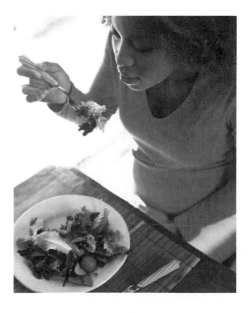

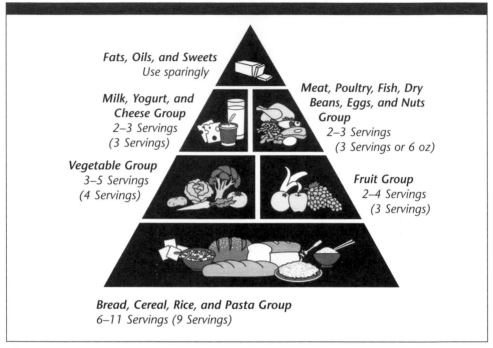

Fats, Oils, and Sweets
Use sparingly

Milk, Yogurt, and Cheese Group
2–3 Servings
(3 Servings)

Meat, Poultry, Fish, Dry Beans, Eggs, and Nuts Group
2–3 Servings
(3 Servings or 6 oz)

Vegetable Group
3–5 Servings
(4 Servings)

Fruit Group
2–4 Servings
(3 Servings)

Bread, Cereal, Rice, and Pasta Group
6–11 Servings (9 Servings)

The food guide pyramid is a guide to help men and non-pregnant women choose foods that will give them the nutrients they need. A pregnant woman needs extra calories and nutrients. You should get at least the number of servings shown in parentheses after the standard servings.

devised by the U.S. Department of Agriculture. It offers guidelines to help you get the nutrients you need. It stresses a diet that is low in fat, sugar, and **cholesterol** (a substance that carries fat through the bloodstream) and high in vegetables, fruits, and grains. If you don't want to measure out each serving to see if you're getting the right amount, follow this rule: a serving size of most food items is about the size of the palm of your hand. The pyramid has six food groups:

1. Bread, cereal, rice, and pasta. This group provides complex carbohydrates (starches). These are a good source of energy, vitamins, minerals, and fiber. Choose whole-grain types of bread and cereal, such as whole-wheat bread, as often as you can. Also look for foods made with little fat or sugar. These amounts equal a serving:

➤ 1 slice of bread

➤ About 1 cup of cold cereal

➤ ½ cup of cooked cereal, rice, or pasta

2. Vegetables. This group provides vitamins such as A, C, and folic acid, and minerals such as iron

and magnesium. Vegetables are low in fat and high in fiber. When you're planning your meals, choose a wide array of vegetables. This will help ensure that you get a variety of nutrients. Women who are worried about pesticides may want to think about buying vegetables and fruit that are grown without chemicals (organic). Pesticides also can be removed from fruit and vegetables by washing them with warm water and a small amount of soap and rinsing them. Eat a mixture of these kinds of vegetables:

➤ Dark-green leafy vegetables (spinach, romaine lettuce, broccoli)

➤ Deep-yellow or orange vegetables (carrots, sweet potatoes)

➤ Starchy vegetables (potatoes, corn, peas)

➤ Legumes (chick peas and navy, pinto, and kidney beans)

These amounts equal a serving:

➤ 1 cup of salad greens

➤ ½ cup of other vegetables—cooked or raw

➤ ¾ cup of vegetable juice

3. Fruits. This group provides vitamins A and C, potassium, and fiber. Choose fresh fruits, fruit juices, and frozen, canned, or dried fruit. Eat plenty of citrus fruits, melons, and berries. Choose fruit juices instead of fruit drinks, which are mostly sugar. A serving consists of:

➤ 1 medium apple, banana, orange, or pear

➤ ½ cup of chopped, cooked, or canned fruit

➤ ¾ cup of fruit juice

➤ ¼ cup of raisins or other dried fruit

4. Milk, yogurt, and cheese. Dairy products are a major source of protein, calcium, phosphorus, and vitamins. Calcium is a key nutrient during pregnancy and breastfeeding. If you don't like the taste of milk, eat dairy products such as yogurt, cottage cheese, or sliced cheese. Choose low-fat, skim, or part-skim items as often as you can. A serving consists of:

➤ 1 cup of milk or yogurt

➤ 1½ ounces of natural cheese (such as cheddar)

➤ 2 ounces of processed cheese (such as American)

5. Meat, poultry, fish, beans, eggs, and nuts. This group provides B vitamins, protein, iron, and zinc. A fetus needs plenty of protein and iron to develop. Choose lean meats and trim off the fat and

skin before cooking. A serving consists of:

➤ 2–3 ounces of cooked lean meat, poultry, or fish

➤ 1 cup of cooked dry beans

➤ 2 eggs

➤ 2½-ounce soy burger

➤ 2 tablespoons of peanut butter (counts as 1 ounce of meat)

➤ ⅓ cup of nuts (counts as 1 ounce of meat)

6. Fats, oils, and sweets. These foods are full of calories and have few vitamins or minerals. No more than 30% of your daily calories should be from fat. Choose low-fat foods as often as you can. Limit butter, margarine, salad dressing, and gravy. Save high-sugar foods such as candy, desserts, and soft drinks for a special treat.

Getting the Nutrients You Need

Every diet should include proteins, carbohydrates, vitamins, minerals, and fat. These fuel your body and help your baby grow. You often can get enough of these nutrients if you eat a healthy diet, but your doctor may suggest you take a supplement or prenatal vitamin to ensure you get the right amount.

To get the right amount of nutrients, you need to know which foods are good sources. Follow these steps to ensure your diet is healthy:

Step 1: Look at the labels on food boxes, cans, and bottles (see box). This will teach you a lot about what's going into your body. These labels list serving sizes, calories, calories from fat, and the amounts of certain nutrients.

You'll also see the words "Daily Value" on most food labels. The daily value is the amount of a nutrient that an average person should eat every day. Keep in mind, though, that pregnant women often need more. Table 6–1 shows the Recommended Dietary Allowances (RDAs) for key nutrients during pregnancy. Daily values are derived, in part, from RDAs.

Step 2: Keep tabs on the nutrients you are getting. The numbers listed below the daily value are the levels of nutrients in one serving of the product. For instance, if the daily value for fat in a granola bar is listed as 10%, that means the bar contains one tenth of the fat you need that day. Reading labels will help you know how to boost your intake of certain nutrients and limit your intake of others.

Step 3: Don't worry about eating the RDA for each nutrient every day. Remember that the "D" stands for dietary, not daily. Your body stores nutrients for later use. Just try to eat a variety of foods and eat enough servings from the Food Guide Pyramid. If you do, chances are good that your diet is healthy and that your baby is getting the right amount of nutrients. Certain nutrients are needed for growth during pregnancy (Table 6–2). During pregnancy, you need more of these nutrients:

➤ Calories to help nourish your growing baby

➤ Iron and folic acid to help make the extra blood needed in pregnancy

➤ Protein to help make blood and build your baby's tissues and muscles

➤ Calcium to help build your baby's bones and teeth

Protein
Protein provides the nutrients your body needs to grow and repair muscles

Reading Food Labels

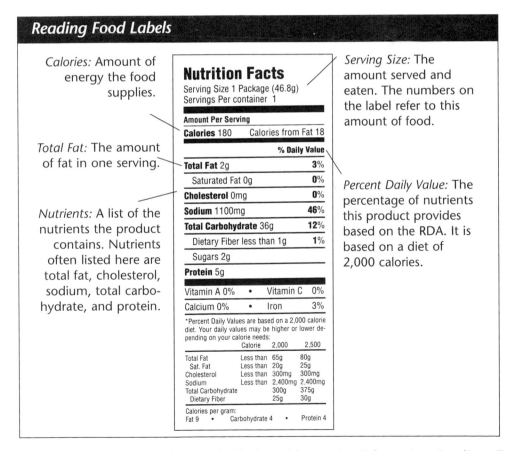

Calories: Amount of energy the food supplies.

Total Fat: The amount of fat in one serving.

Nutrients: A list of the nutrients the product contains. Nutrients often listed here are total fat, cholesterol, sodium, total carbohydrate, and protein.

Nutrition Facts

Serving Size 1 Package (46.8g)
Servings Per container 1

Amount Per Serving

Calories 180   Calories from Fat 18

	% Daily Value
Total Fat 2g	3%
Saturated Fat 0g	0%
Cholesterol 0mg	0%
Sodium 1100mg	46%
Total Carbohydrate 36g	12%
Dietary Fiber less than 1g	1%
Sugars 2g	
Protein 5g	

| Vitamin A 0% | • | Vitamin C | 0% |
| Calcium 0% | • | Iron | 3% |

*Percent Daily Values are based on a 2,000 calorie diet. Your daily values may be higher or lower depending on your calorie needs:

	Calorie	2,000	2,500
Total Fat	Less than	65g	80g
Sat. Fat	Less than	20g	25g
Cholesterol	Less than	300mg	300mg
Sodium	Less than	2,400mg	2,400mg
Total Carbohydrate		300g	375g
Dietary Fiber		25g	30g

Calories per gram:
Fat 9   •   Carbohydrate 4   •   Protein 4

Serving Size: The amount served and eaten. The numbers on the label refer to this amount of food.

Percent Daily Value: The percentage of nutrients this product provides based on the RDA. It is based on a diet of 2,000 calories.

All packaged foods must be clearly labeled with nutrition information. Reading all food labels can help you make smart food choices. The label will tell you how many grams of fat and how many calories are in each serving.

Table 6–1. Recommended Dietary Allowances for Women

Nutrient (unit)	Non-pregnant			Pregnant	Breastfeeding
	14–18 years	19–30 years	31–50 years	19–50 years	19–50 years
Protein (g)	46	46	46	71	71
Calcium (mg)	1,300	1,000	1,000	1,000	1,000
Phosphorus (mg)	1,250	700	700	700	700
Magnesium (mg)	360	310	320	360	320
Iron (mg)	15	18	18	27	9
Zinc (mg)	9	8	8	11	12
Iodine (μg)	150	150	150	220	290
Selenium (μg)	55	55	55	60	70
Vitamin A (μg)	700	700	700	770	1,300
Vitamin C (mg)	65	75	75	85	120
Vitamin D (μg)	5	5	5	5	5
Vitamin E (mg)	15	15	15	15	19
Vitamin K (μg)	75	90	90	90	90
Thiamin (mg)	1.1	1.1	1.1	1.4	1.4
Riboflavin (mg)	1.0	1.1	1.1	1.4	1.6
Niacin (mg)	14	14	14	18	17
Vitamin B_6 (mg)	1.2	1.3	1.3	1.9	2.0
Folic acid (μg)	400	400	400	600	500
Vitamin B_{12} (μg)	2.4	2.4	2.4	2.6	2.8

and other tissues. During pregnancy, protein also is the building block for your baby's cells.

Pregnant women need 60 grams of protein per day. Protein comes from animals—meat, fish, poultry, and dairy products. These animal foods are rich in protein:

➤ Beef, pork, and fish

➤ Chicken

➤ Low-fat milk

Plant products such as grains and legumes also are good sources of protein. For strict vegetarians (called "vegans"), getting enough protein can be a challenge. If you don't eat any meat, dairy products, or eggs, talk to your caregiver about ways to get more protein. He or she may refer you to a nutritionist or a dietitian to help you plan a high-protein vegetarian diet.

Carbohydrates

Food sugar—carbohydrates—is the body's main source of energy. There are two types of sugar: simple sugars and starches.

Simple sugars provide a quick energy boost. That's because they are ready to be used by the body right away. Simple sugars are found in table sugar, honey, syrup, fruit juices, hard candies, and many processed foods.

Starches are a more complex form of sugar. It takes your body longer to process them, so starches provide longer-lasting energy than simple sugars do. Starches are found in bread, rice, pasta, fruits, and starchy vegetables such as potatoes or corn.

Starchy foods also contain fiber. Your body doesn't use fiber the same way it uses other nutrients. Still, you can't live without it. Fiber helps flush out your digestive system and helps prevent constipation. It also helps rid your body of excess fat and cholesterol. Try to eat 20–30 grams (about 1 ounce) of fiber per day. These are good sources of fiber:

➤ Fruits (especially dried fruits, berries, oranges, and apples and peaches with the skin)

➤ Vegetables (such as dried beans and peas)

➤ Whole-grain products (such as whole-wheat bread or brown rice)

Carbohydrates should make up more than half of the food you eat. It's important to have a balance of fruits, vegetables, and grains. Not all starches offer the same benefits, so choose a variety of foods from this group. Because they have other nutrients, fruits and vegetables are better sources of carbohydrates than bread and grains are.

Try to limit simple sugars. They have more calories than they have nutrients, and the energy they provide is used up quickly. Eating a candy bar might give you a brief "sugar high." It doesn't offer much nutrition, though, and you'll soon feel tired again. Starches have lots of nutrients and fiber. They also give you longer-lasting energy.

Fats

Many people have come to think of fat as "bad." Too much fat isn't good for you. The body needs fat to function normally, though.

Fats help your body use vitamins A, D, E, and K, as well as proteins and carbohydrates. Fat that your body doesn't

Table 6–2. Key Nutrients in Pregnancy

Nutrient	Sources
Protein	Meat, fish, eggs, beans, dairy products
Carbohydrates	Bread, cereal, rice, potatoes, pasta
Fat	Meat, eggs, nuts, peanut butter, margarine, oils

Vitamins

A	Green leafy vegetables, deep yellow or orange vegetables (carrots and sweet potatoes), milk, liver
Thiamin (B$_1$)	Whole-grain or enriched breads and cereals, fish, pork, poultry, lean meat, milk
Riboflavin (B$_2$)	Milk, whole-grain or enriched breads and cereals, liver, green leafy vegetables
B$_6$	Beef liver, pork, ham, whole-grain cereals, bananas
B$_{12}$	Animal foods, such as liver, milk, poultry (vegetarians should take a supplement)
C	Citrus fruit, strawberries, broccoli, tomatoes
D	Fortified milk, fish liver oils, sunshine
E	Vegetable oils, whole-grain cereals, wheat germ, green leafy vegetables
Folic acid	Green leafy vegetables, dark yellow or orange fruits and vegetables; liver; legumes and nuts; fortified breads, cereals, rice, and pastas
Niacin	Meat, liver, poultry, fish, whole-grain or enriched cereals

Minerals

Calcium	Milk and dairy products; sardines and salmon with bones; collard, kale, mustard, spinach, and turnip greens; fortified orange juice
Iodine	Seafood, iodized salt
Iron	Lean red meat, liver, dried beans, whole-grain or enriched breads and cereals, prune juice, spinach, tofu
Magnesium	Legumes, whole-grain cereals, milk, meat, green vegetables
Phosphorus	Milk and dairy products, meat, poultry, fish, whole-grain cereals, legumes
Zinc	Meat, liver, seafood, milk, whole-grain cereals

need right away is stored as fat tissue. This tissue is converted into energy when your body needs more calories than you eat. Those fat stores will play a role in making breast milk for your newborn.

You should be aware of different types of fats in your diet:

➤ Saturated fats come mainly from meat and dairy products. They tend to be solid chilled—like butter and lard, for instance. Shortening, palm oil, and coconut oil also are saturated fats.

➤ Trans fats are a kind of saturated fat. Trans fats are made when liquid oils are turned into solid fats like shortening and hard margarine. This is done to make foods last longer and give them better flavor. Vegetable shortenings, some margarines, crackers, cookies, and snack foods like potato chips contain trans fats.

➤ Unsaturated fats tend to be liquid and come mostly from plants and vegetables. Olive, canola, peanut, sunflower, and fish oil are all unsaturated fats.

Too much saturated fat and trans fat can increase your cholesterol level and lead to heart disease. They should make up less than one third of the total fat in your diet, or no more than 10% of the calories you eat each day. The other two thirds of the fat in your diet, or about 20% of your daily calories, should come from unsaturated fat.

Fat also is very high in calories. A gram of fat has more than double the calories as the same amount of protein or carbohydrates.

Fat is found in many foods—from meat and baked goods to nondairy coffee creamer. You can reduce the fat in your diet by changing the way you prepare foods:

➤ Broil, bake, poach, or steam your food instead of frying or sautéing it.

➤ Skim liquid fat from soups.

➤ Trim all fat from meats.

➤ Remove skin from poultry.

➤ Cut back on butter, margarine, cream, oil, and mayonnaise.

➤ Choose unsaturated fats over saturated fats and trans fats as often as you can.

Water

Most people don't think of water as a nutrient. Still, we can't live without it. Water serves many purposes in your body:

➤ Builds new tissue

➤ Allows nutrients and waste products to circulate within and out of the body

➤ Aids digestion

➤ Helps form amniotic fluid around the baby

Nearly three fourths of your body's weight is water. Water is lost through sweat, urine, and even breathing. To replace what's lost, drink water throughout the day—don't wait until you are thirsty. One tip to increase your fluid intake: keep a bottle of water on your desk or in your purse. Drink from it often. Other liquids, such as fruit juice and tea, can stand in for some of the water you need each day.

Iron

Iron is used to make hemoglobin. This protein in red blood cells carries oxygen to your organs, tissues, and baby. Just like the other cells in your body, blood cells die and are replaced in a constant process. The iron from blood cells is used to make more hemoglobin.

When you become pregnant, you may not have enough iron stored in your body to make the extra blood you and your baby need, causing anemia. Women need more iron in their diets during pregnancy to support the growth of the baby and to produce extra blood. Getting plenty of iron when you are pregnant is a must.

Eating certain foods will give you extra iron. Lean beef and pork, organ meats, dried fruits and beans, whole grains, and dark leafy greens are all high in iron.

Vitamin C helps your body absorb the iron in food. However, calcium can block absorption. For this reason iron and calcium should not be taken at the same time. It's a good idea to take iron in the morning and take calcium at night.

Talk with your doctor about whether you need extra iron. An iron supplement or a prenatal vitamin with iron will help boost your intake. Be aware, though, that iron pills can cause constipation, bloating, and black stools. If you are taking an iron supplement, keep it away from children (as with all medication).

Folic Acid

Folic acid is used to make the extra blood your body needs during pregnancy. Not getting enough folic acid in your diet before conception and in the early weeks of pregnancy increases the risk of birth defects such as **neural tube defects** (defects of the spine and skull). Lack of folic acid also may increase the risk of certain other birth defects.

Women who might get pregnant or who are pregnant should consume 0.4 mg of folic acid a day. The government asks food companies to add folic acid to certain products to help lower the rate of neural tube defects. Almost all breads, cereal, pasta, rice, and flour have folic acid added. It also is in some foods such as leafy dark-green vegetables, citrus fruits, and beans. It can be hard to get all of the folic acid you need from food alone. Some women, such as those who are pregnant with twins or have certain medical conditions, may need increased amounts of folic acid.

If you have had a child with a neural tube defect or certain other birth defects, you have increased folic acid needs. You should take 4 mg daily—10 times the amount recommended for most women. This increased amount of folic acid should be taken at least 1 month before conception and through the first 12 weeks of pregnancy. The increased amount of folic acid should be taken separately—not as part of a multivitamin. Otherwise, you would get too many of the other vitamins. If you have had a child with a neural tube defect, talk to your doctor. He or she will prescribe a high-dose folic acid supplement.

Calcium

Calcium is used to build your baby's bones and teeth. If you don't get enough of this mineral from food, your baby will get the calcium it needs from your bones. That can lead to **osteoporosis** (fragile bones). It also may cause you to lose teeth.

Pregnant women should get 1,000 mg of calcium each day (1,300 mg for those younger than 19 years). Drinking about 3 cups of milk a day will fill this quota if you are older than 19 years. Milk and other dairy products such as cheese and yogurt are the best sources of calcium. These foods also are good sources of calcium:

➤ Fortified orange juice

➤ Nuts and seeds

➤ Sardines

➤ Salmon with bones

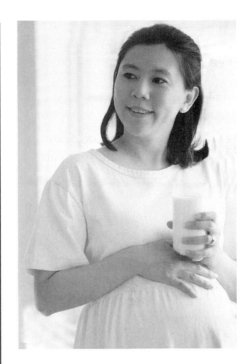

➤ Collard, kale, mustard, spinach, and turnip greens

If you have **lactose intolerance** (trouble digesting milk products), you can get calcium other ways. You may try pills or drops with an enzyme that helps your body break down milk sugar. Taking a daily antacid made with calcium is another simple way to boost your calcium intake. Also, many stores carry low-lactose milk and cheese. Iron prevents calcium from being absorbed, so do not take calcium with iron.

Prenatal Vitamins

Except for iron, folic acid, and possibly calcium, a well-rounded diet should supply all of the nutrients you need during pregnancy. You may need to take a prenatal multivitamin and min-

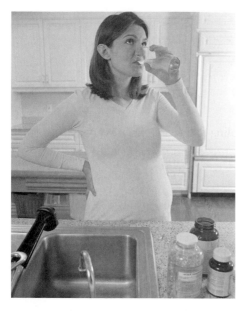

eral supplement to get enough nutrients.

Take prenatal vitamins only as directed. Large doses of anything—even a good thing—can be harmful. Don't take more than the RDA for any vitamin or mineral—especially vitamins A and D—without getting your doctor's approval. Very high levels of vitamin A have been linked with severe birth defects. Your prenatal multivitamin should contain no more than 5,000 IU of vitamin A. If you are already taking a multivitamin, let your doctor know.

Special Nutrition Concerns

For most women, careful meal planning and a daily prenatal vitamin will provide all their nutritional needs. Some mothers-to-be need more nutrients than a normal diet provides. If you have any of these conditions, you may need a special diet or supplements.

Low Stores of Nutrients

Pregnancy demands a lot from your body. Having more than one pregnancy in a short time can wipe out some of the nutrients your body needs to help nourish you and your baby. Iron and calcium, for instance, are minerals that may be low in a woman who has pregnancies close together.

If you have been pregnant more than twice in 2 years (including pregnancies that ended in abortion or miscarriage), you may not have had a chance to replace the nutrients your body has lost. Your stores also may be low if you had complications in a pregnancy, if you had a low-birth-weight baby, or if you are very thin.

Unusual Cravings

Pregnant women often have food cravings. Most often, giving in to these cravings does no harm. Cravings can cause problems if you eat only a few types of food for long periods. They also can be less than healthy if you indulge your cravings for one type of food, for example, and neglect the rest of your diet.

Pica is a strong urge some women feel to eat non-food items such as laundry starch, clay, or chalk. If you feel these urges, don't indulge in them. Eating non-food items can be harmful and prevent you from getting the nutrients you need.

Not Gaining Enough Weight

More than seven million American women have eating disorders, such as *anorexia* or *bulimia*. These disorders starve a woman's body—and her baby—of key nutrients.

Pregnancy raises body-image issues for just about every woman. For a pregnant woman with anorexia or bulimia, anxiety about food and weight gain can cause the disorder to worsen. Eating disorders that were under control before pregnancy may start again during pregnancy. A woman's growing body can make her feel bad and trigger the return of eating problems.

Counseling and medication help control the emotional aspects of eating disorders. If you have an eating disorder, get help for your baby's sake and your own.

Weighing Too Much

Obesity is a major health problem in the United States. Women who are overweight or obese may have problems during pregnancy, such as gestational diabetes or having an overly large baby (macrosomia). Obesity can be related to other health problems for women also, such as high blood pressure. A method for evaluating your weight is "body mass index" (BMI), which compares height to weight. Use Table 6–3 to calculate your BMI. A non-pregnant woman with a body mass index (BMI) of more than 25 is thought to be overweight; more than 30 is thought to be obese. If you are overweight or obese,

pregnancy is not a time to try to lose weight. Popular diets that limit certain food groups may not provide enough nutrients during pregnancy.

Some women with severe obesity have had gastric bypass surgery or gastric stapling to lose weight. If you have had such a procedure, you may need special care to ensure your body is absorbing enough nutrients during pregnancy.

Women With Certain Diseases

Aside from the health problems they cause, some diseases can cause nutrition problems as well. Certain medications that are used to keep a disease under control can affect how your body absorbs food. Conditions such as kidney disease, diabetes, and phenylketonuria (in which a woman lacks an enzyme needed to process certain foods) call for special diets. For women who have such conditions, it can be hard to eat a balanced diet. Your doctor may change your medication, advise another diet, or take other steps to help you get the nutrients you need.

Diet Cautions

Certain items pose special health risks during pregnancy. The risk may be low for the general population but high for the sensitive system of the baby.

Eating Fish

Fish and shellfish can be important parts of a healthy and balanced diet.

Table 6–3. Body Mass Index Chart

To find out your BMI, find your height on the left-hand column of the chart below. Next, read across the column until you find the weight that's closest to yours. Then look at the number at the top of the column. That number is your BMI.

Height (inches)	19	20	21	22	23	24	25	26	27	28	29	30	31	32
						Weight (pounds)								
58	91	96	100	105	110	115	119	124	129	134	138	143	148	153
59	94	99	104	109	114	119	124	128	133	138	143	148	153	158
60	97	102	107	112	118	123	128	133	138	143	148	153	158	163
61	100	106	111	116	122	127	132	137	143	148	153	158	164	169
62	104	109	115	120	126	131	136	142	147	153	158	164	169	175
63	107	113	118	124	130	135	141	146	152	158	163	169	175	180
64	110	116	122	128	134	140	145	151	157	163	169	174	180	186
65	114	120	126	132	138	144	150	156	162	168	174	180	186	192
66	118	124	130	136	142	148	155	161	167	173	179	186	192	198
67	121	127	134	140	146	153	159	166	172	178	185	191	198	204
68	125	131	138	144	151	158	164	171	177	184	190	197	203	210
69	128	135	142	149	155	162	169	176	182	189	196	203	209	216
70	132	139	146	153	160	167	174	181	188	195	202	209	216	222
71	136	143	150	157	165	172	179	186	193	200	208	215	222	229
72	140	147	154	162	169	177	184	191	199	206	213	221	228	235
73	144	151	159	166	174	182	189	197	204	212	219	227	235	242
74	148	155	163	171	179	186	194	202	210	218	225	233	241	249

Adapted from the National Institutes of Health, National Heart, Lung, and Blood Institute. Clinical Guidelines on the Identification, Evaluation, and Treatment of Overweight and Obesity in Adults. Washington, DC: U.S. Government Printing Office, 1998.

They are good sources of high-quality protein and other nutrients. Certain kinds of fish should not be eaten by pregnant women because they have high levels of a certain kind of mercury—methylmercury—that can harm the nervous system of your baby.

You should not eat shark, swordfish, king mackerel, or tilefish during pregnancy. These large fish contain high levels of methylmercury. Albacore tuna also is high in mercury so you may want to choose canned chunk light tuna instead. Other types of fish are fine in limited amounts. You can safely eat up to 12 ounces (two to three meals) of other purchased fish and shellfish per week. Vary the types of fish and shellfish you eat.

Check local advisories about fish caught in your local rivers and streams. If there is no advice about them, it is safe to eat up to 6 ounces (one meal) per week of fish from local waters. During that week, don't eat any other fish. It is safe to eat one to two servings of salmon, sardines, herring, or bluefish per month.

Listeriosis

Listeriosis is caused by bacteria found in certain foods. The foods most likely to have the bacteria are unpasteurized milk, soft cheeses made with unpasteurized milk, hot dogs, luncheon meats, and smoked seafood. Listeriosis causes flu-like symptoms, such as fever and chills. However, there may be no symptoms.

When a pregnant woman is infected, the disease can cause miscarriage or serious problems for the baby. If there is a chance that a newborn is infected, he or she also can be tested and treated.

To prevent listeriosis, wash hands and surfaces often with hot, soapy water; reheat luncheon meats, cold cuts, and other deli-style meat and poultry until they are steaming hot; do not eat unpasteurized milk or soft cheeses or refrigerated smoked seafood.

Calories and Weight Gain

Eating a healthy diet and reaching a healthy weight gain during pregnancy is important for your well-being and that of your growing baby. Different stages of pregnancy can present certain challenges to healthy eating. In the first trimester, morning sickness can affect your eating habits. You may crave certain foods or not feel like eating. You may have heartburn, indigestion, or constipation. Or you may not have any of these. Every pregnancy is different.

Usually, in the second trimester your appetite increases. Keep in mind that "eating for two" doesn't mean eating twice as much. Most women who are not pregnant need between 1,800 and 2,200 calories per day. Pregnant women need about 300 calories more. Those 300 calories add up fast—a glass of skim milk and a half sandwich should do it.

Many women wonder why they gain 30 or so pounds when a baby is only 7 or 8 pounds. Most of the added weight

Table 6–4. Weight Gain During Pregnancy	
Condition Before Getting Pregnant	**Weight Gain (pounds)**
Underweight (BMI less than 20)	28–40
Normal Weight (BMI 20–25)	25–35
Overweight (BMI 26–29)	15–25
Obese (BMI more than 29)	15 or as advised by doctor

Where Does the Weight Come From?

The average newborn weighs about 7½ pounds. Yet, most mothers-to-be are advised to gain 25–35 pounds when they are pregnant. Where do the other pounds come from? Here's a break-down of the weight gain for a normal-weight woman who gains 30 pounds during pregnancy.

Baby	7½ pounds
Amniotic Fluid	2 pounds
Placenta	1½ pounds
Uterus	2 pounds
Breasts	2 pounds
Body Fluids	4 pounds
Blood	4 pounds
Maternal Stores of Fat, Protein, and Other Nutrients	7 pounds

is for your body to nurture the baby (see box).

A woman who gains too few pounds is more likely to have a small baby (less than 5½ pounds). These babies often have health problems after birth. Women who gain too much weight also are at risk for health problems. These problems include diabetes, high blood pressure, and a baby that's too large (see Chapter 14).

How many pounds should you gain? That depends on how much you weighed before getting pregnant. Table 6–4 gives a general guide for weight gain.

Ask your doctor about the right amount of pregnancy weight gain for you.

Eating for Two

Eating well during pregnancy is important. If healthy eating is an old habit for you, keep it up now. If it's not, having a baby is a great reason to improve your diet. In many cases, small changes can make a big difference in your health and your baby's. Many women often stick with better eating habits long after the baby's born. Try to follow a healthy, balanced, and varied diet as often as you can.

CHAPTER 7

Changes During Pregnancy

During pregnancy, your uterus grows from the size of your fist to a size able to hold a baby up to 10 pounds. In fact, your uterus grows to about 60 times its normal size.

Other parts of your body also are changing. Many of these changes are triggered by pregnancy hormones. These hormones nurture your fetus and prepare your body for childbirth and breastfeeding. They also can cause physical and emotional changes. By understanding these changes, you can better prepare for and cope with them.

Physical Changes

Backache

Backache is one of a pregnant woman's most common problems, especially in the later months. Back pain during pregnancy has many causes. One cause is the strain on your back muscles from carrying extra weight. Another is the posture women often assume during pregnancy to offset the weight. Stretched and weakened abdominal muscles (which support the spine) are yet one more reason. Exercises to stretch and strengthen your back muscles can help reduce this pain.

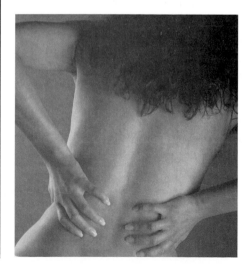

A Healthy Back

The following exercises strengthen and stretch the muscles of the back, abdomen, hips, and upper body. These muscles support the back and legs and promote good posture. The exercises will help ease back pain as well as help prepare you for labor and delivery.

Upper Body Bends

This exercise strengthens the muscles of your back and torso.

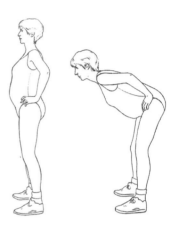

➤ Stand with your legs apart, knees bent slightly, with your hands on your hips.

➤ Bend forward slowly, keeping your upper back straight. You should feel a slight pull along the back of your thighs.

➤ Repeat 10 times.

Diagonal Curl

This exercise strengthens the muscles of your back, hips, and abdomen. If you have not already been exercising regularly, skip this exercise.

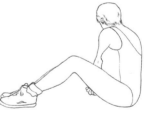

➤ Sit on the floor with your knees bent, feet on the floor, and hands clasped in front of you.

➤ Twist your upper torso to the left until your hands touch the floor.

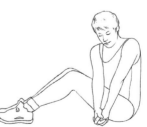

➤ Do the same movement to the right.

➤ Repeat on both sides five times.

(continued)

A Healthy Back (continued)

Forward Bend

This exercise stretches and strengthens the muscles of your back.

➤ Sit in a chair in a comfortable position. Keep your arms relaxed.

➤ Bend forward slowly, with your arms in front and hanging down.

➤ If you feel any discomfort or pressure on your abdomen, do not bend any farther.

➤ Hold this position for a count of five, then sit up slowly without arching your back.

➤ Repeat five times.

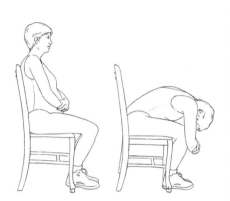

Trunk Twist

This exercise stretches the muscles of your back, spine, and upper torso.

➤ Sit on the floor with your legs crossed, with your left hand holding your left foot and your right hand on the floor at your side for support.

➤ Slowly twist your upper torso to the right.

➤ Do the same movement to the left after switching your hands (right hand holding right foot and left hand supporting you).

➤ Repeat on both sides 5–10 times.

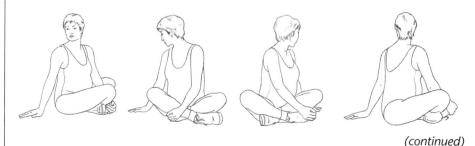

(continued)

A Healthy Back (continued)

Backward Stretch

This exercise stretches and strengthens the muscles of your back, pelvis, and thighs.

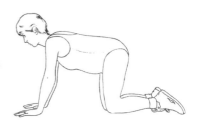

➤ Kneel on hands and knees, with your knees 8–10 inches apart and your arms straight (hands under your shoulders).

➤ Curl backward slowly, tucking your head toward your knees and keeping your arms extended.

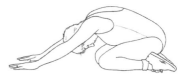

➤ Hold this position for a count of five, then come back up to all fours slowly.

➤ Repeat five times.

Leg Lift Crawl

This exercise strengthens the muscles of your back and abdomen.

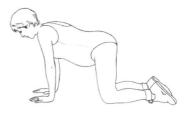

➤ Kneel on hands and knees, with your weight distributed evenly and your arms straight (hands under your shoulders).

➤ Lift your left knee and bring it toward your elbow.

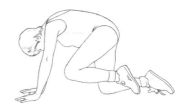

➤ Straighten your leg without locking your knee.

➤ Extend your leg up and back.

➤ Do this exercise to a count of five. Move slowly—don't fling your leg back or arch your back.

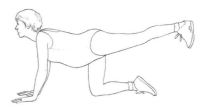

➤ Repeat on both sides 5–10 times.

(continued)

A Healthy Back (continued)

Rocking Back Arch

This exercise stretches and strengthens the muscles of your back, hips, and abdomen.

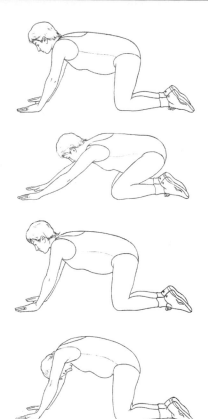

➤ Kneel on hands and knees, with your weight distributed evenly and your back straight.

➤ Rock back and forward, to a count of five.

➤ Return to the original position and curl your back upward as much as you can.

➤ Repeat 5–10 times.

Back Press

This exercise strengthens the muscles of your back and torso and promotes good posture.

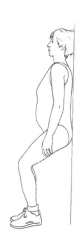

➤ Stand with your back against a wall and your feet 10–12 inches away from the wall.

➤ Press the lower part of your back against the wall.

➤ Hold this position for a count of 10, then release.

➤ Repeat 10 times.

Here are some other tips to help lessen back pain:

➤ Wear low-heeled (but not flat) shoes with good arch support. High heels tilt your body forward and strain your lower-back muscles.

➤ Avoid lifting heavy objects. Heavy lifting puts even more strain on your back.

➤ Don't bend at the waist to pick something up. If you must lift something (like a bag of groceries or a small child), squat down, bend your knees, and keep your back straight.

➤ Get off your feet. If you have to stand for a long time, rest one foot on a stool or a box to take the strain off your back.

➤ Sit in chairs with good back support, or tuck a small pillow behind your lower back.

➤ Keep things within reach. Put objects that you use often in close reach. This way, you won't have to bend or stretch to grab them.

➤ Sleep on a firm mattress. If your bed is too soft, have someone put a board between the mattress and box springs to make it firm.

➤ Sleep on your side rather than on your back. Tucking a pillow between your legs will give your back added support.

➤ Buy an abdominal support garment (for sale in maternity stores and cata-logs). It looks like a girdle and helps take the weight of your belly off your back muscles. Also, some maternity pants come with a wide elastic band that fits under the curve of your belly to help support its weight.

➤ Apply a heating pad using the lowest temperature setting, warm-water bottle, or cold compress to ease the pain. Be sure to use a towel for wrapping to avoid burns.

Breast Changes

Early in pregnancy, your breasts begin changing to get ready for feeding the baby. For many women, tingling, tender, swollen breasts are the first clue that they are pregnant. By 6 weeks of pregnancy, in fact, breasts may grow a whole bra-cup size. There are many changes that take place:

➤ Fat builds up in the breasts, making your normal bra too tight.

➤ Blood flow increases, causing bluish veins to appear just under the skin.

➤ The number of milk glands increases as your body gears up for making milk.

➤ The nipples and *areolas* (the pink or brownish skin around your nipples) darken.

➤ Your nipples may begin to stick out more, and the areolas will grow larger.

➤ Small glands (called Montgomery's tubercles) on the surface of the areo-

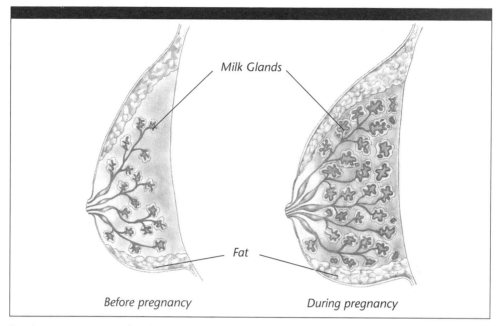

Milk Glands

Fat

Before pregnancy   *During pregnancy*

During pregnancy, the fat layer of your breasts thickens, and the number of milk glands increases. This makes your breasts larger than they were before pregnancy.

las become raised and bumpy. These glands produce an oily substance that keeps the nipples and areolas soft and supple.

Your breasts may keep growing in size and weight during the first 3 months of pregnancy. If they are very tender, wearing a good bra that fits well will help provide relief.

A maternity bra is a good choice for pregnant women. These bras have wide straps, more coverage in the cups to protect tender breasts, and extra rows of hooks so you can adjust the band size as your baby grows. You also might want to buy a special sleep bra for nighttime support.

Most women's nipples stick out more when they are pregnant. But some women have nipples that are flat or even recessed (***inverted nipples***). For these women, when the breast is squeezed just behind the nipples, the nipples stay flat or are drawn in rather than sticking out. This can make it hard for the baby to nurse.

If you have flat or inverted nipples and want to breastfeed, there are things you can do ahead of time to correct the problem, such as special exercises. Talk to your doctor or a lactation consultant (breastfeeding specialist) about this early in pregnancy. (See Chapter 10 for more detailed information on breast-feeding.)

By the end of your first trimester, your breasts may start leaking. This fluid, called *colostrum*, is normal—it shows that your breasts are getting prepared. Colostrum nourishes your newborn until your breasts start making milk a few days after birth. It is rich in fat and calories and contains water, proteins, minerals, and antibodies that protect against disease.

Early in pregnancy, colostrum is thick and yellow. As birth draws near, it becomes pale and has almost no color. Colostrum may leak on its own or dribble out when your breasts are massaged. It also can leak when you are sexually aroused.

Don't worry if your breasts don't leak during pregnancy. Leaking doesn't happen to all women, and it doesn't mean that you won't be able to breastfeed later.

Congestion and Nosebleeds

During pregnancy, your hormone levels increase, and your body makes extra blood. Both of these changes cause the mucus membranes inside your nose to swell up, dry out, and bleed easily. This may cause you to have a stuffy or runny nose. You also may get nosebleeds from time to time. Here are suggestions to deal with the problem:

➤ Try saline drops to relieve congestion. (Never use other types of nose drops, nasal sprays, or decongestants without your doctor's approval.)

➤ Drink liquids to help keep your nasal passages moist.

➤ Use a humidifier to moisten the air in your home.

➤ Dab petroleum jelly around the edges of your nostrils to keep the skin moist.

Constipation and Gas

Most pregnant women get constipated at some point. When that happens, gas can build up in your belly and cause bloating and pain.

Constipation occurs when you have infrequent bowel movements with stools that are firm or hard to pass. Constipation (and the gas that results) can occur for many reasons. The hormone progesterone may slow digestion. Iron supplements may worsen constipation. Toward the end of pregnancy, the weight of the uterus puts pressure on your rectum, adding to the problem. If you are constipated and have gas, these tips may help:

➤ Drink plenty of liquids. Drinking eight glasses of liquid per day will help you. Drinking prune or other fruit juice also can help relieve constipation.

➤ Eat high-fiber foods. Raw fruits, vegetables, beans, whole-grain bread, and bran cereal are good choices.

➤ Exercise. Walking or doing another safe activity every day aids your digestive system.

➤ Ask your doctor about taking a bulk-forming agent. These products absorb water and expand inside your body. That adds to the moisture in stool and makes it easier to pass. Don't take laxatives during pregnancy.

Leg Cramps

During late pregnancy, a sharp, painful cramp or "charley horse" in the calf may be a bother—especially at night. Although these cramps were once thought to be caused by the amount of calcium or potassium in a woman's diet, this is no longer thought to be true. It is not clear what causes leg cramps during pregnancy.

Stretching your legs before going to bed can help relieve cramps. Avoid pointing your toes when stretching or exercising. If a painful spasm in your calf muscles wakes you up at night, try massaging the calf in long strokes downward. Straighten you leg and flex (bend) your foot, keeping the heel down and the toes up. Do not point your toes; instead bend your entire foot.

Frequent Urination

Many pregnant women have a frequent need to urinate. There are a number of reasons:

➤ During pregnancy, the kidneys work harder than ever to flush waste products out of your body. Hence, frequent trips to the bathroom.

➤ As your uterus grows, it puts pressure on the bladder. Your bladder may be nearly empty but still feel like it's full. In mid-pregnancy some of the pressure should be relieved when your uterus no longer presses down on your bladder.

➤ In the last weeks of pregnancy (later for second pregnancies), the fetus "drops" into your pelvis. When that happens, the baby's head moves down in the uterus and presses against your cervix and bladder. This is called *lightening*. During this time, you may feel the need to urinate even more frequently. Your need to urinate may wake you up in the middle of the night, too.

There's not much you can do for relief except cut down on coffee, tea, and cola. These drinks have caffeine,

Warning Signs of a Urinary Tract Infection

Call your doctor if you have any of these warning signs of a urinary tract infection:

➤ Pain when you urinate

➤ Feeling like you must urinate right away

➤ Blood in your urine

➤ Fever

➤ Back pain

Kegel Exercises

Kegel exercises strengthen the muscles that surround the openings of the vagina, anus, and urethra (the tube that carries urine out of the body). If they are done often enough, Kegel exercises will help stop urine leaks. They may even lower the chance that you'll need an episiotomy (a cut to widen the opening of the birth canal) when you give birth.

Here's how to do Kegel exercises: squeeze the muscles that you use to stop the flow of urine. Hold for 10 seconds, then release. Do this 10–20 times in a row at least three times per day. You can do Kegel exercises anywhere—while talking on the phone, reading, or riding in the car, for example.

which makes you urinate more. Don't cut back on liquids. Drinking less to try to reduce those bathroom trips will rob your body of vital fluids.

The weight of your uterus on your bladder may even cause you to leak a little urine when you sneeze or cough. You can wear sanitary pads or panty shields for protection. Doing *Kegel exercises* (see box) will help improve your bladder control.

Hemorrhoids

Pregnant women who are constipated often have hemorrhoids. These are painful and itchy *varicose veins* in the rectal area. The main causes are the extra blood in the pelvic area and the pressure the growing uterus puts on veins in the lower body.

Constipation can make these swollen, itchy veins worse. That's because straining during bowel movements traps more blood in the veins. Talk to your doctor about using creams and suppositories to provide relief.

Even if hemorrhoids improve during pregnancy, straining during delivery can bring them back. Hemorrhoids often go away for good after the baby is born. In the meantime, try these tips for a little relief (or to avoid the problem in the first place):

➤ Eat a high-fiber diet and drink plenty of liquids.

➤ Don't gain too much weight. Extra pounds can worsen hemorrhoids. Keep your weight gain within the limits your doctor suggests.

➤ Get moving. Standing or sitting for a long time puts pressure on the veins in your pelvic area. Get up and move around to shift the weight of your uterus off these veins.

➤ If you get hemorrhoids, apply an ice pack or witch hazel pads to the area to relieve pain and reduce swelling. Your pharmacist can help you find an over-the-counter witch hazel product.

➤ Try soaking in a tub a few times a day.

Headache

Headaches are common during pregnancy. Pregnancy hormones are one cause. Hunger and stress also can be factors. Also, some women cut back on caffeine during pregnancy. This can cause caffeine withdrawal headaches.

For some women, pregnancy headaches are a minor bother. For others, very painful headaches (called migraine headaches) can affect their daily lives.

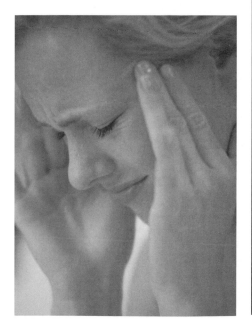

If you get headaches, ask your doctor what pain relief is safe to use when you're pregnant. You also may want to try placing a cold washcloth on your forehead for relief. Gently massage your temples. Rest in a dark, quiet room.

Call your doctor if headaches are a constant problem. Also call if a headache doesn't go away, is very severe, causes blurred vision or spots in front of your eyes, or makes you feel sick to your stomach.

Mouth and Tooth Changes

Pregnancy hormones can make your gums swell and bleed. Don't let this keep you from brushing and flossing. Switching to a softer brush may help lessen irritation.

You also may notice that your mouth waters more during pregnancy. No one knows why this occurs.

Don't cancel your regular dental visit just because you are pregnant. A dental checkup early in pregnancy will help ensure that your mouth stays healthy. Putting off dental work can lead to further problems. Pregnant women are at an increased risk for cavities and gum disease.

When you go to the dentist, be sure to let him or her know that you are pregnant. Don't worry if you need local anesthesia or dental X-rays, but ask for a guard to protect your thyroid. Neither anesthesia nor X-rays pose a risk as long as they are done with your baby's safety

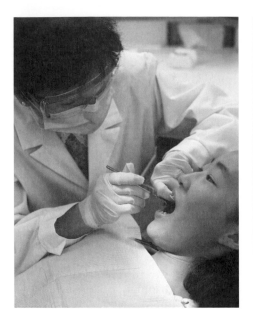

in mind. If your dentist has concerns, ask him or her to contact your doctor.

Heartburn and Indigestion

The words "heartburn" and "indigestion" often are thought to mean the same thing. They are not. Indigestion is what happens when a sluggish stomach takes hours to empty. Women with indigestion feel very full, bloated, and gassy.

Heartburn is a burning feeling in the throat and chest. It is common among pregnant women. Heartburn doesn't mean that something is wrong with your heart. Pregnancy hormones, which relax the muscle valve between your stomach and esophagus (the tube leading from the throat to the stomach), are a main cause of heartburn. When the valve doesn't close, stomach acids leak into the esophagus. As your uterus grows, it adds to the problem by pressing up against your stomach.

Follow these tips to help relieve (or prevent) indigestion and heartburn:

➤ Eat six small meals per day instead of three big ones.

➤ Eat slowly and chew your food well.

➤ Don't drink a lot of liquid with your meals. Drink fluids between meals instead.

➤ Stay away from fried, greasy, and fatty foods.

➤ Avoid foods that bother your stomach. If heartburn is a problem, avoid fizzy drinks, citrus fruits or juices, and spicy or fatty foods.

➤ Don't eat or drink within a few hours of bedtime. Don't lie down right after meals, either.

➤ Try raising the head of your bed. Prop a few extra pillows under your shoulders or stick a couple of books or wood blocks under the legs at the head of your bed.

➤ Ask your doctor about using antacids or other medications.

Insomnia

After the first few months of pregnancy, you may find it hard to sleep at night. As your abdomen grows larger, it may be hard to find a comfortable position. These suggestions may help you get the rest you need:

➤ Take a shower or warm bath at bed-time.

➤ Try the relaxation tips you learned in childbirth classes.

➤ Lie on your side with a pillow under your abdomen and another pillow between your legs.

➤ Limit your daytime rest.

Lower-Abdominal Pain

As the uterus grows, the round liga-ments (bands of tissue that support the uterus on both sides) are pulled and stretched. You may feel this stretching as either a dull ache or a sharp pain on one side of your belly. The pains are most common between 18 and 24 weeks of pregnancy.

Try the following steps to prevent or relieve these pains:

➤ Avoid quick changes of position.

➤ Don't turn sharply at the waist.

➤ When you do feel a pain, bend toward it to help relieve it.

➤ Rest or change your position.

If abdominal pain doesn't go away or gets worse, call your doctor. It could be a sign of a problem.

Fatigue

Most women feel very tired when they are pregnant—mostly during early and late pregnancy. Your body is working hard to create and support a new life.

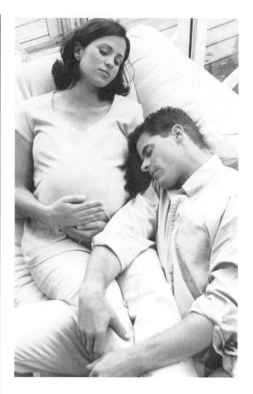

The pregnancy hormone progesterone also may make you feel tired.

There's not much you can do about fatigue, other than try to get as much rest as you can. Exercise and a healthy diet may help boost your energy.

Nausea and Vomiting

Nausea and vomiting are common dur-ing pregnancy, especially during the first part of pregnancy. This often is called "morning sickness," although it can occur at any time of the day. Although no one is certain what causes the nausea and vomiting, increasing levels of hor-mones during pregnancy may play a role.

The early months of your pregnancy may be spent fighting against nausea triggered by certain food odors. You also may have trouble keeping down the food you have just eaten. Most mild cases of nausea and vomiting do not harm you or your baby's health. Morning sickness does not mean your baby is sick.

Nausea and vomiting should lessen by about 14 weeks of pregnancy. Until the nausea and vomiting go away, there are some things you can do that might help you feel better:

➤ Take a supplement of vitamin B_6.

➤ In the morning, sit on the side of the bed for a few minutes and then get up slowly.

➤ Eat dry toast or crackers before you get out of bed in the morning.

➤ Get plenty of fresh air. Take a short walk or try sleeping with a window open.

➤ Drink fluids often during the day. Cold drinks that are bubbly or sweet may help.

➤ Eat five or six small meals each day. Try not to let your stomach get empty, and sit upright after meals.

➤ Avoid smells that bother you.

➤ Eat foods that are low-fat and easy to digest. The "BRATT" diet (bananas, rice, applesauce, toast, and tea) may help. This diet will provide vital nutrients that will replace those you have lost.

Prenatal vitamins and iron can cause nausea for some women. A children's chewable vitamin with folate (folic acid) taken at the end of the day may help. Acupressure, ginger, motion sickness bands, or hypnosis also may help relieve symptoms. Talk with your doctor before taking any medication or trying any treatment.

Morning sickness can become a more serious problem if you can't keep any foods or fluids down and begin to lose weight. If your nausea and vomiting are severe, call your doctor. You may have a condition called **hyperemesis gravidarum**. It can lead to loss of weight and body fluids.

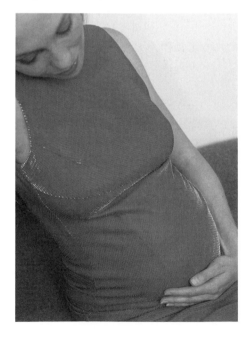

If your nausea and vomiting are severe, you may need medical treatment. If you have hyperemesis gravidarum, you may need to stay in the hospital for awhile. You may be given fluids through an intravenous (IV) line. You also may be treated with anti-nausea medications. In most cases, you will not be allowed to eat any food until the vomiting stops. You may get relief from resting in a dimly lit room where it is quiet and private. This type of treatment in the hospital often relieves symptoms.

Numbness and Tingling

Some women have pain, numbness, or tingling in certain parts of their bodies during pregnancy. These feelings can be caused by a number of changes in your body.

As your uterus grows, it presses on some of the nerves connecting your legs to your spinal cord. This may cause chronic pain in the hip or thigh (sciatica).

Nerves also can get pressed if your legs swell during pregnancy (see "Swelling"). This pressure can cause your legs or toes to tingle or feel numb. Most often, these symptoms are minor and go away after the baby is born.

Your arms or hands also may tingle as a result of tissue swelling. For instance, a condition called **carpal tunnel syndrome** is common in pregnant women. It causes a burning, tingling feeling in one or both hands. It also may make your fingers numb. Wearing a special wrist splint can help.

Another cause of numbness and tingling in some women is hyperventilating (overbreathing). You may feel short of breath, either from anxiety or simply from pregnancy (see "Shortness of Breath"). This shortness of breath makes you breathe deeper and faster to try to get some air. When you hyperventilate, you may feel sweaty and dizzy and your heart may pound. If you get these symptoms, breathe into a paper bag for about 1 minute. This restores the balance of oxygen and carbon dioxide in your body.

Shortness of Breath

Early in pregnancy, you may feel short of breath because of the increase of progesterone in your body. This feeling may stop when you become used to the progesterone.

Later in pregnancy, a new cause of shortness of breath occurs. Your uterus is starting to take up more room in your abdomen. By about 31–34 weeks of pregnancy, the uterus is so large that it presses the stomach and the diaphragm (a flat, strong muscle that aids in breathing) up toward the lungs. Although you may feel short of breath, this does not mean your baby is not getting enough oxygen. The following tips may help you breathe easier:

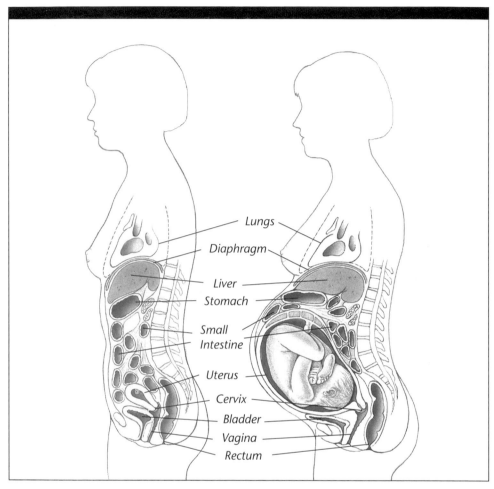

Lungs
Diaphragm
Liver
Stomach
Small
Intestine
Uterus
Cervix
Bladder
Vagina
Rectum

As the uterus grows from the beginning (*left*) to the end (*right*) of pregnancy, it takes up more room in your abdomen. This presses the digestive organs and the diaphragm up toward the lungs.

➤ Slow down. When you move more slowly, your heart and lungs don't have to work so hard.

➤ Sit (or stand) up straight. This gives your lungs more room to expand.

➤ Sleep propped up. This gives your lungs more space.

Skin and Hair Changes

During pregnancy your body produces more melanin, the pigment that gives color to skin and hair. This increase in pigment is the reason your nipples become darker, for example. These changes are temporary and harmless.

You also may notice other changes in your hair and skin:

➤ *Acne.* Some women find that their faces break out more during pregnancy. To treat breakouts, wash your face a few times a day with a mild cleanser. You may want to buy a good, water-based cover-up, too. Some acne products are not safe to take during pregnancy. Accutane (isotretinoin) causes birth defects and should not be taken by a pregnant woman. Tetracycline also should not be used. Tretinoin (Retin-A) and benzoyl peroxide (Benzamycin), which come in gels or lotions, are a few of the prescription treatments that are safe to use during pregnancy.

➤ *Chloasma.* This "mask of pregnancy" gives some women brownish marks around their eyes and on their noses and cheeks. This is one of the changes caused by your body's increase in the pigment melanin. Spending time in the sun can worsen chloasma. Protect yourself from the sun. Wear a hat with a brim and use sun block. Limit the time you spend in the sun, especially from 10 AM to 2 PM. These marks will fade after delivery, when hormone levels return to normal. In the meantime, make-up can be used to cover the chloasma.

➤ *Linea nigra.* In many women, the extra pigment produced in pregnancy causes the faint line running from the belly button to the pubic hair to darken during pregnancy. This line has always been there, but before pregnancy it was the same color as the skin around it. It will fade after delivery.

➤ *Red palms and spider veins.* You may have red, itchy palms and tiny red veins that show up under the skin of your face or legs. Again, the redness should fade after delivery.

➤ *Skin tags.* Skin tags are little flaps of skin on your breasts, neck, or armpits that may show up during pregnancy. Skin tags will not go away after the baby arrives, but they can be removed easily.

➤ *Stretch marks.* As your belly and breasts grow, they may become streaked with reddish lines. These stretch marks happen when skin stretches quickly to support the growing fetus. Don't waste your money on any of the "miracle" creams or lotions sold to prevent stretch marks. There's little you can do to keep them from appearing or to make them go away. Once your baby is born, these red streaks will slowly fade. Some marks may remain.

➤ *Thicker hair.* Your hair may become thicker, and you may sprout new hairs where you never had them before—usually on your face and arms, or sometimes on your belly. Most likely, your hair will thin out after the baby's born. Your hair should return to normal in 3–6 months.

Swelling

Some swelling (called *edema*) in the hands, face, legs, ankles, and feet is normal during pregnancy. It's caused by the extra fluid in your body. It tends to be worse in late pregnancy and during the summer.

For relief, put your feet up often and sleep with your legs propped up on pillows. This keeps fluid from pooling in the lower half of your body. Also, standing neck deep in a swimming pool for 30 minutes a day may help reduce leg swelling. Don't take water pills or other medications to reduce swelling without your doctor's consent.

Let your doctor know if you are badly swollen or if you have sudden swelling in your face or hands (hint: your rings will be too tight). This could signal a problem such as high blood pressure.

Vaginal Discharge

Vaginal discharge often increases during pregnancy. A sticky, clear, or white discharge is normal, and it's nothing to worry about. Let your doctor know if the discharge has blood in it, is watery, has a bad odor, or has changed from normal. Also, tell the doctor if you have pain, soreness, or itching in the vaginal area. Never douche when you're pregnant.

Varicose Veins

The weight of your uterus pressing down on a major vein can slow blood flow from your lower body. The result may be sore, itchy, blue bulges on your legs called varicose veins. These veins also can appear near your vagina, and rectum (see "Hemorrhoids"). In most cases, varicose veins are not a problem.

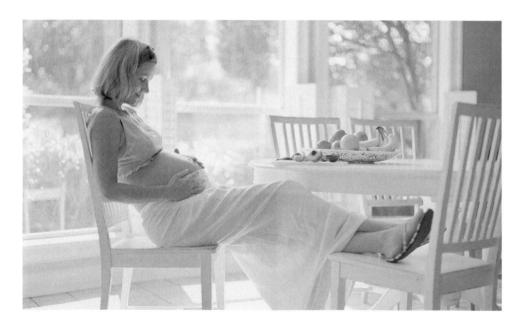

You are more likely to have varicose veins if someone in your family has had them. You can't prevent varicose veins. However, taking these steps will help relieve swelling and soreness and may stop varicose veins from getting worse:

➤ If you must sit or stand for long periods, be sure to move around from time to time.

➤ Don't sit with your legs crossed.

➤ Prop up your legs—on your desk, a couch, a chair, or a footstool—as often as you can.

➤ Exercise—walk, swim, or ride an exercise bike.

➤ Wear support hose.

➤ Don't wear stockings or socks that have a tight band of elastic around the legs.

Emotional Changes

Your body's going through big changes now, and so are your emotions. Don't blame yourself if you are sad or moody. The emotions you are feeling—good and bad—are normal. Ask loved ones to support you and be patient. Rest and relax as often as you can. You'll feel better, emotionally and physically, if you do.

Feelings and Concerns

Pregnant women and their partners often have fears about pregnancy, labor and delivery, the effect a child will have on their lives, and whether they'll be good parents. Some people have strange or scary dreams during pregnancy. This is normal.

Most often, there's nothing to worry about. Still, there are things you can do to ease your mind. Here are some common fears and what you can do about them:

➤ *"I'm worried that something will be wrong with the baby."* Keep in mind that most children are born healthy. Calm your fears by doing all that you can to ensure that your baby is healthy: eat right, exercise, avoid risky behavior, and get early and regular prenatal care. If you smoke, stop.

➤ *"I've never given birth before. I'm scared of the pain and afraid that I won't be able to stand it."* Know what to expect during labor and delivery. Take a childbirth class to learn relaxation methods, ways to ease labor pain, and the options you have for pain relief. For instance, if you plan to give birth without pain relief, remind yourself that you won't "fail" if you decide you need some relief. Often, medication helps a woman relax enough to help labor along.

➤ *"I'm worried that I'll forget the pain-management techniques I learned in class."* Practice makes perfect. Rehearse the methods taught in childbirth class until they become second nature to you. Keep in mind, too, that your health care team will be there to support you.

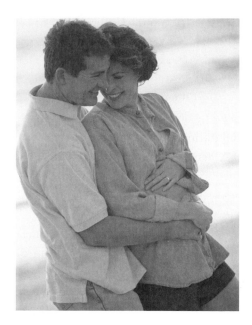

➤ *"I just know that something will go wrong in the delivery room."* Remind yourself that having a baby is a natural event. Even if your birth doesn't go just as planned, chances are that you and your baby will be fine.

➤ *"I don't know how to take care of a baby."* Feeding, bathing, changing diapers, and dressing a baby are easy to learn. You may feel better prepared if you take a newborn-care class before your due date. Many hospitals offer these 1- or 2-day courses. Also, read up on infant care before your baby arrives. To pick up a few tips, spend some time with a friend or family member who has just had a baby. After your baby is born, ask the nurses at the hospital to help you practice baby-care basics before you leave. Once you're home, ask family and friends for advice.

There are good books at libraries and bookstores that contain advice on caring for your newborn. Ask your doctor or your baby's doctor about the books they suggest.

➤ *"My life will never be the same again."* You are right—but that doesn't have to be a bad thing. Having a baby means big changes. Your relationships will change. Hanging out with friends or spending time alone with your partner may be harder. Your interests may shift. Having a baby doesn't mean you have to give up everything you enjoy. You can still do many of the same things you did before. You just need to alter them to include your baby. Keep in mind, too, that a whole new world—with new people, new places, and new things to do—will open up to you now.

Body Image

Mixed feelings about your pregnant body are normal. Your growing body is a sign of a new life growing inside you. There still may be days when you'll feel fat and wonder if your body will ever be the same.

Eating a healthy diet and exercising will help keep these feelings at bay. Regular workouts will help you feel better about how you look. Eating right and keeping a healthy weight are an important part of health. If you're in good shape and don't gain more than the suggested weight during pregnancy, you'll have an easier time losing weight after delivery.

The Second Time Around

Women who are pregnant for the second time (or third or fourth time) know what to expect throughout pregnancy to labor and delivery. Still, this pregnancy may not be like the last one.

Keep in mind, too, that just as every pregnancy is different, so is every baby. This child may not be at all like your first. The tricks and tips that worked the first time may not work with this baby.

Physical Differences

You may not have had any nausea during your first pregnancy. That may not be the case this time. You may have been active right up until the end then, but this time you feel tired all the time. There's no way to know ahead of time what a second (or later) pregnancy will be like.

One thing that is almost always true of a later pregnancy is that you will be more tired this time. There are a few reasons for this. You are older than you were during your first pregnancy. You may not have had a chance to get back in shape after giving birth. Also, you have a child who needs care.

You'll "show" earlier this time, too. In fact, you may need to start wearing your maternity clothes before your fourth month of pregnancy. That's because your abdominal muscles were stretched by your prior pregnancy. They may not have regained their former strength. As a result, these muscles won't hold the growing uterus in or up as well as they did during the first pregnancy.

Chances are, you'll feel this baby move weeks earlier than you felt your first baby. The fetus isn't really moving sooner. You just know what to look for this time. You also may notice **Braxton Hicks contractions** sooner than you did during your first pregnancy. These "practice" contractions may show up during the second trimester rather than the third, for instance.

Women who have nursed a baby before may not notice the breast changes that first-time mothers do. That's because much of the work needed to prepare for breastfeeding has already taken place. Breasts that have been primed by prior nursing may begin to leak earlier in pregnancy, too. Your breasts may not be as tender or grow as much as they did in the first pregnancy.

Some women, though, find that their breasts grow bigger and sag more in a second pregnancy. This can happen because the tissue that supports the breasts is stretched out from prior growth and nursing.

Your first baby most likely dropped into your pelvis weeks before you went into labor. This time, though, lightening may not take place until delivery day. No one knows for sure why this happens.

Although second-time moms more or less know what's going to happen next, it's still vital to pay attention to your body's signals. If something doesn't seem quite right to you, ask your doctor.

Your Other Children

Children can have very different reactions to your pregnancy and to a new baby in the family. Small children may have lots of questions about where babies come from, or they may not want to talk about the baby at all. Some children are eager to be a big brother or sister. Others resent losing center stage to the new baby. A teen, busy with his or her own life, may show little interest in the baby. He or she also may be embarrassed by your pregnancy.

When should you share your news with them? That depends on your child. Tell your school-aged children before you tell anyone outside your family. If you don't, they might resent being the last to know. With young children, it's a good idea to wait until they ask about your changing body. The idea of a baby growing inside you may be too hard for a small child to grasp before they can see your expanded belly.

No matter how your children act when you tell them about the baby, be sure to remind them that you love them and will always be there for them. Also

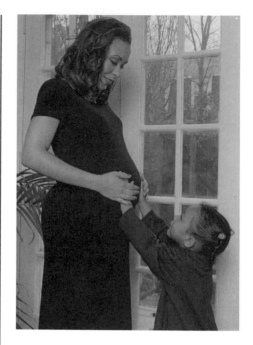

assure your children that delivering the baby won't harm you. Let them know that even though you will be in the hospital, it's not because you're sick.

To prevent your children from feeling left out, involve them in your pregnancy as much as you can. Ask your kids to help you get ready for the baby's arrival. Take them shopping and let them pick out items for their new brother or sister. Have them help you sort through hand-me-downs. Let them vote for the name they like best. The relationship between siblings is one of the longest and most important ones in life. Here are some tips to help promote this bond right from the start:

➤ Tell your child about the role he or she can play in guiding and teaching the new baby.

➤ Read books together about pregnancy, childbirth, babies, and being a big brother or sister.

➤ If "sibling prep" classes are offered in your area, sign your child up for one.

➤ Let your child feel the baby move.

➤ Take your child along on prenatal visits and let him or her hear the baby's heartbeat.

➤ Take your child on a tour of the hospital where you'll be giving birth.

➤ Show your child pictures and videos from when he or she was a newborn. Use photos of you and your partner caring for your child as a baby to talk about the kinds of care the new baby will need.

➤ Set up the baby's sleeping area well in advance. This way, your child won't feel displaced if he or she must share a room with the baby or give up his or her crib.

Some families even invite their children into the delivery room to witness a sibling's birth. Only you can tell if this option is right for your child—or for you. If you would like to make your baby's birth a family affair, talk to your doctor first. Also, check to see what the hospital policy is on siblings being present at births. Arrange to have an adult look after your child during delivery. If your child isn't with you during delivery, there's no reason he or she can't meet a new sibling shortly after birth.

A Look Ahead

Your pregnancy is heading for its conclusion. Your baby is about to arrive. With your labor day close at hand, the day-to-day changes of your pregnancy soon will be a distant memory.

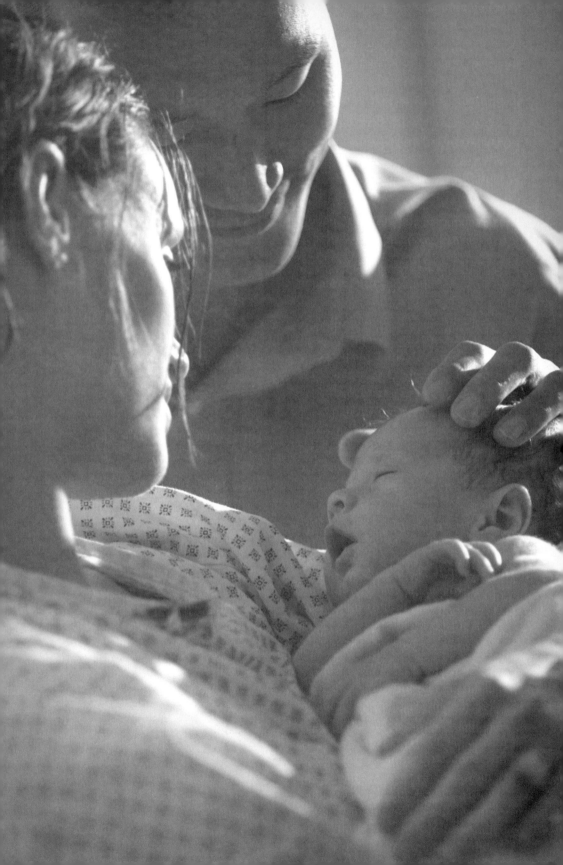

LABOR, DELIVERY, AND POSTPARTUM

For the past 40 weeks, your body has been changing as your baby grows. Now, as you near the end of pregnancy, you are eager to meet your new baby.

Still, you may be nervous about what's ahead and wonder what your life will be like after the baby arrives. You also may feel anxious about labor and delivery. This may be even more true if you have never given birth before.

The best way to approach labor, delivery, and the postpartum period is to be informed. Knowing what to expect and being prepared for the experience will help you get the most out of birth and being a new mother.

CHAPTER 8

Labor

Your body has gone through some big changes during the past 40 weeks. It will go through a few more as you near birth. Sometimes it's hard to tell if labor is starting or if it is simply a false alarm. There may be times when you wonder, "Is this it?"

Rest assured, when labor happens, you will know. Plenty of women think they are in labor when they are not. However, very few women think they are not in labor when they are in labor.

Once labor really starts, things may move quickly. Your water may break, your contractions will come faster and more often, and your baby may be born within hours. The more you know in advance about what to expect during labor, the better prepared you will be for the actual event.

Getting Ready

Your labor may go more smoothly if you plan for it ahead of time. Practice the exercises from your childbirth classes, such as breathing, relaxation, stretching, or meditation. Make a list of the phone numbers of people you or your partner will want to call after the baby is born. The more details you handle in advance, the more relaxed you will be when labor starts.

Planning Your Hospital Trip

For the trip to the hospital, plan the route you will take so you know how much time to set aside. Map out a backup route. It will come in handy if you run into a delay. Consider the following items ahead of time to ensure that your trip to the hospital is smooth:

➤ *Transportation.* How will you get there? Is your car reliable? (Be sure to keep the gas tank filled.) Can someone drive you? Is there someone who can take you at any hour, day or night? How can you reach your partner at different times of day?

➤ *Distance.* How long does it take to drive to the hospital? Try a practice run to see how long it takes to get there from your home or your workplace.

➤ *Time of day.* Find out how much time the drive will take at different times of day, such as during traffic rush hours.

➤ *Time of year.* Don't forget to allow for bad weather. The trip to the hospital may take longer in a snowstorm than it will on a spring day.

Getting Ready for Delivery

To plan for your baby's birth, be sure you have the answers to these questions well before delivery day:

➤ What number do I call if I have an emergency during pregnancy?

➤ What maternity benefits does my job offer?

➤ Have I filled out all the paperwork needed to begin my maternity leave and collect disability pay?

➤ Do I need to register at the hospital before I check in for delivery? If so, have I done this?

➤ Is there anything special I should—or shouldn't—do when I think labor has started?

➤ When should I call the doctor's office if I think I'm in labor?

➤ What number do I call when I go into labor?

➤ At what point in my labor should I leave for the hospital?

➤ Should I go straight to the hospital or call the doctor's office first?

➤ Who will drive me to the hospital?

➤ How will I get in touch with my driver when I'm ready to go?

➤ Where can we park the car?

➤ Can the birth be videotaped?

➤ When can family and guests visit me?

➤ *Other concerns.* Do you have children who will need to be taken to a friend's or a family member's home? Do you need someone to take care of a pet while you are in the hospital? Is there anything else that will need to be arranged in advance?

Pack Your Hospital Bag

The last thing you want to be doing once labor starts is tossing items into a suitcase in a panic. To avoid this, pack your bag a few weeks before your due date. Leave it in a handy place, such as a hall closet or the trunk of your car.

You can't pack everything ahead of time—you will need some things in the meantime, such as your glasses and slippers. Make a list of these last-minute items that need to be packed before you leave for the hospital and tape it to your suitcase as a reminder.

It's a good idea to pack two bags: a small one with supplies you will want during labor and a larger one for your hospital stay (see box). You can grab the small bag on your way out the door. After your baby's born, someone can bring you the larger bag.

Don't worry if you forget something. The hospital will have most of the things you need. To find out what the hospital supplies, call the childbirth educator or nurse's desk in the labor-and-delivery department.

Labor

Certain changes in your body signal that labor is near (see Table 8–1). But some women do not have any of these signs before labor begins.

Most people think of "labor" as the period when the mother has contractions in her uterus and her cervix changes before the baby is born. In fact, the medical term "labor" includes that period, plus the baby's birth and the delivery of the placenta.

The first stage of labor begins with the cervix beginning to thin out (efface) and open (dilate). You also feel the first contractions of your uterus at this stage. During contractions, you may feel pain or pressure that starts in your back and moves around to your lower abdomen. When this happens, your belly will tighten and feel hard. Between contractions, the uterus relaxes and your belly softens.

These contractions are doing vital work. They help open (dilate) the cervix. They also help push your baby lower into the pelvis. As labor proceeds, the contractions last longer, become more intense, and occur closer together. Your doctor may examine you to see how ready you are for birth. Certain physical changes are key signs of progress toward birth.

The first stage of labor is almost always the longest. For a woman's first

Things You May Want to Pack

For labor:

___ Your health insurance card, ID, and hospital registration forms

___ Lotion or oil for massage

___ A picture or a treasured object to use as a focal point during contractions

___ An old nightgown or nightshirt (if you don't want to wear a hospital gown)

___ Your favorite pillow

___ A bathrobe

___ Slippers

___ Socks

___ A barrette or band to pull back your hair

___ Glasses, if you wear them (you may not be allowed to wear contact lenses)

___ Lollipops or hard candies to keep your mouth moist

___ A cassette or CD player and some soothing music

___ A camera with film and fully charged batteries, if you plan to take pictures (check the hospital policy in advance if you want to use a video camera during delivery)

For your hospital stay:

___ Two or three nightgowns (be sure the gowns open at the front if you plan to nurse)

___ Two or three nursing bras and a dozen or so nursing pads

___ A few pairs of socks and panties

___ Shampoo, lotion, deodorant, lip balm, and other toiletries

___ A toothbrush and toothpaste

___ A hair brush or comb

___ Barrettes or hair ties

___ Contact lenses, if you wear them

___ A notepad and pen

___ Your cell phone or a long-distance calling card

___ Change for the vending machines

___ Phone numbers of people you want to call after the birth

___ Magazines or other reading material

___ A receiving blanket and clothes for your newborn to wear home

___ Loose-fitting clothes for you to wear home

___ A car seat (see "A Car Safety Seat" in Chapter 11)

Table 8–1. Signs That Labor Is Near		
Sign	**What It Is**	**When It Happens**
Feeling as if the baby has dropped lower in your belly	*Lightening.* The baby's head has dropped down into your pelvis.	From a few weeks (for first-time moms) to a few hours (for later births) before labor starts
Vaginal discharge (clear, pink, or slightly bloody)	***Show.*** Thick mucus seals off the cervix during pregnancy. When the cervix starts to open, this mucus plug is released into the vagina.	Anytime from a few days before labor starts to the onset of labor
Fluid leaking from your vagina in a trickle or a gush	***Rupture of membranes*** (your "water breaks"). The fluid-filled amniotic sac that surrounds your baby during pregnancy breaks.	At the start of labor or during labor
Strong, periodic cramps that feel like a bad menstrual cramps	*Contractions.* Your uterus tightens and relaxes. These contractions open the cervix and help push the baby into the birth canal.	At the onset of labor (although Braxton Hicks backache or contractions—"false labor"—can happen weeks or even months before labor starts)

baby, the "average" first stage of labor lasts 6–12 hours. With births after a woman's first baby, the first stage of labor is often much shorter—on average, about 4–8 hours.

The first stage of labor has two different phases: 1) early labor (sometimes called "latent labor"), when the cervix dilates to 4 centimeters; and 2) active labor, when the cervix dilates from 4 to 10 centimeters. At the end of this stage of labor your body is ready for the baby's birth and you will start pushing.

True Versus False Labor

During the last month or two of pregnancy, many women have periods of "false" labor. False labor pains are called Braxton Hicks contractions. They tend to occur more often as your due date draws near—during the last month of pregnancy.

Sometimes Braxton Hicks contractions are very mild. They can barely be felt or feel like a slight tightness in your abdomen. Other times, they can be painful. These contractions help your body gear up for birth, but do not do

The First Stage of Labor

The first stage of labor, before the delivery, has two distinct phases:

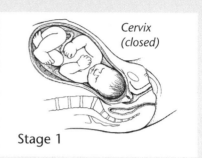

Cervix (closed)

Stage 1

Early Labor (your cervix dilates from 0 to 4 centimeters)

What Happens:

➤ Mild contractions begin. They are 5–15 minutes apart, and each one lasts 60–90 seconds.

➤ Contractions gradually get closer together. Toward the end of early labor, they are less than 5 minutes apart.

How Long It Lasts:

➤ The length of early labor varies quite a bit. For some women, it's a few hours. For others, it's a day or more. But the average for first-time moms is 6–12 hours.

What You Can Do:

➤ Go for a walk with your partner or labor coach.

➤ Take a shower or bath (as long as your water hasn't broken).

➤ Try to rest and relax.

➤ Practice relaxation exercises or meditation.

➤ If you can, sleep.

Active Labor (your cervix dilates from 4 to 10 centimeters)

What Happens:

➤ Contractions get stronger. They come as often as 3 minutes apart, and each one lasts about 45 seconds.

➤ Your water may break. If it does, your contractions will get much more intense.

➤ You'll bleed a little from your vagina as your cervix opens.

➤ If the baby's head seems to press down on your backbone during contractions, you'll have back pain.

➤ Your legs may cramp.

➤ You may feel anxious and tired.

➤ You may have trembling legs, nausea, or vomiting.

➤ You may feel the urge to push.

The First Stage of Labor (continued)

How Long It Lasts:

➤ About 4–8 hours, on average

What You Can Do:

➤ If you feel like it and your doctor says it's OK, walk the halls.

➤ Urinate often. An empty bladder gives your baby's head more room to move down.

➤ Work with your labor coach through each contraction.

➤ Take your contractions one at a time. Focus on your breathing.

➤ Try to relax between contractions and don't think about the next one.

➤ Use the pain-management methods you learned in childbirth class.

➤ Ask someone to massage your back.

➤ If you have leg cramps, ask to have your feet flexed.

➤ Try different positions to find the one that works best for you.

➤ If you feel like lying down, lie on your side. Being flat on your back will add to your pain and cut down on the oxygen your baby gets.

➤ Ask for pain relief if you want it.

➤ If you feel the urge to push, tell your doctor. Don't give in to the urge just yet—your cervix isn't fully dilated. Pant or blow to keep yourself from bearing down.

much to open the cervix. Braxton–Hicks contractions often occur in the afternoon or evening, after physical activity and sexual intercourse. They are more likely when a woman is tired or dehydrated. Be sure you drink enough fluids to stay hydrated.

If you have contractions, time them. Note how long it is from the start of one contraction to the start of the next. Keep a record for an hour and also jot down how your contractions feel. You can walk around or do household tasks while you are timing your contractions.

The time between contractions will help tell you if you are in true or false labor (see Table 8–2).

Painful contractions don't always signal true labor. Painless ones don't always mean false labor, either. Each woman feels pain differently, and it can differ from one pregnancy to another.

It's easy to be fooled by false labor. Even a doctor, midwife, or a nurse can have a hard time telling false labor from the real thing. He or she may need to observe you for a few hours to decide. A

Labor Defined

Four terms are used to measure a woman's progress before and during labor:

Ripening—the softening of the cervix. The cervix must be ripe before it can begin to thin or open.

Effacement—the thinning out of the cervix. It is measured in percentages, from 0% (no effacement) to 100% (fully effaced).

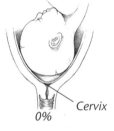
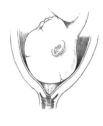
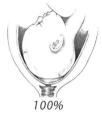

0%   Cervix   100%

Dilatation—the amount that the cervix has opened. It is measured in centimeters, from 0 centimeters (no dilatation) to 10 centimeters (fully dilated).

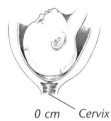
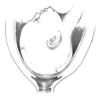

0 cm   Cervix   10 cm

Station—where the baby's head is in relation to the *ischial spines*, bony parts that stick out on each side of the pelvis. When doing a pelvic exam, your doctor or nurse can feel where the baby's head is compared to these spines protruding from the walls of the pelvis. The station is measured in numbers, from -5 (the baby's head is floating above the pelvis) to 0 (the baby's head has dropped into the pelvis) to +5 (the baby's head is *crowning* at the opening of the vagina).

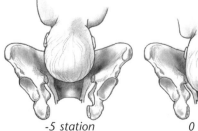
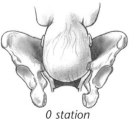
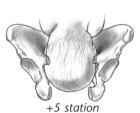

-5 station   0 station   +5 station

Table 8–2. Are You Really in Labor?

Hint	False Labor	True Labor
Timing of contractions	Contractions often are irregular; they don't get closer together as time goes on.	Contractions come at regular intervals and get closer together. They last 30–90 seconds.
Change with movement	Contractions may stop when you walk, rest, or change position.	Contractions keep coming no matter what you do.
Strength of contractions	Contractions often are weak, and they tend to stay that way; or strong contractions are followed by weaker ones.	Contractions steadily get stronger.
Pain of contractions	Pain usually is felt only in the front.	Pain usually starts in the back and moves to the front.

vaginal exam also will be done to see if your cervix is opening.

No matter what your watch says about the timing of contractions, it's better to be safe than sorry. If you think you may be in labor, call your doctor or midwife's office or hospital. These are other signs that should prompt a call:

➤ You have symptoms of labor before 37 weeks of pregnancy.

➤ Your water (the fluid-filled amniotic sac that surrounds the baby during pregnancy) breaks.

➤ You have vaginal bleeding.

➤ You have constant, severe pain, with no relief between contractions.

➤ You have a fever or chills.

➤ The baby seems to be moving less.

Admission

Once you're in labor, it's time to check into the hospital. Each hospital has its own procedures. After you are admitted, the next steps may vary. These are the actions that take place in most cases:

➤ *Consent form.* These forms vary, but most spell out who will be taking care of you, why a procedure is being done, and the risks involved. Read this form and be sure to ask about anything that's not clear. Signing the consent form means that you understand your medical condition and agree to the care described. You may need to sign separate consent forms for anesthesia and for cesarean delivery.

➤ *Room assignment.* You'll be taken to a hospital room. In some hospitals

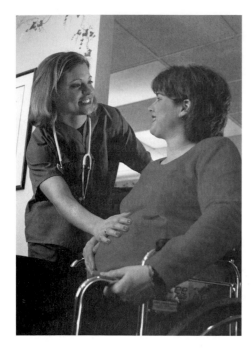

you will stay in the same room for both labor and delivery. Other hospitals have a separate delivery room.

➤ *Changing clothes.* You'll be asked to put on a hospital gown. If you'd rather wear your own nightgown or nightshirt, just ask. It may get stained or ruined, however.

➤ *Vital signs.* Your pulse, blood pressure, and temperature will be checked.

➤ *Lab tests.* A urine or blood sample may be taken.

➤ *Physical exam.* You'll eventually be given a vaginal exam to see how much your cervix has dilated.

➤ *IV line.* An IV line may be started in your arm or wrist. A needle is placed

in your vein, a narrow plastic tube is threaded over it, and the needle is removed. Medications and fluids can be given through the IV if you need them. An IV may limit your activity a bit during labor, though. If you'd rather not have an IV, talk to your doctor or midwife. He or she may be willing to wait and see if one is needed.

➤ *Fetal monitoring.* You may be hooked up to an *electronic fetal monitor* to measure your contractions and check the baby's heart rate.

Once you are in your room at the hospital, a labor-and-delivery nurse will be checking on you from the time you check in until after your baby is born. (If your labor goes on for a long time or if a shift change happens in the middle of your labor, you may have more than one nurse.) These nurses are well trained to help women through the physical and emotional demands of labor. In teaching hospitals, a resident doctor, student nurse, or medical student also may be a part of your birth team.

Your own doctor or midwife may be there from start to finish, or he or she may arrive shortly before you give birth. Even if they are there only while you are pushing the baby out, he or she will check on your progress by telephone often during labor. These are the conditions that your doctor, midwife, or nurse will keep close tabs on before delivery:

➤ *Your heart rate and blood pressure.* This will give clues to how well your body is handling the stress of labor.

➤ *Your contractions.* The time and length of contractions help to monitor the progress of your labor.

➤ *Dilatation of your cervix.* From time to time the doctor, midwife, or nurse will examine your cervix to see if it has dilated.

➤ *Fetal heart rate.* If an electronic fetal monitor is not in place, the nurse will use a special stethoscope called a **fetoscope** to check your baby's heartbeat often during labor (see the "Monitoring" section).

If you haven't done so, talk to your doctor, midwife, or nurse about the sort of birth you hope to have and the options available (see Chapter 2). They are there to answer your questions. You already have learned a lot about labor and delivery during your prenatal care and childbirth classes. Still, lots of new questions may occur to you now. Ask them.

Helping Labor Along

Sometimes your body needs a little help to start labor. Using medications or other methods to bring on labor is called **labor induction**. If continuing the pregnancy is more risky than delivering the baby, the doctor might induce labor. Some of the methods used to induce labor also can speed up a labor that's not going forward as it should. Labor may be induced if:

➤ Your water has broken.

➤ Your pregnancy is postterm (more than 42 weeks).

➤ You have high blood pressure caused by your pregnancy.

➤ You have health problems such as diabetes that could affect your baby.

➤ You have **chorioamnionitis** (an infection in the uterus).

➤ Your baby has growth problems.

Labor induction carries some risks, especially if your cervix hasn't started to dilate or efface. Your baby may be monitored with electronic fetal monitoring if labor is induced (see the "Monitoring" section).

There are four methods for inducing labor:

1. *Stripping the membranes.* Your doctor inserts a gloved finger through your cervix. Next, he or she sweeps a finger over the thin membranes that connect the amniotic sac to the wall of your uterus. You may feel some intense cramping and have spotting when this is done. Stripping the membranes causes your body to release **prostaglandins.** These are hor-

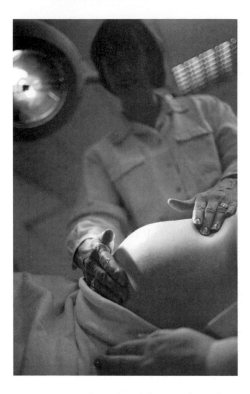

mones that ripen the cervix and may cause contractions.

2. *Ripening or dilating the cervix.* If your cervix is not ready for labor, the doctor may give you some medication or insert a device in the uterus to help make the cervix soft and able to stretch for labor. This is called ripening the cervix. The medication may be given to you through an IV tube or by placing a tablet, gel, or drug-releasing device in your vagina.

3. *Rupturing the amniotic sac (breaking your water).* If your water has not broken already, breaking it can get contractions started or

make them stronger. Your doctor may make a small hole in the amniotic sac. This is called an amniotomy. You may feel discomfort as this is done with a special instrument. Usually, you will feel a warm sensation when the fluid flows out. Most women go into labor within hours of their water breaking. If labor does not begin, another method may be used to bring on contractions. That's because you and your baby are at risk for infection once the amniotic sac has broken.

4. *Giving **oxytocin.*** This is a hormone that causes contractions or makes contractions stronger. If your doctor decides to use oxytocin, it will be given to you through an IV tube in your arm. A pump hooked up to the IV controls the amount you are given.

Monitoring

To see how the baby is doing during labor, your doctor or nurse will check the fetal heart rate often. A normal fetal heart rate is between 110 and 160 beats a minute. A rate that's not in that range can signal a problem.

Monitoring can't stop a problem from happening, but it can alert your doctor or nurse to warning signs. The doctor or nurse then can take steps to help the baby. These steps might include the following:

➤ Asking you to change positions

➤ Giving you oxygen through a mask

➤ Giving you IV fluids

➤ Stopping the use of oxytocin

➤ Putting extra fluid around your baby

➤ Giving you medicine to weaken contractions and relax your uterus

Fetal monitoring is done by *auscultation* or with an electronic fetal monitor. Sometimes auscultation and electronic fetal monitoring can be used together. The method used depends on the following:

➤ The equipment on hand

➤ The number of nurses on duty

➤ The hospital's policy

➤ Your risk of problems

➤ How your labor is going

Auscultation

Auscultation means listening to the baby's heartbeat at set times during labor. The timing depends on how well labor is going and whether there are any risk factors. The doctor or nurse will place his or her hands on your abdomen to feel the contractions. Auscultation has no known risks. Two devices can be used to detect the heart-

beat: a fetoscope or a *Doppler* ultrasound:

1. A fetoscope is a type of stethoscope. Your doctor or nurse presses one end of the scope to your belly and listens to the baby's heartbeat through earpieces.

2. A Doppler ultrasound is a small, hand-held device that's placed on your belly. It uses sound waves to create a signal of the baby's beating heart (see "Ultrasound" in Chapter 3).

Electronic Fetal Monitoring

The other type of monitoring measures the baby's heart rate with electronic equipment. It provides an ongoing record and often is used in high-risk pregnancies. Usually, you will be asked to stay in bed if electronic monitoring is used.

Electronic fetal monitoring can be done from the outside (external), inside (internal), or both:

➤ *External monitoring:* Two belts are wrapped around your belly. Each belts holds a small device in place. One device uses ultrasound to detect the fetal heart rate. The other measures the length of contractions and the time between them.

➤ *Internal monitoring:* Internal monitoring can be done only after the amniotic sac has broken. A small

Monitoring

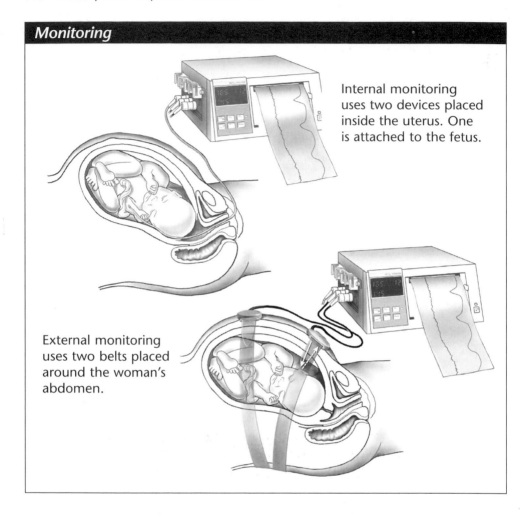

Internal monitoring uses two devices placed inside the uterus. One is attached to the fetus.

External monitoring uses two belts placed around the woman's abdomen.

device called an **electrode** is inserted through your vagina and placed on the baby's scalp. The electrode records fetal heart rate. A thin tube called a **catheter** also may be put in your uterus to gauge the strength of contractions. Most women report only minor pain when the devices are put in place about the same as a routine pelvic exam.

➤ *Combined internal and external monitoring:* Sometimes, both methods are used. The internal electrode is used to record the fetal heart beat. One external belt is wrapped around your belly to record contractions.

No matter which type of electronic monitoring is used, the information recorded is sent to a machine where a needle traces how the fetal heart rate reacts to contractions.

There are pros and cons to each type of electronic monitoring. One benefit of external monitoring is that the amniotic sac around the fetus can be left intact. Another one is that it can be used even if the cervix is not dilated. Internal monitoring has the benefit of giving a slightly more precise picture of the baby's condition and actually measuring the strength of contractions. But there is a small risk with an internal monitor that the spot where the electrode is placed on the baby's head can get injured or infected. This is rare.

The Support Person's Role

Your childbirth partner who attended childbirth classes with you will be helpful to you emotionally and physically during labor. He or she can help you use the relaxation and pain-management methods you learned in childbirth class. This person also can cheer you on when the going gets tough.

These are some of the things your support person can do during labor:

➤ Help distract you in early labor: play cards or other games with you, tell stories, read aloud, or take short walks with you

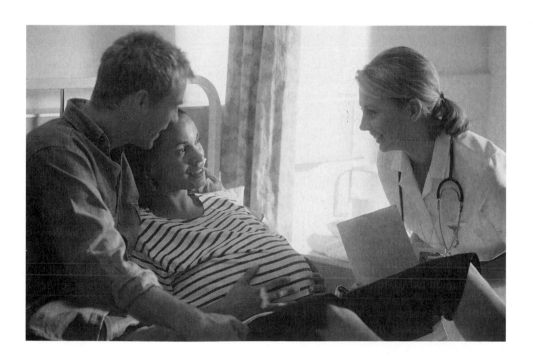

➤ Keep the room soothing by dimming the lights and keeping the noise level low

➤ Massage your back and shoulders, if that helps you relax

➤ Time your contractions

➤ Talk you through contractions

➤ Act as a focal point during contractions

➤ Guide you in breathing or other relaxation exercises

➤ Help you get into different labor positions

➤ Offer comfort and support

Some mothers hire a professional labor coach, called a doula. A doula is a woman who provides physical and emotional support to women and their partners during labor and birth. A doula offers help and advice on breathing, relaxation, and positioning. Doulas are there for your support. They do not diagnose medical conditions, give medical advice, or perform clinical tasks, such as vaginal exams or fetal heart rate monitoring.

If there's an emergency during labor or delivery, your support person may need to leave the room. The hospital staff doesn't always have time to explain why. If your partner is asked to leave, he or she should do so right away. This is in the best interests of you and your baby.

Easing Discomforts

Following are some ways to ease discomfort you may feel during labor:

➤ Do relaxation and breathing techniques taught in childbirth class.

➤ Have your partner massage or firmly press on your lower back.

➤ Change positions often.

➤ Take a shower or bath, if permitted.

➤ Place an ice pack on your back.

➤ Use tennis balls for massage.

➤ When contractions are closer together and stronger, rest in between and take slow, deep breaths.

➤ If you become warm or perspire, soothe yourself with cool, moist cloths.

Pain Relief During Labor

Each woman's labor is unique. The amount of pain a woman feels during labor may differ from that felt by another woman. Pain depends on many factors, such as the size and position of the baby and the strength of contractions.

Some women take classes to learn breathing and relaxation techniques to help cope with pain during childbirth. Others may find it helpful to use these techniques along with pain medications.

There are two types of pain-relieving drugs—*analgesics* and *anesthetics*. Analgesia is the relief of pain without total loss of feeling or muscle movement. Analgesics do not always stop pain completely, but they do lessen it.

Anesthesia is blockage of all feeling, including pain, as well as blockage of muscle movement. Some forms of anesthesia, such as *general anesthesia*, cause you to lose consciousness. Other forms, such as regional anesthesia, remove all feeling of pain from parts of the body while you stay conscious. In most cases, analgesia is offered to women in labor or after surgery or delivery, whereas anesthesia is used during and right after a surgical procedure such as *cesarean delivery*.

Not all hospitals are able to offer all types of pain relief medications. However, at most hospitals, an *anesthesiologist* will work with your health care team to pick the best method for you.

Systemic Analgesics

Systemic analgesics often are given as injections into a muscle or vein. They lessen pain but will not cause a loss of consciousness. They act on the whole nervous system rather than a specific area. Sometimes other drugs are given with analgesics to relieve the tension or nausea that may be caused by these types of pain relief.

Like other types of drugs, this pain medicine can have side effects. Most are minor, such as feeling drowsy or having trouble concentrating. Systemic analgesics are not given right before delivery because they may slow the baby's reflexes and breathing at birth.

Local Anesthesia

Local anesthesia provides numbness or loss of sensation in a small area. It does not, however, lessen the pain of contractions.

A procedure called *episiotomy* (a cut to widen the opening of the birth canal) may be done by the doctor before delivery. Local anesthesia is helpful when an episiotomy needs to be done or when any vaginal tears that happened during birth are repaired.

Local anesthesia rarely affects the baby. There usually are no side effects after the local anesthetic has worn off.

Regional Analgesia

Regional analgesia tends to be the most effective method of pain relief during labor and causes few side effects. Epidural analgesia, spinal blocks, and combined spinal–epidural blocks are all types of regional analgesia that are used to decrease labor pain.

Epidural Analgesia

Epidural analgesia, sometimes called an **epidural block**, causes some loss of feeling in the lower areas of a woman's body, yet she remains awake and alert. An epidural block may be given soon after contractions start, or later as labor progresses. An epidural block with more or stronger medications (anesthesia, not analgesia) can be used for a cesarean delivery or if a vaginal birth requires the help of **forceps** or **vacuum extraction**. The anesthesiologist and obstetrician will help to determine the proper time to give the epidural.

An epidural block is given in the lower back into a small area (the epidural space) below the spinal cord. During the procedure, a woman will be asked to sit or lie on her side with her back curved outward. When the procedure is completed, a woman may be allowed to move, but may not be allowed to walk around.

Before the block is performed, the skin will be cleaned and local anesthesia will be used to numb an area of the lower back. After the epidural needle is placed, a small tube (catheter) usually is inserted through it, and the needle is withdrawn. Small doses of the medication can then be given through the tube to reduce the discomfort of labor. The medication also can be given continuously without another injection. Low doses are used because they are less likely to cause side effects for the mother and the baby. In some cases, the catheter may touch a nerve. This may cause a brief tingling sensation down one leg.

Because the medication needs to be absorbed into several nerves, it may take a short while for it to take effect. Pain relief will begin within 10–20 minutes after the medication has been injected.

Although an epidural block will make a woman more comfortable, she still may be aware of her contractions. She also may feel her doctor's exams as labor progresses. The anesthesiologist will adjust the degree of numbness for your comfort and to assist labor and delivery. This may cause a bit of temporary numbness, heaviness, or weakness in the legs.

Although rare, complications or side effects, such as decreased blood pressure or headaches, can occur. To help prevent a decrease in blood pressure, fluids will be given through a vein by a tube in the arm. This may increase the risk of shivering. However, a woman may shiver during labor and delivery even if

Side Effects and Risks

Although most women do not have problems with an epidural, there may be some drawbacks to using this pain relief method:

➤ An epidural can cause your blood pressure to decrease. This, in turn, may slow your baby's heartbeat. To prevent this, you'll be given fluids through an IV before the drug is injected. You also may need to lie on your side to improve blood flow.

➤ After delivery, your back may be sore from the injection for a few days. However, an epidural should not cause long-term back pain.

➤ If the covering of the spinal cord is pierced, you can get a bad headache. If it's not treated, this headache may last for days. This is rare.

➤ When an epidural is given late in labor or a lot of anesthetic is used, it may be hard to bear down and push your baby through the birth canal. If you cannot feel enough when it is time to push, your anesthesiologist can adjust the dosage.

Serious complications are very rare:

➤ If the drug enters a vein, you could get dizzy or, rarely, have a seizure.

➤ If anesthetic enters your spinal fluid, it can affect your chest muscles and make it hard for you to breathe.

As long as your analgesia or anesthesia is given by a trained and experienced anesthesiologist, there's little chance you'll run into trouble. If you think a regional block may be the choice for you, bring up any concerns or questions you have with your doctor.

an epidural is not given. Keeping warm often helps to stop the shivering.

Some women (less than 1 out of 100) may get a headache after the procedure. A woman can help decrease the risk of a headache by holding as still as possible while the needle is placed. If a headache does occur, it often subsides within a few days. If the headache does not stop or if it becomes severe, a simple treatment, which involves placing another epidural needle and injecting your own blood, may be needed to help the headache go away.

The veins located in the epidural space become swollen during pregnancy. There is a risk that the anesthetic medication could be injected into one of them. Signs that this has occurred include dizziness, rapid heartbeat, a funny taste, or numbness around the mouth when the epidural is placed. If this happens, let your doctor know right away.

Spinal Block

A *spinal block*—like an epidural block is an injection in the lower back. For this procedure, a woman must sit or lie on her side in bed while a small amount of a drug is injected into the spinal fluid to numb the lower half of the body. It brings good relief from pain and starts working fast, but it lasts only an hour or two.

A spinal block can be given using a much thinner needle in the same place on the back where an epidural block is placed. The spinal block uses a much smaller dose of the drug, and it is injected into the sac of spinal fluid below the level of the spinal cord. Once this drug is injected, pain relief occurs right away.

A spinal block usually is given only once during labor, so it is best suited for pain relief during delivery. A spinal block with a much stronger medication (anesthesia, not analgesia) often is used for a cesarean delivery. It also can be used in a vaginal delivery if the baby needs to be helped out of the birth canal with forceps or by vacuum extraction. A spinal block can cause the same side effects as an epidural block, and these side effects are treated in the same way.

Combined Spinal–Epidural Block

A combined spinal–epidural (CSE) block has the benefits of both types of pain relief. The spinal part helps provide pain relief right away. Drugs given through the epidural provide pain relief throughout labor. This type of pain relief is injected into the spinal fluid and into the space below the spinal cord. Some women may be able to walk around after the block is in place. For this reason this method sometimes is called the "walking epidural." In some cases, other methods, such as an epidural or a spinal block, also can be used to allow a woman to walk during labor.

General Anesthesia

General anesthetics are medications that cause a woman to lose consciousness. With general anesthesia, a woman is not awake and does not feel pain. General anesthesia often is used when a regional block anesthetic is not possible or is not the best choice for medical or other reasons. It can be started quickly and causes a rapid loss of consciousness. Therefore, it often is used when an urgent delivery (vaginal or cesarean) is needed.

A major risk during general anesthesia is caused by food or liquids in the woman's stomach. Labor usually causes undigested food to stay in the stomach. During unconsciousness, this food could come back into the mouth and go into the lungs where it can cause damage. To avoid this, eating or drinking may not be allowed once labor has started. In some cases, the anesthesiologist may place a breathing tube into the woman's mouth and windpipe after she is asleep. During a cesarean delivery, an antacid also may be given to reduce stomach acid. In some cases, small sips of water or ice chips are allowed during labor. Talk to your doctor about what is best for you.

Anesthesia for Cesarean Births

Whether you have general, spinal, or epidural anesthesia for a cesarean birth will depend on your health and that of your baby, as well as why the cesarean delivery is being done. In emergencies or when bleeding occurs, general anesthesia may be needed.

If you already have an epidural catheter in place and then need to have a cesarean delivery, most of the time your anesthesiologist will be able to inject a much stronger drug through the same catheter to increase your pain relief. This will numb the entire abdomen for the surgery. Although there is no pain, there may be a feeling of pressure.

Many women worry that receiving pain relief during labor will somehow make the experience less "natural." The fact is, no two labors are the same, and no two women have the same amount of pain. Some women need little or no pain relief, and others find that pain relief gives them better control over their labor and delivery. Talk with your doctor about your options. In some cases, he or she may arrange for you to meet with an anesthesiologist before your labor and delivery. Be prepared to be flexible. Don't be afraid to ask for pain relief if you need it.

The Reward for Labor

Although you can't predict when labor will begin, understanding the signs and symptoms can help you better manage your labor. Knowing what happens during labor will make it easier for you to relax, do what you can to help the process along, and focus on your baby's arrival when the time comes.

CHAPTER 9

Birth

Many women are nervous about the prospect of delivery. In most cases, the birth of a baby occurs without a problem. However, if the baby's health is at risk special procedures may be required. For instance, if the baby is has a problem exiting the birth canal, a cesarean delivery may be needed. Keep in mind, no matter how the birth proceeds, a healthy baby is the main goal.

Delivery

The second stage of labor, as the baby's birth is called, starts when the cervix has opened fully—to 10 centimeters. During this time, you'll notice a change in the way contractions feel. With each contraction, you'll have an urge to bear down. This can feel like the urge to move your bowels, but much stronger.

Tell your doctor or nurse as soon as you feel like pushing. He or she will check your cervix to make sure it's dilated all the way. (If you start pushing before you are fully dilated, you can damage your cervix as well as exhaust yourself.)

If your doctor tells you to avoid pushing, controlling your breathing can help. Blowing air out in short puffs, for instance, stops many women from bearing down. If you took a childbirth class, you may have learned controlled breathing methods. If not, your nurse will guide you in breathing exercises.

If you have been in a standard labor room, you'll be moved to a delivery room now. If you are in a labor/delivery/recovery room, your doctor and nurse will help you get into a good delivery position.

Many women give birth to their babies while propped up in bed, with their legs braced against foot rests. There are other birth positions you can try (lying on your side, for instance) as long as your doctor approves. There are various techniques used to make labor and delivery more comfortable (see box).

The Second Stage of Labor

Once your cervix is fully dilated, you can begin to push your baby out. After your baby is born, the placenta will be expelled.

The Second Stage

What's Happening:

➤Contractions may slow. They are 2–5 minutes apart and last 60–90 seconds.

➤Contractions usually are regular.

➤You feel the urge to push or bear down with each contraction.

➤You feel great pressure on your rectum from the baby's head.

➤You feel pressure and stinging in your vagina as the baby's head crowns.

➤The baby's head emerges.

➤Your doctor guides the baby's shoulders and body out of the birth canal.

How Long It Lasts:

➤20 minutes to 3 hours or more

What You Can Do:

➤Ask for a mirror so you can see your baby being born.

➤Find a pushing position that works for you.

➤If you are not comfortable or pushing has stalled, change positions.

➤Push when you feel the urge or when you are told to.

➤Rest between contractions.

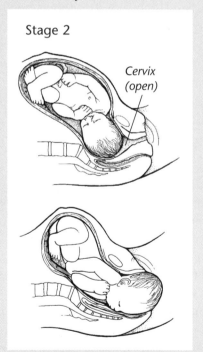

Stage 2

Cervix (open)

➤Ask the nurse to hold a warm cloth to your perineum. This will focus your pushing efforts and help your skin stretch.

The Third Stage of Labor: Delivery and Afterbirth

The Third Stage

What's Happening

➤ Contractions keep coming. They are less painful, though.

➤ The placenta peels away from the wall of the uterus.

➤ The placenta and amniotic sac are pushed out through the vagina.

➤ Contractions cause the uterus to get smaller.

➤ Your doctor or your labor coach cuts the umbilical cord.

➤ If you had an episiotomy or tear, it's stitched closed.

➤ You may shake or shiver.

How Long It Lasts:

➤ From a few minutes to about 20 minutes

What You Can Do:

➤ Push when you feel the urge or you are asked. This will help expel the placenta and amniotic sac.

➤ Ask for a warm blanket if you are cold.

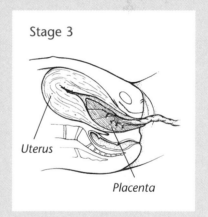

Stage 3

Uterus

Placenta

Tell your childbirth coach where you want him or her to stand. By standing at your shoulder, he or she can offer emotional and physical support as you push your baby into the world. From this spot, your coach will have the same view that you do of the baby's birth. The presence of others in the delivery room and use of video-tapes often are dictated by hospital policy.

Once your doctor gives you the go-ahead, bear down with each contraction or when you are told to push. As the baby moves down the birth canal, your doctor will track the progress and tell you how to help your baby along. The vagina is a very elastic organ. It can eas-

Labor and Childbirth Options

Following are some of the options that you may have at your hospital or birthing center:

➤ *Birthing bed/birthing chair.* A bed that can be adjusted for numerous positions for the mother, such as squatting, sitting on the end of the bed with her feet supported, or lying on her side.

➤ *Birthing stool.* A frame that allows the mother to squat. It stabilizes and supports her while she does so.

➤ *Birthing ball.* A large rubber ball that a woman can sit on during labor. It allows the woman to rock back and forth on a soft surface.

➤ *Squatting bar.* The mother squats while holding onto a bar securely attached to the bed.

➤ *Birthing pool/tub.* During labor the mother gets in a large tub or pool with water that is at body temperature. The tub is large enough for both the mother and childbirth partner, if desired. It is not recommended to give birth in water.

ily stretch to make way for a 7- or even a 10-pound newborn.

Sometimes, a few good pushes is all it takes before a baby is born. Other times, it may take hours before the baby is born.

When the baby's head appears at the opening of your vagina, you'll feel a burning or stinging feeling there as the **perineum** stretches and bulges. This is normal. Sometimes it is hard for the baby's head to fit through without tearing the skin at the opening to the vagina.

To help prevent these tears, your doctor may perform an episiotomy (see box). This is a small cut to widen the opening of your vagina. The doctor also may do an episiotomy if the baby needs

to be delivered quickly. The area is numbed with a local anesthetic before the cut is made. (An episiotomy will hurt as it heals.) However, most women will not need an episiotomy.

After the head emerges from the birth canal, the baby's body turns. First one shoulder slips out, and then the other. After the shoulders are delivered, the rest of the baby's body follows quickly.

Afterbirth

After your newborn is delivered, one more part of labor remains. Delivery of the placenta (often called the afterbirth) is called the third stage of labor. This last stage of labor is the shortest of all. It will likely last from just a few minutes to about 20 minutes.

During this stage, you will still have contractions. They will be closer together than they were when you were pushing out the baby and usually will cause less pain.

These contractions help the placenta separate from the wall of the uterus. Then the contractions move the placenta down into the birth canal. Once there, a push or two by you will help expel the placenta from the vagina.

These contractions also help your uterus return to its smaller size. As the uterus shrinks, the blood vessels that

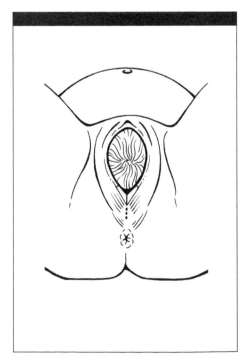

For an episiotomy, a cut is made in your vagina and perineum to widen the opening of the vagina.

brought nutrients and oxygen to the placenta and took waste products away are sealed, which helps control blood loss.

Forceps and Vacuum Extraction

No one can predict just how the birth of a baby will proceed. Sometimes the birth of the baby occurs fairly quickly and there are no problems. With some births, though, the woman may push for hours without making much progress.

In some cases, your doctor may need to help delivery along by using forceps or vacuum extraction. This is done in about 1 in 10 vaginal deliveries for various reasons. The baby's heartbeat may become slow or erratic or the woman may become too tired to push or the baby's position makes delivery harder.

Forceps look like two large spoons. They are inserted into the vagina. Next, the doctor places the forceps around the baby's cheeks and jaw (the fat there provides a cushion). The doctor then uses the forceps to gently guide the baby's head out of the birth canal.

Vacuum extraction is another way the doctor can help the baby's birth. Using this method, the doctor inserts a special suction cup into the vagina and presses it to the baby's head. Suction holds the cup in place. A handle on the cup allows the doctor to assist the baby through the birth canal while the woman continues to push.

Forceps and Vacuum Extraction

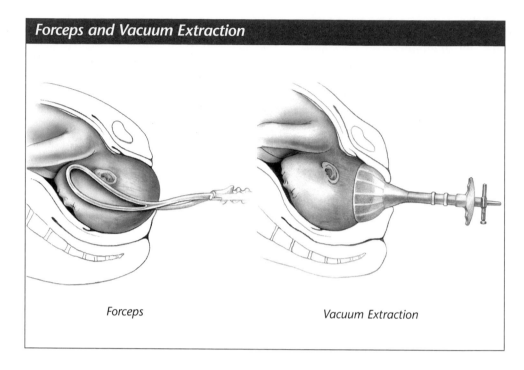

Forceps   Vacuum Extraction

In most cases, using special tools to help delivery causes no major problems. But there is some risk that forceps or vacuum extraction can bruise the baby's head or tear the vagina or cervix.

Cesarean Birth

Most babies enter the world through the birth canal. However, in about 1 in 4 cases, a baby is born by cesarean delivery. This means the baby is delivered through an incision in the mother's abdomen and uterus.

A cesarean birth may be planned ahead of time because of certain problems. Also, issues may come up in labor that make a cesarean birth a safer choice than a vaginal birth.

A cesarean delivery may be needed in the following situations:

➤ *Previous cesarean birth.* A previous cesarean birth may mean that you'll need cesarean delivery this time, too. But some women who have had cesarean birth can try to deliver vaginally. (For details, see "Vaginal Birth After Cesarean Delivery.")

➤ *Certain medical conditions.* An active genital herpes infection, for instance, may make a vaginal birth risky, but most women with these conditions may not need cesarean birth.

➤ *Multiple pregnancy.* Many women having twins can give birth vaginally. The risks of vaginal birth go up with the number of fetuses. As a result, women carrying more than two babies usually have a cesarean delivery.

➤ *Large baby or a small pelvis.* Sometimes, a baby is too big to pass safely through a woman's pelvis and vagina. This is called **cephalopelvic disproportion.**

➤ *Breech position.* If you are in labor and your baby is **breech** (with buttocks or feet closest to the vagina), your doctor may feel that a cesarean birth is the safest way to deliver the baby (see box). If the baby is transverse (lying sideways in the uterus rather than head-down), a cesarean birth is the only choice for delivery.

➤ *Umbilical cord problem.* Sometimes, the umbilical cord becomes pinched or compressed. If this happens, the baby may not get enough oxygen and an emergency cesarean delivery may be needed.

➤ *Placenta problems.* Placenta previa is a condition in which the placenta is below the baby and covers part or all of the cervix. This will block the baby's exit from the uterus. This condition can cause heavy bleeding.

➤ *Labor fails to progress.* About 1 in 3 cesarean births is done because labor slows down or stops. You may have contractions, but they don't open the cervix enough for the baby to move through the vagina, for instance. If medication doesn't speed things up (see "Helping Labor Along" in Chapter 8), a cesarean delivery may be needed.

➤ *Labor is too stressful for the baby.* Cesarean births often are needed in cases where fetal monitoring detects signs of problems.

Sometimes a cesarean birth is planned, and in other cases it maybe done quickly because a problem arises. The process can vary depending on the reason. In most cases, a cesarean birth proceeds as follows:

1. To numb pain during surgery, an epidural, a spinal block, or general anesthesia is given. The anesthesiologist will talk to a woman about her pain relief choices and take her wishes into account. (For more information on pain relief, see Chapter 8.)

2. A woman will be monitored to track her breathing, heart rate, and blood pressure. Her nose and mouth will be covered with an oxygen mask or a tube will be placed in her nostril to make sure she gets plenty of oxygen during surgery.

3. The labor coach puts on a clean mask and gown so he or she can be at the woman's side in the operating room. (If an emergency cesarean birth is needed, her partner most likely won't be allowed to join her.)

4. A nurse prepares the woman for surgery. Her abdomen will be washed and, if needed, hair between the pubic bone and navel

Breech Presentation

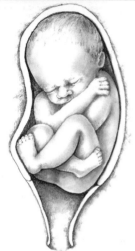

Complete breech: The buttocks are down, with the legs folded at the knees and the feet near the buttocks.

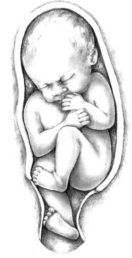

Footling breech: One or both of the baby's legs are extended and the feet are pointing down.

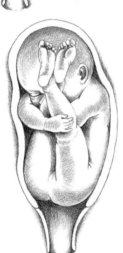

Frank breech: The baby's buttocks are at the top of the birth canal, and the legs extend straight up in front of the body, with the feet up near the head.

may be trimmed. A catheter will be inserted into the bladder. This keeps the bladder empty so that it's not injured during surgery. The abdomen will be swabbed with an antiseptic, and sterile drapes will be placed around the area of the incision.

5. A 4- to 6-inch incision is made through the skin and the wall of the abdomen. This cut usually goes from side to side, just above the pubic hairline (transverse).

6. The doctor gently spreads apart the abdominal muscles and cuts through the lining of the abdomi-

nal cavity. The abdominal muscles usually are not cut.

7. When the doctor reaches the uterus, another cut is made in the uterine wall. This also can be transverse or vertical. In most cases, a transverse incision is made. This type of cut is done in the lower, thinner part of the uterus. It causes less bleeding and heals with a stronger scar. A vertical incision may need to be done if a woman has had placenta previa or if the baby is in an unusual position. A woman should ask her doctor what type of incision was made in her uterus, so she will know if she will be able to give birth to her next baby vaginally.

8. The doctor lifts the baby out through the incisions. The umbilical cord is cut, and the baby is passed to the nurse. The placenta is removed from the uterus.

9. The uterus and abdominal wall are repaired with stitches that dissolve in the body. The skin incision is closed with stitches or surgical staples. A dressing is placed on it.

As with any surgery, a cesarean birth involves risks. Although the following risks can occur in any type of delivery, a

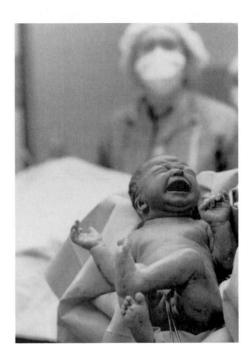

cesarean delivery may include increased risks of:

➤ Infection in the uterus, pelvic organs, or abdominal incision

➤ Blood loss, but rarely enough to require a blood transfusion

➤ Blood clots in the legs, pelvic organs, or lungs

➤ Injury to the bowel or bladder

Vaginal Birth After Cesarean Delivery

Some women who have had a cesarean delivery can give birth through the vagina in a later pregnancy. This is called vaginal birth after cesarean (VBAC)

delivery. It is not the right choice for all women and there are some risks.

Of women who try VBAC, 60–80% succeed and are able to give birth vaginally. The success rate varies depending on the reason for the previous cesarean delivery. Other women may try VBAC but need to switch to a cesarean birth. There are some reasons why a woman may want to try VBAC over cesarean delivery:

➤ No abdominal surgery

➤ Shorter hospital stay

➤ Lower risk of infection

➤ Less blood loss

➤ Less need for blood transfusions

Risks of VBAC

VBAC has risks as well as benefits. However, having more than one cesarean delivery also has risks. With VBAC, there is a very small, but serious, risk of rupture of the uterus. Although it does not occur often, a rupture of the uterus may be harmful to you or your baby. Your doctor will let you know if VBAC is an option.

Sometimes, when a woman chooses VBAC, she may have to switch to a cesarean delivery during the course of labor. This can happen if problems arise or worsen during childbirth. The hospital or other facility where your baby will be delivered should be equipped to han-

dle an emergency cesarean delivery should the need arise. There is a higher risk of infection in the mother and baby in women who try VBAC and then give birth by cesarean delivery.

Is VBAC Right for You?

In deciding if VBAC is an option, a key factor is the type of incision used in the uterus for a previous cesarean birth. Some types are more likely to rupture than others.

For cesarean birth, one incision is made in your abdomen and another incision is made in your uterus. Any incision makes a scar. You can't tell what kind of incision you had in your uterus by looking at the scar on your skin. Your doctor should be able to tell which kind of incision was used by looking at your medical records. There are three types of incisions:

1. *Low transverse*—A side-to-side cut made across the lower, thinner part of the uterus

2. *Low vertical*—An up-and-down cut made in the lower, thinner part of the uterus

3. *High vertical (also called "classical")*—An up-and-down cut made in the upper part of the uterus

Women with high vertical incisions have a much higher risk of rupture. Women who have had more than one previous cesarean delivery also have an increased risk of rupture. Women who have had at least one vaginal delivery, in addition to the previous cesarean delivery, are more likely to succeed with VBAC.

Other Factors to Consider

Other factors may affect whether VBAC is an option. These include problems with the placenta, problems with the baby, or certain medical conditions during pregnancy.

For example, a woman can still try VBAC when her pregnancy is postterm (her pregnancy continues past the due date). But VBAC may not be a good option if the doctor decides that there is a need to induce labor (use drugs to help labor begin).

In some cases, VBAC may be an option for women carrying twins. VBAC is not performed in some hospitals because they are not equipped for emergency cesarean delivery. Talk to your doctor to find out what is best for you.

After Delivery

Once your baby's born, your doctor and nurse will monitor you both to make sure there are no problems. The health care team will care for the baby after vaginal delivery in the following ways:

➤ The baby will be held with his or her head down to keep fluids from getting into the lungs. The baby may be placed on your lower abdomen while these fluids drain.

Uterine Incisions

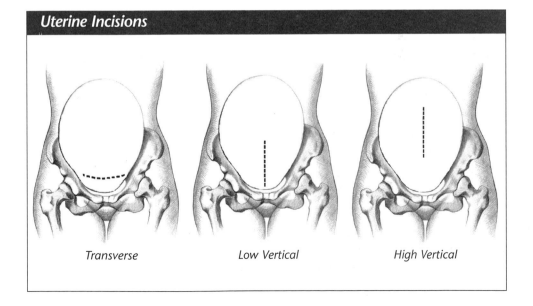

Transverse   Low Vertical   High Vertical

➤ The baby's mouth and nose are cleared of fluid with a small bulb syringe.

➤ The doctor will put a clamp on the umbilical cord close to the baby's abdomen. The cord then will be cut. If you wish to store or donate cord blood, it will be collected now (see box).

➤ In most cases, you will be given the baby to hold. This helps you bond with your baby. Close body contact also helps the baby maintain a good body temperature. If you are going to nurse, put your baby to your breast. (Chapter 10 will cover breastfeeding in more detail.)

➤ One minute after delivery, the baby's *Apgar score* will be checked (see Chapter 11 for Apgar scoring). This is used to assess a newborn's health and to see if extra care is needed. The test is done again 5 minutes after delivery.

➤ When you are ready to part with your new baby, the nurse will weigh and measure the baby, give him or her a bath, slip identification bands around the baby's ankle and wrist, and perhaps take handprints and footprints.

➤ Within a few hours of birth, the baby will have a head-to-toe exam and a few standard procedures to assess the newborn's health.

Banking Cord Blood

The blood in a baby's umbilical cord contains stem cells. These cells can be transplanted into persons with matching genes to treat diseases such as leukemia and other forms of cancer. The cord blood is collected after your baby is born and the umbilical cord has been clamped.

There are two types of cord blood banks: private and public. When cord blood is donated to a public bank, it is listed in a registry for patients all over the world who are searching for a match. The identity of the donor is not disclosed. There is no cost for donating cord blood to a public cord blood bank.

When cord blood is stored at a private bank, it is for the future use of your family only. Private cord blood banks will store blood for a yearly fee. It is highly unlikely your child will ever need stem cells (1 in 1,000 and 1 in 200,000 by age 18), and there is a significant cost involved in storing the blood. You may want to consider cord blood banking if there is a family member with a current or potential need to have stem cells transplanted.

Use of cord blood in stem cell transplants is a new area in medicine. There are many unknowns and some concerns. Ask your doctor if you have questions.

You also will be watched to make sure there are no problems. If you had a vaginal delivery, these steps will be taken:

➤ The doctor will examine your vagina, cervix, and perineum to make sure that it all looks normal.

➤ If you had an episiotomy or a tear, it will be repaired with stitches. These stitches will dissolve on their own and do not need to be removed.

➤ A nurse will take your blood pressure, pulse, and temperature often and massage your uterus. The nurse also will check for heavy vaginal bleeding or signs of infection.

If you had a cesarean delivery, you will be taken to a recovery room or straight to your hospital room. There, nurses will do the following:

➤ Give you medicine to relieve pain or nausea (the anesthetic used for surgery may leave you feeling sick to your stomach)

➤ Check your incision, blood pressure, pulse, breathing, and temperature

➤ Bring your baby to you to hold and nurse.

➤ Take your IV out when you are ready to eat and drink again

➤ If you don't feel up to being with your newborn right away, you can wait a while. Let your doctor or nurse know if you have discomfort.

Your Hospital Stay

Hospitals vary in how mothers and their babies are cared for after delivery. If you had a vaginal delivery, you should move around—with the nurse's help—as soon as you can.

Your baby may "room-in" with you until you go home. This is a good way to get to know your new baby. It's also the best way to get started breastfeeding. Otherwise, the baby can be brought to your room for feedings. Many hospitals allow your partner to stay with you, too.

If you feel unsure about newborn care (and many new parents do), now is the perfect time to get tips and advice from the hospital staff. Ask your nurse to help you with breastfeeding, teach you the best ways to hold and soothe your baby, or show you how to diaper your newborn—whatever advice you need. Maternity nurses are experts at infant care. This is a good chance to learn from them.

Before you gave birth, you may have pictured yourself cradling a plump, rosy-cheeked infant. The way your newborn really looks can come as quite a surprise—the baby's body is scrunched up, the head is long and pointy, the genitals appear too large for such a small body, and the skin is covered with a greasy whitish coat, called vernix, and also may bear traces of blood and other materials. Most of the time, nothing is wrong. If something about the way your

Recovering From a Cesarean Delivery

If you had a cesarean delivery, it may take a while for you to feel like yourself again. You are not just recovering from labor and delivery. You also are recovering from major surgery.

On top of all the normal postpartum aches and pains (see Chapter 12), you'll have a few more symptoms that need care. Here's what to expect after a cesarean birth:

➤You may be very tired. Why? You lost blood during surgery. This can sap your energy for a few days or weeks. You may be even more tired if you went through hours of labor before the surgery began.

➤You have to stay in bed for at least several hours after the surgery. When you are ready to get out of bed, you'll need help.

➤The incision in your abdomen will be very sore for the first few days or even weeks. Your doctor can give you medication to ease the pain. (It is safe to use over-the-counter pain relievers, even if you are breastfeeding. As always, use these medications as directed.) You may need to nurse your baby while lying on your side. You have to avoid heavy lifting and driving for a few weeks, too. This keeps excess pressure off the incision while it heals.

➤You may have painful gas and constipation. Anesthesia and surgery slow digestion. This causes your bowels to get bloated from trapped food gases. Walking should get things moving again.

➤You may stay in the hospital for 3–4 days after a cesarean birth. Even after you check out, you will have to take it easy for a while. You will need extra help at home for a few weeks. Ask someone to bring the baby to you for feedings and to help change the baby's diaper. Also ask friends and relatives to help with cooking, cleaning, errands, or older children.

➤You should be on the lookout for fever or incision pain that gets worse. Both can signal an infection.

Bonding With Your Baby

For many women, love doesn't come at first sight. A baby may be whisked away shortly after birth to get special medical care. A woman may be tired from hours of labor, fuzzy from pain medication, or coping with the effects of a cesarean birth. Lots of new moms are simply too overwhelmed by the responsibility that's just been thrust into their arms to feel much emotion at all. This is normal, and it doesn't mean you won't form a loving bond with your baby.

If you feel up to it, take time after birth to hold your newborn. Don't feel guilty if your first

Jane Levine

moments or even days with your baby aren't as close as you thought they would be.

Bonding takes months not minutes. Give yourself time to warm up to your baby. Your connection may take a little while, but it'll be strong enough to last a lifetime.

baby looks or acts worries you, though, be sure to ask about it. The doctors and nurses at the hospital can answer your questions and set your mind at ease.

A federal law called the Newborn's and Mother's Health Protection Act required managed care plans and health insurers that offer hospital childbirth coverage to pay for at least 48 hours in the hospital after a vaginal delivery and at least 96 hours after a cesarean birth. The 48- or 96-hour period applies independently to women and their newborn children. A mother's length-of-stay may not be the same as her child's. The length of time the mother and infant need to stay in the hospital is deter-

mined by the doctor in consultation with the mother. Some women may need to stay longer if problems come up during labor or after delivery.

If you are discharged early, your insurance may pay for follow-up home care. Many insurance plans pay for a nurse to visit you at home a day or two after your hospital discharge.

Visits From Older Children

If you have other children, they'll be eager to meet their new brother or sister. They can visit you and the baby in the hospital. The more involved siblings feel, the better they'll respond to the new baby.

Are You Ready To Go Home?

You should be able to answer yes to these questions before checking out:

____   Do you know how to hold, bathe, diaper, and dress your baby?

____   Do you know the best ways to put your baby down to sleep?

____   Do you know how to care for the baby's umbilical stump?

____   If your son was circumcised, do you know how to care for his penis?

____   If you are breastfeeding, has your baby latched on and nursed well at least twice?

____   Do you know how to tell if your baby is getting enough milk?

____   Do you know how to get in touch with a lactation consultant (breast-feeding expert) if you run into nursing problems?

____   If you are bottle-feeding, has your baby taken at least two bottles?

____   Has your baby urinated and passed stool?

____   If you are checking out within 48 hours of giving birth, have you arranged for a follow-up home visit to take place within the next couple of days?

____   Has your baby had all of his or her newborn tests, procedures, and vaccines?

____   Do you know how to spot signs of common problems, such as jaundice?

____   Do you know the warning signs that should prompt a call to your baby's doctor?

____   Have you scheduled your newborn's first visit to the pediatrician within a few weeks of birth?

(continued)

Are You Ready To Go Home? (continued)

_____ Have you filled out the paperwork for your baby's birth certificate and Social Security card?

_____ Do you have a rear-facing infant safety seat correctly installed in the back seat of your car?

_____ Do you know how to care for yourself (such as keeping stitches clean and managing pain)?

_____ Is your blood pressure normal?

_____ Have you urinated?

_____ Can you walk without help?

_____ Can you eat and drink without trouble?

_____ Do you know the warning signs that should prompt a call to your doctor?

_____ Have you asked your doctor when it's safe to resume sex?

_____ Have you picked a birth control method? (See Chapter 12 for details on postpartum birth control.)

Jane Levine

_____ Have you scheduled your postpartum visit (often 4–6 weeks after delivery)?

_____ Do you have help (from your partner, family, friends, a postpartum doula, or a baby nurse) lined up for your first few days at home?

Home Care

A home nurse can provide the following care:

➤ Give you and your baby a thorough exam to make sure you are both doing well

➤ Find out how you are recovering from delivery and check you for signs of infection

➤ Look your baby over for conditions such as newborn jaundice. This often doesn't show up until a few days after birth

➤ Make sure your milk has come in if you are breastfeeding and that your baby is latching on and nursing is going well

➤ Find out how you are doing with the basics of newborn care and ask how you and your baby are settling in

If a home visit is an option for you, don't pass it up even if all seems to be going fine.

Before an older child's visit, be sure to check the hospital's policies and hours for visitors. Make sure the child is prepared for the visit in the following ways:

➤ The child hasn't been exposed to any known viruses, such as chicken-pox.

➤ The child is healthy. If your child has a fever, a cough, or other symptoms, wait until he or she is feeling better before meeting the new baby.

➤ A partner or a family member has talked to the child about the visit and told him or her how to behave and what to expect.

➤ An adult is there to keep an eye on the child during the visit.

Visits From Friends

Greeting visitors can be tiring. Having your children and other close relatives drop by is fine. You may want to hold off on other visits so you have more time to rest and get to know your baby.

There will be plenty of time for people to wish you well and to see the new baby after you are settled in at home. It may be best to suggest that well wishers visit you at home after a few weeks.

Going Home

The idea of leaving the hospital after your baby's birth may make you a little nervous. Let the hospital staff know you really don't feel ready to go home or if you are worried about your baby. You can (and should) call your doctor, the hospital nursery, or your baby's doctor with any questions that arise. Before heading home, you should be prepared to care for yourself and your baby.

If Your Baby Needs To Stay in the Hospital

If your baby has health problems, he or she may need to stay in the hospital after you go home. It may be hard to leave your newborn behind. Keep in mind that this is the best place for your baby to be cared for until his or her health improves.

In most cases, you'll be able to spend much of each day in the hospital nursery. If you are breastfeeding, the nurses there can set you up with a breast pump and teach you how to express milk for your baby when you go home.

Some hospitals may allow you to remain with your newborn around the clock after you have been discharged. If your baby needs to stay in the hospital for a while, find out what you can do to spend time with him or her.

Your New Family

The birth of your baby may be the most exciting time of your pregnancy. It also may be the most challenging part of your pregnancy. Know that support is there for you—the hospital staff, your doctor, your baby's doctor, friends, and family—if you need it. As soon as you see your new baby you will know that all your work and effort was worth it.

CHAPTER 10

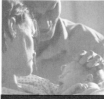

Breastfeeding

Breastfeeding is the best way to feed your new baby. It protects against many illnesses. It also creates a bond between mother and baby and provides the best nutrition for your infant. One of the most special times in a mother's life is when she is breastfeeding her baby.

To help you decide how to feed your baby, talk to your doctor, your baby's doctor, your partner, family members, and friends who have breastfed their babies. You also may find it helpful to talk with a *lactation specialist*. They can tell you more about methods of breastfeeding and how to pump your breast milk. You can find one of these breastfeeding experts through your doctor or hospital. Also, find out if your local hospital or parents' resource center offers breastfeeding classes for mothers-to-be.

How you feed your newborn is a personal choice. However, even if you are not sure breastfeeding (also called nursing) is right for you, think about giving it a try. You can switch to formula later, if necessary. Bottle-fed babies can be well nourished, and a combination of bottle feeding and breastfeeding works for some mothers. However, many women who aren't sure about breastfeeding find that, once the baby arrives, they love the sense of closeness it gives them.

Benefits

Breast milk is nature's perfect baby food. Your milk has just the right nutrients, in just the right amounts, to nourish your baby completely. The protein and fat in breast milk are better used by the baby's body than the protein and fat in formula.

Breast milk has hormones, proteins, and other things that help a baby grow and develop the way he or she should. As the baby grows, breast milk changes to supply the baby's needs at that stage of life. Breast milk has antibodies that help your baby's *immune system* fight off sickness. Breastfed children are less likely to have the following:

➤ Ear infections

➤ Allergies

➤ Diarrhea

➤ Pneumonia, wheezing, and respiratory infections

➤ Meningitis

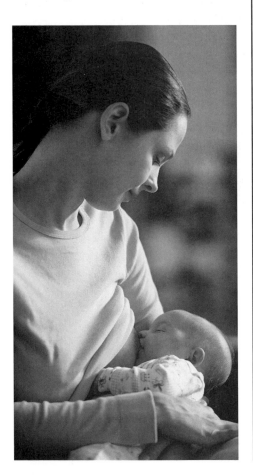

Breast milk is easier than formula for babies to digest. Infants who are breastfed have less gas, fewer feeding problems, and often less constipation than those given formula. Some studies show that breastfeeding may reduce the chance of sudden infant death syndrome (SIDS) and diabetes. Breastfeeding also may help your baby's brain develop.

Breastfeeding isn't just good for babies—it's also good for women. Breastfeeding provides the following benefits:

➤ Breastfeeding releases the hormone oxytocin, which makes the uterus contract. This helps the uterus return to its normal size more quickly and cuts down on bleeding after delivery.

➤ Nursing burns calories. You are likely to return to your pre-pregnancy weight faster than you would if you were bottle feeding.

➤ Breastfeeding has been associated with a decreased risk of ovarian cancer and breast cancer.

➤ Breastfeeding is easier and cheaper than bottle feeding. You don't need to go to the grocery store to pick up formula or to stock up on bottles and nipples. You also don't have to heat a bottle when your baby is hungry or keep bottles cool when you go out for the day.

➤ Nursing helps you bond with your baby. When you nurse, you hold your baby close to you and have skin

Your Support System

The support of your partner is important to your breastfeeding success. To help promote this support, talk to your partner about why you want to breastfeed. Explain that it is good for the baby's health.

Also, ask your partner to come with you to a prenatal breastfeeding class. The more he or she knows about the benefits (and challenges) of nursing, the more likely he or she is to support you in your efforts.

What if your partner agrees, but some of your friends or family members don't agree with your choice to breastfeed? Simply tell them that your doctor says it's best for the baby.

If you are going to succeed at breastfeeding, you need to feel that you have support. If your loved ones don't offer this support, find it elsewhere. Ask your doctor for suggestions. Join a new mothers' group that has lots of nursing moms. Seek out a local La Leche League chapter or other breastfeeding support group.

contact. You also learn to pick up and respond to his or her signals. Both of these things help strengthen the bond between you.

Facts About Breastfeeding

After delivery, your breasts at first produce colostrum, a thin, yellowish fluid. This is the same fluid that leaks from some women's breasts during pregnancy. The colostrum that your breasts make for the first few days after birth helps your newborn's digestive system grow and function. It is rich in protein and is all your baby needs for the first few days of life. It is especially high in ingredients that help make your baby immune to diseases.

Within 3 or 4 days your body sends a signal to your breasts to start making milk. At first this milk is thin, watery, and sweet. This quenches the baby's thirst and provides sugar, proteins, minerals, and the fluid the baby needs. Over time, the milk changes. It becomes thick and creamy. This milk will satisfy hunger and give your baby the nutrients he or she needs to grow.

When your baby is breastfeeding, the nerves in your nipples send a message to your brain. In response, your brain releases hormones that tell the ducts in your breasts to "let down" their milk so that it flows through your nipples. This

Common Questions About Breastfeeding

Pregnant women often have lots of questions about nursing. Here are answers to a few of the questions asked most often. If you have a question that isn't addressed here, be sure to ask your doctor or a lactation specialist.

Are my breasts too small for breastfeeding?
It may seem logical that well-endowed women would make more milk than their less well-endowed peers. However, breast size doesn't matter. The amount of milk your breasts make has to do with your health and how well your breasts are stimulated. It has nothing to do with their size or shape.

Will nursing make my breasts sag?
Breastfeeding alone won't cause your breasts to sag. Aging is mostly to blame for that. Your breasts will get heavier during pregnancy and nursing as they enlarge and make milk. This extra weight can stretch the ligaments that support them. Wearing a good support bra will help.

How do I get ready to nurse my baby?
You don't need to do anything to prepare. If you are concerned about your nipples or breasts, discuss it with your doctor or a lactation consultant.

Will I be able to make enough milk?
In most cases, making enough milk to nourish your baby is a simple matter of supply and demand. In other words, your body supplies as much as your baby demands. Nurse as often as your baby needs to and for as long as the baby wants. Your body will respond by making just the right amount of milk. You also can prevent a milk shortage by getting enough to drink each day, eating well, and getting plenty of rest. Using formula to make up for a shortfall may cause you not to make as much milk. That's because skipping feedings tells your body to cut down on milk production.

What if I couldn't breastfeed last time?
If you have given birth before and had trouble breastfeeding, that doesn't mean you can't nurse now. Whatever caused the problem last time most likely won't happen again. Even if it does, getting expert help early on will boost your chance of nursing success. To help prevent problems, talk with your doctor, childbirth educator, a lactation specialist, and other nursing mothers about what happened before. Sometimes a change in technique is all it takes to solve the problem.

is called the **let-down reflex**. Some women barely notice let-down. Others have a pins-and-needles feeling in their breasts 2–3 minutes after their babies start nursing.

Sometimes, let-down is slowed if you are in pain or feeling anxious or stressed. Other times, it is triggered simply by looking at your baby, thinking about your baby, or hearing your baby cry. For some women, hearing any baby cry will trigger the let-down reflex. When your milk lets down, your breasts will feel full, and you will want to breastfeed very soon. (See "Engorgement" for details on what you can do if your breasts are so full you have trouble nursing or if they remain full and tender.)

Many nursing mothers learn how to express breast milk by hand. This is a good skill for any breastfeeding mom to have. Still, most women find it easier to use a breast pump to empty their breasts for storing milk. This is even more true for working mothers who need to express milk several times a day.

There are dozens of breast pumps on the market, with many features to choose from. How do you know which one to pick? That depends on your needs. If you plan to stay home with your baby until he or she is weaned, a simple manual pump may be fine. If you are going back to work full time soon after your baby is born, an electric pump likely is the best choice.

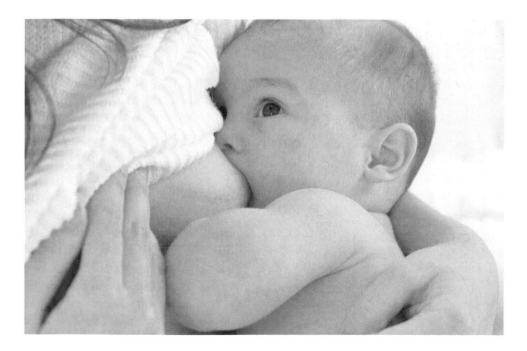

Choosing a Breast Pump

Talk to your doctor or a lactation specialist before you rent or buy a pump. Some pointers:

➤ If you plan to pump only for a short time, you may want to rent. You can rent a high-quality breast pump from a medical supply store or hospital for as little as $1 per day. Some programs also loan out breast pumps. If you rent, you'll need to buy a kit with tubing for the pump, cups that fit over your breasts, and collection bottles.

➤ If you think you'll pump for more than a few months, buying a breast pump is a good idea. Compare rental costs to purchase price before you decide.

➤ If the cost of renting or buying a pump seems high, just think about all the money you'll save by not having to buy formula or not having to buy as much. You'll also help maintain your baby's health.

➤ Pick a pump that has two tubes and kits. This cuts your pumping time in half by letting you empty both breasts at once.

➤ You may want to choose a pump with automatic cycling. This closely mimics a baby's natural sucking rhythm as it draws milk out of your breasts. It also means you don't have to keep pushing a button or roll your finger over a hole, as semiautomatic pumps require you to do.

➤ Look for quick cycling times. The more often a pump cycles (or sucks), the less time it takes to empty your breasts and the more milk you'll get. Cycling times range from about 12–60 cycles per minute.

➤ Choose a pump that lets you adjust the suction level. Otherwise, you may find the suction so strong that it hurts your breasts or so weak that you can't get much milk out.

➤ Look for a lightweight, portable model if you are going to be on the road for work or if you need to bring your pump home with you each night.

➤ If you want a manual pump to use at home, avoid the kind with a rubber bulb at one end. Your milk can flow back into the bulb. This type of pump is hard to clean and can harbor bacteria.

Breastfeeding Know-How

Breastfeeding is the natural way to nourish a newborn. Still, not all mothers and babies get the hang of it right away. It takes learning, practice, and patience for both of you to master this skill. Some pointers will give you a good start.

Be Prepared

Take a breastfeeding class before your baby is born. These classes are offered at many hospitals and parents' centers. A breastfeeding class will teach you what you need to know to get started. It also will help you avoid some common problems.

Talk With Your Doctor

During your pregnancy, tell your doctor that you plan to breastfeed your baby. He or she can give you advice and answer any questions you may have. When you get to the hospital, remind the doctor and nurses that you want to breastfeed. They can help you get started right after delivery.

Nurse Right After Your Baby Is Born

Someone in the delivery room can help you find a good position and put your baby to your breast. This is a great way to greet your new baby. This also is the time that your newborn is most alert and ready to suck. Later, your baby may be too sleepy to nurse well.

If you are positioned right when you breastfeed, you'll be able to hold the baby for some time without feeling cramped or stiff. Also, the baby will be able to get a good grasp on your breast. No matter which position you use, make sure the baby's whole body (not just his or her face) is turned toward you. To avoid back and neck strain, use pillows or folded blankets to place the baby at the level of your breast. Tuck pillows behind your back, under your arms, and on your lap (if you are sitting up) for extra support. You may want to prop your feet on a stool to raise your knees so your baby is closer to your breast.

Get the Baby Latched On

A baby is born with the instincts he or she needs to nurse. For instance, the rooting reflex is a baby's natural instinct to turn toward the nipple, open his or her mouth, and suck. When you and your baby are ready to begin nursing, cup your breast in your hand and stroke your baby's lower lip with your nipple. The baby will open his or her mouth wide (like a yawn). Quickly center your nipple in the baby's mouth, making sure the tongue is down, and pull him or her close to you. You need to bring your baby to your breast—not your breast to your baby.

Good Breastfeeding Positions

Finding a good position will help the baby latch on. It also will help you relax and be comfortable. Use pillows or folded blankets to help support the baby.

Cradle hold. Sit up as straight as you can and cradle your baby in the crook of your arm. The baby's body should be turned toward you and his or her belly should be against yours. Support the baby's head in the bend of your elbow so that he or she is facing your breast.

Cross-cradle hold. As in the cradle hold, nuzzle your baby's belly against yours. Hold the baby in the arm opposite the one you are using to nurse. For instance, if the baby is nursing from your right breast, hold him or her with your left arm. Place the baby's bottom in the crook of your left arm and support the baby's head and neck with your left hand. This position gives you more control of the baby's head. It's a good position for a newborn who is having trouble nursing.

Football hold. Tuck your baby under your arm like a football. Hold the baby at your side, level with your waist, so he or she is facing you. Support the baby's back with your upper arm and hold his or her head level with your breast. The football hold is good for nursing twins. It's also good if you had a cesarean birth because the baby doesn't lie on your abdomen.

Side-lying position. Lie on your side and nestle your baby next to you. Place your fingers beneath your breast and lift it up to help your baby reach your nipple. This position is good for night feedings. It's also good for women who had a cesarean birth because it keeps the baby's weight off the incision. Rest your head on your lower arm. You may want to tuck a pillow behind your back to help hold yourself up.

Check the Baby's Technique

If the baby is latched on right, he or she will have all of your nipple and a good deal of the areola (the dark area around the nipple) in his or her mouth. The baby's nose will be touching your breast. The baby's lips also will be curled out around your breast. The baby's sucking should be smooth and even. You should hear him or her swallow. You may feel a slight tugging. You may feel a little discomfort for the first few days. You shouldn't feel any severe pain, though.

Keep Trying

Start again if any of these things occur:

➤ The baby's mouth grasps only your nipple.

➤ The baby's lips are curled under.

➤ You hear clicking sounds as he or she sucks.

➤ Nursing hurts.

A newborn who doesn't latch on well won't get a good meal. To break the suction, gently insert one of your fingers (make sure it is clean) between your breast and your baby's gums. When you hear a soft pop, carefully pull your nipple out of his or her mouth. Try nursing again and keep trying until your baby is latched on well.

Don't Watch the Clock

Experts used to think that newborns should nurse for just a few minutes at each breast. They now know that this may make babies stop eating before they are full. Cutting back on nursing time also keeps your breasts from making enough milk. Let your baby set his or her own nursing pattern. Many newborns nurse for 10–20 minutes on each breast. (A baby who wants to nurse for a very long time—say, 30 minutes on each side—may be having trouble getting enough milk. If this happens each time you breastfeed, tell your doctor.) When your baby is full, he or she will let go of your breast. If not, gently break the suction.

Switch Sides

When your baby empties one breast, offer the other. Don't worry if he or she doesn't latch onto it. You don't have to nurse at both breasts in one feeding. You may want to put a safety pin on your bra strap to mark the side your baby nursed from last. At the next feeding, offer the other breast first.

Nurse On Demand

When your baby's hungry, he or she will nuzzle against your breast, make sucking motions, or put hands to mouth. Crying is a late sign of hunger. (Rooming in with your baby at the hospital will help you pick up on these cues.) Follow your baby's signals—not the clock. Using a schedule for feeding times will deprive your baby of nourishment and tell your body to make less milk. During the first few weeks, your baby should be fed at least 8–12 times in 24 hours (every 2–3 hours). Some newborns are happy to go 3 hours between feedings. Others need to nurse once an hour for the first few weeks. Over time, you and your baby will set your own schedule.

Do Not Supplement

The colostrum your breasts make for the first few days after birth is all your baby needs at that time. Your newborn has extra stores of fat and body fluids to draw on until your milk comes in. Even if you plan to combine breast milk and formula when your baby is older, breast-feed without supplements for at least the first 6 weeks of your baby's life if you can. This will help you make enough milk. It also will help your baby get used to sucking your breast. Sucking from a bottle isn't the same as sucking from a breast. If a baby gets used to bottle nipples, he or she may forget how to draw milk out of your nipples. For the same reason, it may be best not to give your baby a pacifier until he or she is used to nursing.

When your breastfeeding baby is about 2 months old, he or she should begin taking a vitamin D supplement. When your baby is about 6 months old, you should gradually start adding iron-enriched solid foods to the breast milk diet. Some babies may need to take an iron supplement before then. A baby should not drink cow's milk until he or she is older than 12 months. Talk to your baby's doctor about what is best for you and your baby.

Special Challenges

Most women can breastfeed, given support and guidance. You may wonder if a certain health condition, past surgery, or your type of breasts will keep you from nursing. Talk with your doctor about your questions.

Chronic Illness

In most cases, you can nurse if you have a chronic illness (for exceptions, see "When Women Should Not Breast-feed"). Sometimes it's not the illness itself that's cause for concern. Rather, it's the medications a woman takes to control a health problem.

Certain prescription and over-the-counter medications can pass through breast milk and harm the baby. In such cases, your doctor may advise you to switch to another medicine, take the medication just after breastfeeding, or lower your dose until your baby is no longer breastfeeding. Most of the time, medications are not harmful.

There are some drugs that you should not take while nursing. Prescription drugs that can pass into breast milk and harm a baby include ergotamine (used to treat migraine headaches), lithium (used to treat mental illness), some drugs used to treat high blood pressure, and chemotherapy drugs (used to treat cancer). Be sure any doctor treating you knows that you are breastfeeding. If you have a chronic illness or take medication for an ongoing health condition, before your baby is

How Can I Get Help?

If you and your baby are having trouble nursing, don't give up—get some help. Ask the nurses at the hospital to assist you with nursing positions or getting the baby latched onto your breast. Let your doctor know if you are worried the baby isn't getting enough to eat. Also seek help if nursing hurts. Breastfeeding may be a little uncomfortable at first, but it should never hurt.

Find out if the hospital or your pediatrician's office employs a licensed, certified lactation specialist. These breastfeeding experts offer telephone advice or hands-on help for a small fee (some health insurance companies will cover this cost).

Even if nursing seems to be going fine, don't leave the hospital without getting a phone number to call for breastfeeding help. If you forget, these are organizations that will help you:

➤ The International Lactation Consultant Association at 919-787-5181 or www.ilca.org. This group can direct you to certified lactation specialists in your area.

➤ La Leche League International at 800-525-3243 or www.lalecheleague.org. This support network for breastfeeding mothers can help with questions and concerns. Local chapter leaders offer free phone advice and run support groups for nursing moms.

➤ Women, Infants, and Children (WIC) federal program at 703-305-2746 or 2286 or www.fns.usda.gov/wic. WIC helps low-income, nutritionally at-risk pregnant and breastfeeding women through pregnancy and up to 1 year after birth. One in four new mothers participates in WIC.

born talk to your doctor about breastfeeding. Also, if you need to be treated for an illness or health condition after giving birth, be sure to tell the doctor that you are breastfeeding.

Cesarean Delivery

If you have had a cesarean birth, you will still be able to breastfeed. You may have certain challenges, though. Sometimes after a cesarean delivery there may be a delay before breastfeeding

starts. The mother may be groggy or in pain, for instance. Be sure the nurses at the hospital know you want to breastfeed as soon as possible.

After a cesarean birth, certain breastfeeding positions may be more comfortable than others. These are some positions that you can try:

➤ Sit up with the baby resting on a pillow or two. This will help protect your incision.

➤ Lie on your side with your baby facing you.

➤ Use a "football hold" (see box).

Being comfortable will help you relax. This helps you succeed at breastfeeding.

Breast Surgery

Surgery to remove cysts and other benign breast lumps rarely causes problems with future breastfeeding. If you have had surgery on your breasts, talk to your ob-gyn or surgeon before your delivery date to help plan for breastfeeding.

Many women who have had their breasts enlarged are able to nurse their babies. But some women with **breast implants** may have problems if the implants rupture. A rupture may cause scarring that affects milk production and release. If you are worried about your breast implants, talk to your doctor.

Likewise, women who have had surgery to reduce the size of their breasts may have breastfeeding problems. This is because breast-reduction surgery can cut into milk ducts and prevent a nursing mother from making enough milk. If you have had this surgery, talk with your doctor to be sure your nipples, the areolas, and the ducts were left intact.

Inverted or Flat Nipples

It is very common for a woman to have one or both nipples that do not protrude fully. In most cases, women with flat or inverted nipples can breastfeed.

During the first feedings after birth is the time when inverted or flat nipples are most likely to present problems. This is because it may be hard for the baby to latch on at first. Ask for help from your doctor or a lactation expert. You may be advised to use a breast pump just before breastfeeding or to stimulate the nipple in other ways. Breastfeeding will be easier as the baby grows bigger and stronger.

Preterm Babies

A baby born early will benefit from your breast milk. It is higher in protein and other nutrients that a preterm baby needs than the milk made when the baby is born at full term. If your baby is born preterm, make sure your doctor knows that you want to breastfeed. The nurses or a lactation expert at the hospital will help work out the feedings for your baby.

A preterm baby may not be able to leave the neonatal nursery. Even if your baby is able to be with you, he or she may be too small to learn to latch on to your breast. In either case, you should use a breast pump as soon after the birth as you are able. Use a high-quality double pump. Pumping both breasts at once will save you time. Many hospitals have these pumps for you to use. If not, ask your doctor to help you get one.

You will need to use the pump every 2–3 hours. This will mimic your baby's feeding needs and bring in a good milk supply.

Multiple Births

If you have more than one baby, you can still breastfeed. Breastfeeding works by supply and demand. The more your babies breastfeed, the more milk your body will make. Using formula as a supplement may not be necessary for twins or even triplets. Usually, supplemental feeding is needed with four or more, though.

It may seem hard to breastfeed more than one baby, but bottle feeding them also would be hard. Many mothers of multiple babies say it is much easier to breastfeed because you don't have to fix double batches of bottles every day.

Breastfeeding both babies at once can give you more time to rest between feedings. One position to try is to let their legs overlap in front of you, across your lap. Another is the football hold. Be sure the babies' entire bodies are facing you.

Some multiple births also are preterm. (See "Premature Babies" for more information about breastfeeding in this case.)

When Women Should Not Breastfeed

As good as breastfeeding is, it is not for every woman. There are some situations in which a woman should not breastfeed her baby.

Infections

If you have certain infections, they can be passed to your baby through breast milk. You should not breastfeed if you have human immunodeficiency virus (HIV) or active tuberculosis (TB). If TB is treated and is no longer contagious, the baby can be breastfed. If you have the hepatitis B virus infection, your baby should be immunized within the first few hours after birth. (Chapter 17 has details on the infections that can be passed to your baby.)

Smoking and Substance Abuse

Mothers who use illegal drugs, abuse alcohol, or smoke should not breastfeed. Drug use and heavy drinking (more than two drinks per day on a regular basis) may be harmful both to you and your baby. These substances can be passed to the baby through breast milk.

If you smoke regularly, breastfeeding may harm your baby. Even cigarette smoke from other people can be harmful to a baby. For your own health and that of your baby, ask your doctor for help with quitting smoking and ask people not to smoke around your baby.

Is Your Baby Getting Enough Milk?

When an infant is fed formula, it's simple to figure out how much he or she is drinking. All you have to do is add up those empty bottles. Not so with breast-feeding. There are other ways to tell if your baby is well nourished:

➤ Your baby nurses often. A newborn should nurse at least 8–12 times in 24 hours. The bigger your baby is, the more his or her stomach will hold and the less often he or she will need to eat. Even so, a newborn shouldn't go more than 3 hours without nursing (even at night). Each nursing session should last 20–45 minutes.

➤ Your baby is full after nursing. A baby who's just had a good meal will be drowsy and content.

➤ Your breasts fill and empty. Your breasts should feel full and firm before feedings. After, they should be less full and feel softer.

➤ The baby goes through lots of diapers. After your milk comes in, your baby should soak at least six diapers per day. His or her urine should be nearly clear. During the first month, your baby should have at least three bowel movements per day. (In fact, most breastfed newborns pass a stool after each feeding.) The stool should be soft and yellow.

➤ Your baby is gaining weight. Most newborns lose a little weight at first. After 2 weeks, your baby should be

Warning Signs

Call the doctor right away if your baby:

➤ Has trouble latching on or staying latched on

➤ Cries when you offer your breast or cries after 1–2 minutes of nursing

➤ Refuses the breast

➤ Often falls asleep after only a few minutes of nursing or is often too sleepy to nurse

➤ Has fewer than six wet and three soiled diapers per day

➤ Has dark green stools or stools with mucus in them

➤ Has a sunken soft spot on the top of his or her head (this can be a sign of dehydration)

➤ Feeds less than six times every 24 hours in the first month of life

➤ Looks yellow (jaundice) below the navel and is groggy

back up to his or her weight at birth. The doctor will weigh your baby at each visit and let you know if he or she isn't gaining enough weight. If you are worried that your baby isn't getting enough milk, tell the doctor.

What To Wear

Unlike bottle feeding, breastfeeding requires little in the way of supplies. Still, buying a few good nursing bras is well worth it. You can find nursing bras, pads, and clothes in maternity shops, baby supply stores, and mail-order catalogs. You can save money by asking friends or relatives to lend you their nursing clothes or by shopping for used clothing at exchange or consignment shops.

Nursing bras have cups that open (with snaps, hook-and-eye closures, or peel-away hook-and-loop closures) for easy access at feeding time. Some cups open from the top. Others open from the side.

No matter which style you choose, you should be able to open the cups quickly and with one hand (the other hand will be holding your baby). Be sure to test this feature before you buy the bra.

Some nursing bras also have cups that can be made bigger or smaller. These bras allow you to adjust the size of the cup by closing it at a higher or lower point. Why? Your breasts will grow and shrink as they fill with milk

and your baby empties them. Your breasts also will be larger in the early weeks of nursing, and smaller once the breasts adjust to nursing. By 3 months of nursing, there may seem to be little change between feedings.

It's a good idea to pick up a nighttime nursing bra as well. These bras give breasts a little support while you sleep. The cups can be opened for feedings.

When you are choosing nursing bras, stock up on nursing pads, too. Many women find that their breasts leak between feedings. One nipple also may dribble a little milk while your baby nurses on the other side. Wearing pads inside your bra will soak up the excess.

You can wear just about anything to breastfeed—as long as you can lift it up or unbutton it. Clothes that are designed for nursing mothers will help you feed your baby quickly. Some of these clothes have openings that you can spread apart to get your baby latched on, and still cover your breast once your baby's nursing. Nursing clothes make many breastfeeding mothers feel even more comfortable feeding their babies in restaurants, at the mall, while traveling, or wherever they go.

A Healthy Diet

When you are pregnant, your body stores extra nutrients and fat to prepare

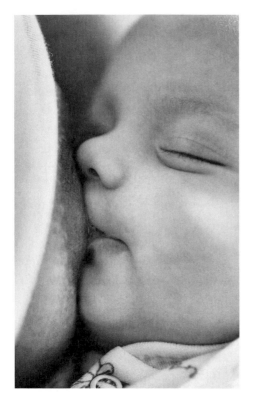

you for breastfeeding. Even so, once your baby is born you need more food and nutrients than normal to fuel milk production. Don't panic if your diet isn't always perfect. Your baby still can get the nutrients he or she needs. Do the following when you are nursing:

➤ Eat more. During breastfeeding you need about 200 calories per day more than you did during pregnancy. That's 500 more calories than you needed before you got pregnant. (A government program called the Special Supplemental Food Program for Women, Infants, and Children provides vouchers so that low-income nursing mothers can get the extra food they need).

➤ Eat a well-balanced diet. Eat a variety of healthy foods, as outlined in the Food Guide Pyramid (see Chapter 6). That means daily servings of fruits and vegetables, whole-grain breads and cereals, milk and milk products, and high-protein foods such as fish, beans, meat, and poultry.

➤ Get the right nutrients. Nursing moms need 1,000 mg of calcium per day, for instance. You can get that by eating plenty of dairy products like milk, yogurt, and cheese. If you can't digest milk products, ask your doctor about taking a calcium supplement. When you are nursing, you also need an extra serving of protein each day— four servings instead of the three you needed during pregnancy. Be sure to get folic acid each day, too. This will help you maintain good health and ensure that you have plenty of folic acid stores. Your doctor may suggest that you keep taking a daily prenatal vitamin until your baby is weaned. (Chapter 6 details nutritional needs during breastfeeding.)

➤ Skip foods that bother the baby. Some nursing infants are sensitive to certain foods in their mothers' diet. If your baby acts fussy or gets a rash, diarrhea, or congestion within a couple hours of nursing, let his or her doctor know. This can signal a food allergy. Cut out that food for a few days and see if your baby seems better. You also may want to keep a food diary. This will help you spot links between what you eat and how your baby reacts.

➤ Drink up. Breastfeeding uses up lots of fluid. That's why nursing mothers often are thirsty. You need at least eight glasses of liquid per day. If you get dehydrated, it can affect your milk supply. To prevent this, make sure you have a drink within easy reach each time you sit down to nurse. Do not force fluids, though. Drinking more will not increase your milk supply if you already drink enough for your body's normal use and to replenish fluid the baby drinks.

➤ Don't diet. Be patient about losing the weight you may have gained during pregnancy. If you eat a well-balanced diet, you'll be close to your normal weight within a few months. Start an exercise routine once your doctor gives you the go-ahead. This will keep your muscles toned.

Birth Control

Breastfeeding has pros and cons when it comes to your sex life. Round-the-clock nursing may reduce your desire for sex. However, some breastfeeding women notice an increase in desire. In some cases, you may have the desire, but prefer a hands-off policy to protect sore or leaking breasts.

Breastfeeding delays ovulation, which means your estrogen levels will stay low while you are breastfeeding. This may result in vaginal dryness that can make sex difficult. An over-the-counter lubricant will help with these problems. (See Chapter 12 for more tips.)

When you are breastfeeding, you are temporarily less likely to get pregnant. You may not ovulate or have your period for as long as you exclusively breastfeed. To become pregnant, ovulation (the release of an egg to be fertilized) must occur.

It's best not to rely on breastfeeding as birth control. Women's periods return at different times after delivery. Thus, it is hard to predict when you will begin to ovulate again. You could get pregnant before you even know you are fertile.

You should think about an additional method of birth control and discuss it with your doctor before your baby is born. Afterwards, review your plan. If your baby is about 6 months old, getting any food or drink other than breast milk, or if you do not nurse frequently during every 24-hour period, you could get pregnant even before you have a period.

If you are not ready for another baby right away, talk to your doctor about which method of birth control is good for you. What you were using before pregnancy might not be a good choice now. Combination birth control pills contain the hormone estrogen and *progestin*, a synthetic version of the hormone progesterone. Estrogen can cut down on your milk supply. As a result, combination pills should not be used until milk flow is steady. Until then, use progestin-only birth control methods, such as minipills or injections without estrogen, or barrier methods such as condoms or a diaphragm with spermicide. (Chapter 12 has more details on birth control after delivery.)

Work

Going back to work—whether it's a few weeks or many months after your baby is born—doesn't have to mean the end of breastfeeding. Many mothers keep nursing their babies after their maternity leave ends.

If you want to breastfeed when you go back to work, decide on your plan. Will you pump breast milk to leave for the feedings you miss? If you work close to home or childcare, would you be able to arrange breaks and lunch hours around your baby's feeding times? Ask your doctor, your lactation consultant, and other working women who have breastfed for tips and advice.

If you plan to express your milk while you are at work, practice with

Storing Breast Milk

Store breast milk in clean glass or plastic bottles or special milk collection bags. Store it in small amounts (2–4 ounces) to avoid wasting it. Mark the bottles or bags with the date the milk was pumped. If you are going to freeze it, leave a 1-inch space at the top of the container.

You can keep breast milk in the refrigerator (40°F or below) for up to 2 days. Do not store milk in the door of the refrigerator—the temperature can vary there. If you need to store milk longer than 2 days, you can keep it in a deep freeze (0°F or below) for up to 3 months.

If there is not a refrigerator to use at work, keep the milk you have just pumped in a small cooler with a few ice packs. Don't leave breast milk at room temperature for more than 8 hours—the enzymes will begin to digest the fat.

Never thaw frozen milk at room temperature. To thaw frozen milk, hold it under cool running water. Once it has begun to thaw, use warm running water to finish. You also can let frozen milk slowly thaw in the fridge. Once milk is thawed, use it within 24 hours. Never refreeze milk that has been thawed.

You can add freshly expressed milk to breast milk that was pumped before. Always cool the fresh milk first.

Warm chilled breast milk by placing it in a bowl of very warm water. Don't heat bottles on the stove or in the microwave. This destroys breast milk's disease-fighting qualities.

the pump a few weeks before your return. Pump any milk that's left in your breasts after a feeding. Give some of this milk to your baby in a bottle. This will help your baby get used to drinking your milk from something other than your breasts. (You may want to have someone else feed the baby with a bottle of your milk. Breastfed babies often do not want to take a bottle from their mothers.) Also, store a few bottles of milk in the freezer for later use.

If you plan to pump milk while you are at work, talk to your employer about your plans. Ask if there's a clean, private place for you to pump—such as a mother's lounge, an empty office, or a meeting room that's rarely used. Feeding your baby breast milk may even cut down on future absences from work. That's because breastfed babies have fewer illnesses than those who are given formula. That means you'll need less time off to care for a sick baby or to take him or her to the doctor.

Express your milk at least twice a day. It may take a while to get used to your new routine. Give yourself time. Once you get it down and fit pumping into your workday, it will become easier.

Breast Health

As they start to breastfeed, some women may have a few minor problems. Most often, though, they are easy to treat.

However, if you notice a lump in your breast that lasts for more than a few days, your doctor should check it. It could be a problem that is not related to breastfeeding.

Engorgement

Engorgement may occur when your milk comes in a few days after delivery. Engorged breasts feel full and tender. You may even run a low fever. If the fever exceeds 101°F or if you are in severe pain, call your doctor. If your breasts are very engorged, it can be hard for your baby to latch on.

Once your body figures out just how much milk your baby needs, the problem should go away. This often takes a week or so. In the meantime, you can do the following:

➤ Increase feedings. This will help drain your breasts.

➤ Express a little milk with a pump or by hand to soften your breasts before nursing.

➤ Before feedings, massage your breasts, take hot showers, or apply hot packs to your breasts. This will help your milk flow.

➤ After feedings, apply cold packs to your breasts to relieve discomfort and reduce swelling.

Sore Nipples

It's normal for your nipples to feel a little tender during the first few days of nursing. However, if breastfeeding is painful or your nipples are cracked or bleeding, get expert help. Try the following tips to relieve soreness and prevent it from getting worse:

➤ Make sure your baby has your entire nipple and a good portion of your areola in his or her mouth.

➤ Check that the baby's lips are curled out around your breast and that his or her tongue is beneath your nipple.

➤ Before you remove your breast from your baby's mouth, use your finger to break the suction.

➤ Change positions at each feeding so the baby's mouth doesn't always put pressure on the same part of your nipple.

➤ Gently pat your nipples dry with a clean cloth after feedings. You may also want to expose them to air and dry heat (such as a hairdryer on low or sunlight streaming through a window).

➤ Use only cotton bra pads, and change them as soon as they get wet.

➤ Don't wash your nipples with harsh soaps or use perfumed creams.

➤ Check for thrush. This is a yeast infection in your baby's mouth that can spread to your breasts. Suspect thrush if your baby has diaper rash and white patches in his or her mouth. Other signs of thrush include a cracked, itchy, red, and burning nipple or shooting pains in your breasts during or after nursing. In this case, call your doctor.

➤ Nurse often. Your baby sucks harder if you wait until he or she is really hungry. This can make sore nipples hurt even more.

➤ If one nipple is tender, offer the other breast first. Save your sore side for when your baby is less hungry.

Blocked Ducts

If a duct gets clogged with unused milk, a hard, tender knot will form in your

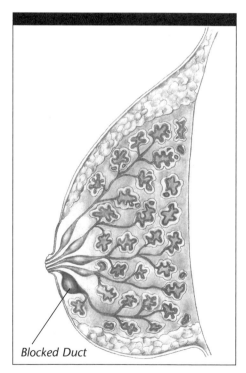

Blocked Duct

While breastfeeding, it is common a woman to have a blocked milk duct in one of her breasts.

breast. Call your doctor if the knot doesn't go away within a few days or if you run a fever. In the meantime, try these methods to drain the duct:

➤ Let your baby nurse long and often on the breast that is blocked.

➤ Offer the breast with the blocked duct first.

➤ If there's any milk left in your breast after a feeding, pump it out or hand express it.

➤ Take a hot shower or apply a hot pack to the lump before nursing.

➤ Massage the lump while your baby nurses to help the milk drain.

Mastitis

If a blocked duct doesn't drain, it may become inflamed. A breast infection, called mastitis, can result.

If your breast is swollen, painful, streaked with red, and feels hot to the touch, you may have mastitis. Women with mastitis often feel like they are coming down with the flu. They run a fever and feel achy and tired.

If you think you have mastitis, call your doctor right away. He or she will prescribe an **antibiotic** to treat the infection. You should feel better within a day or two of starting treatment, but keep taking the treatment for the full prescription.

Until then, do the same things you'd do to treat a blocked duct. Get plenty of rest and drink lots of fluids. Your doctor

may suggest you take ibuprofen to ease your discomfort, too.

Don't stop nursing. Breastfeed your baby often to help drain your breast. (The baby cannot catch the infection.) If you stop nursing, the clogged duct will get more inflamed, your milk supply will go down, and recovery will take longer.

When to Stop

You can breastfeed for as long as you and your child want. Any amount of breastfeeding—even a few days—is good for the baby. The longer you stick with it, the better off your baby will be. Women should try to nurse their babies for at least 6 months.

Breastfeeding doesn't have to be an all-or-nothing thing. Some women give their baby only breast milk for the first few weeks or months and then combine breastfeeding and bottle feeding. However, this can cause your milk supply to decrease and you may have trouble continuing to breastfeed.

When you want to stop breastfeeding, there are a few ways to do it. Some women slowly drop feedings as their baby eats more food and starts drinking from a cup. This can be a long process. It's a gradual change for both of you.

Other women decide to wean their baby when he or she reaches a certain age. In this case, it's still best to take it slow. A sudden stop in breastfeeding can cause you physical pain as your breasts fill with unused milk. It also can be hard for your baby.

One approach is to replace one nursing session with a bottle or cup feeding every few days. Start by cutting out the feedings your baby seems to enjoy the least. Slowly work your way up to the more important ones. Most often, the feeding before bedtime is the last to go—and the hardest to give up. As you reduce the amount you nurse, your milk supply will decrease slowly.

A Unique Bond

Breastfeeding creates a special bond between you and your child. Even if you nurse for only a short while, you'll know that you gave your baby a healthy start in life.

CHAPTER 11

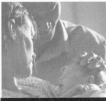

The Newborn Baby

You'll never forget the first time you see your new baby. For 40 weeks, you sheltered and nurtured the baby growing inside you. Now, you must learn to care for this life in a new way. Your baby, nestled safely in your uterus for so long, also must learn to adapt.

As a new mother, you may have lots of questions about the way your newborn looks and acts. Chances are, you'll also wonder how to best care for him or her.

Knowing what's normal and what to expect from this time in your baby's life will help you relax and enjoy watching your baby grow. Relish this special time in your baby's life—it will be over before you know it.

At Birth

How well did your baby fare during labor and delivery? To find out, your doctor will look over your newborn at 1 minute and at 5 minutes after birth. The baby will be assigned a score to measure his or her well-being. The score—called the Apgar score—is named after Dr. Virginia Apgar. She had a strong interest in babies' responses to birth and life outside the uterus.

The Apgar score rates five features:

1. Heart rate

2. Breathing

3. Muscle tone

4. Reflexes

5. Skin color

Each is given a score of 0, 1, or 2 (see Table 11–1). The total of all scores is the Apgar score. Most babies have an Apgar score of 7 or more at 5 minutes after birth. Few babies score a perfect 10.

The Apgar score is a good measure to check the baby's condition right after delivery. It's also a good way to see how

Table 11–1. The Apgar Score

Component	Score		
	0	1	2
Heart rate	Absent	Fewer than 100 beats per minute	More than 100 beats per minute
Respiration	Absent	Weak cry or hyperventilation	Good, strong cry
Muscle tone	Limp	Some flexing of arms and legs	Active motion
Reflexes	No response	Grimace	Cries or withdraws feet
Color*	Blue or pale	Body pink; hands and feet blue	Pink all over

*In babies with dark skin, the mouth, lips, palms, and soles are examined.

the baby adjusts to the outside world in the minutes after birth. But the Apgar score doesn't show how healthy your baby was before birth or what the future will hold.

Your Baby's First Breath

During pregnancy, your baby got oxygen through the placenta and umbilical cord. In the moments after birth, your newborn takes his or her first breath of air.

This is a huge step. It's not just the lungs that must be able to fill with air seconds after delivery. All the related structures—such as muscles around the lungs and airways leading from the mouth and nose—also must be ready to start working.

After birth, there's more pressure outside the lungs than there is inside them. This pressure causes the lungs to expand and fill with air. As a result, the baby draws breath and may start crying.

Many babies cry on their own at birth. Others don't cry right away. Instead, they simply start breathing. (That doesn't mean these babies won't cry later.)

After birth, the doctor and nurses watch your baby's breathing closely. If the baby isn't breathing well, they take steps to help. Often, this simply means rubbing the baby's body to wake him or her up a bit. Sometimes, the baby may be given a little oxygen.

Temperature

The temperature inside your uterus is fairly stable. There, your baby was kept warm by your body. After birth, your baby enters a place that's much cooler. Your newborn also is wet with amniotic fluid. As a result, the baby can lose a lot of heat as the moisture on his or her skin evaporates. If the baby is given to you right after birth, hold the baby close to your skin. A nurse will dry off your baby and snugly wrap him or her in a blanket to keep warm.

Just like you, your newborn has controls to keep body temperature even. These controls don't work as well as yours do. A newborn can easily get too hot or too cold. To keep your newborn warm, dress him or her in a cotton shirt or gown and wrap a light blanket around his or her body

Nervous System

Right from birth, your newborn responds to people, sound, light, and touch. You may not pick up on all of these responses right away. As your baby matures, they'll become easier to notice.

Babies are born with certain reflexes, or automatic responses:

➤ *The Moro (startle) reflex.* This happens when there's a loud noise, or when someone nearby makes a sudden movement. In response, your baby will throw out his or her arms, extend his or her neck, and then draw his or her arms back to the chest.

➤ *The rooting (sucking) reflex.* This is an instinct to search for the breast. If you stroke your baby's cheek or lip, he or she will turn toward you with pursed lips, ready to suck. This helps the baby find your nipple at feeding time. A newborn also has the reflex to suck when he or she feels pressure on the roof of the mouth, behind the upper gums.

➤ *The grasp reflex.* If you stroke your baby's palm, his or her fingers will close tightly around yours.

Digestive System

For 40 weeks, the placenta was your baby's main food source. Nutrients from your blood crossed the placenta and entered your baby's bloodstream through the umbilical cord.

Shortly after delivery, your baby can suck and swallow milk. This milk moves through the digestive tract, where carbohydrates, proteins, and fats are broken down and absorbed into your baby's blood.

Once the milk gets to your baby's intestines, it mixes with **meconium.** This is the greenish-black, sticky sub-

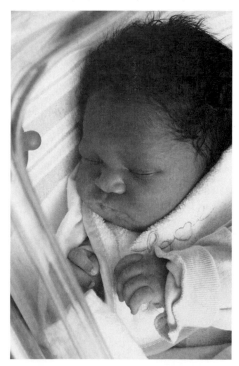

stance that formed in the baby's bowels during pregnancy. In most cases, you see meconium in the baby's first bowel movement. This often occurs within 24 hours of birth. During the first few days of your baby's life, the color of his or her stools will slowly change as the greenish meconium is replaced by yellowish digested milk.

How Your Newborn Looks

Magazines and TV shows often use babies who are a few months old to depict newborns. Unless you have seen a real newborn, you may be surprised by the way your baby really looks:

➤ Your newborn's body may seem scrunched up. That's because a new baby draws his or her arms and legs up close, into the so-called "fetal position." This is the way he or she fit into the close confines of your uterus. Even though the baby has more room now, it'll take a few weeks for him or her to stretch out a bit.

➤ Your baby's face may be slightly swollen, and the area around his or her eyes may be a little puffy for a few days.

➤ The baby's head may be long and pointy at first. Why? Babies have two soft spots on the top of their heads. This is where the skull bones haven't yet joined. These soft spots make the head flexible enough to fit through the birth canal. If your baby's head is pointy at first, it will round out in a few days or weeks.

➤ Your newborn's genitals may look swollen or very large for such a small body. In boys, the scrotum may be red. Girls may have a slight discharge from their vagina. This can be bloody, clear, or white. Both boys and girls may have puffy-looking breasts. Some babies' nipples may leak a few drops of milk. These signs are the result of the high levels of hormones your baby was exposed to in the uterus. They go away a few days after birth, once the hormones work their way out of your baby's system.

Skin, Hair, and Eyes

A baby who has just been born often is covered with a greasy, whitish coating called vernix. There also may be traces of blood and other material on your baby's skin at birth. After he or she is cleaned up, a baby may have some of these features:

➤ *Delicate skin.* A newborn's skin is new and fragile. Don't use harsh soaps or scented creams on it.

➤ *Peeling skin.* After the protective layer of vernix is washed away, the skin may peel slightly.

➤ *Hair covering.* Fine hair called lanugo often appears on a baby's shoulders and back. It will shed within 1 or 2 weeks.

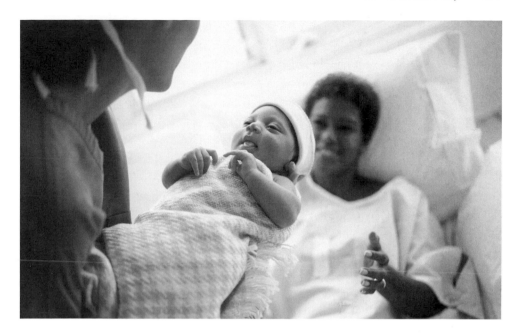

➤ *Blotchy skin.* The skin on some new-borns' hands, feet, and mouth area has a bluish or grayish cast. This is caused by early changes in the baby's circulation. Most often, it goes away.

➤ *Coloring.* A baby's skin color may change somewhat as he or she grows older. This is even more true of babies whose racial or ethnic groups tend to have dark skin. Hair and eye color often change, as well.

➤ *Yellowish skin.* This coloring, called **jaundice**, is caused by a buildup of **bilirubin** in the blood. This green-ish-yellow substance forms when old red blood cells break down. During pregnancy, the placenta (and then your liver) removes bilirubin from your baby's blood. The baby's liver won't start remov-ing bilirubin until a few days after birth. Therefore, bilirubin can build up and cause your baby to have a yellowish tint to the skin. Although too much bilirubin can be harmful, normal levels won't cause a prob-lem. If your baby has jaundice, the doctor will check the level of biliru-bin in his or her blood. If it's high, special treatment will bring the level down.

Your Baby's Weight

One of the first questions people ask after a baby arrives is how much he or she weighs. In fact, that's one of the first things doctors and nurses at the hospi-tal want to know, too.

There's no such thing as a "right" weight for a newborn. Even so, there is a range that is thought to be normal for most babies. The hospital staff notes your baby's weight in grams (2.2 pounds = 1,000 grams = 1 kilogram).

They'll give you the figure in pounds and ounces, though. Most full-term babies weigh between 5½ and 9½ pounds. The average weight is 7½ pounds (about 3,400 grams).

The weight often depends on how close a baby is born to his or her due date. Babies born early tend to weigh less than those born at term (37– 42 weeks after your last period). Babies born late tend to weigh more. In the first 3 days after birth, it is normal for a baby to lose a very small amount of weight before beginning to gain.

How Your Newborn Acts

Most newborns' basic needs and responses to the outside world are the same. Even so, each baby has a unique personality right from the start.

The way one baby behaves and interacts with people can be very different from the way another newborn acts. Some babies are quiet and calm. This is likely to be true of babies who seemed quiet in the uterus. Other babies are bundles of energy from the start. They cry and kick with vigor and demand round-the-clock attention.

After the stress of birth, most newborns are very alert for the first hour or so. This is a good time to nurse, talk to, or just hold your new son or daughter.

When this alertness fades, the baby will get sleepy. Don't worry if your newborn seems very drowsy or sleeps a lot for the next few hours or even days. After all, you are not the only one who needs to recover from the birth.

Many babies do little else besides sleep at first. Most newborns spend 14–18 hours a day sleeping—although not all at once. Short stretches of sleep broken up by brief alert periods are normal. But again, it depends on the baby. Some newborns sleep less and are fussy when they wake up. Others sleep for long stretches and are quiet and calm when they are awake.

Medical Care for Your Baby

Your baby will receive a complete physical exam in the hospital. A doctor or nurse will look your baby over from head to toe, listen to the breathing and heartbeat, check the pulse, feel the belly, and look for normal newborn reflexes.

Newborns have certain things done to prevent disease and to check for conditions that can be treated (see box). Some states have laws requiring certain tests or procedures.

Hearing test

Most hospitals do routine hearing tests on newborns. Unless a baby has these

Newborn Tests and Procedures

Before the baby leaves the hospital, a doctor or nurse will do the following:

➤ Take a blood sample from his or her heel to check for certain diseases. One of these is phenylketonuria (PKU). A baby with this defect can't break down a substance in food called phenylalanine. Another disease the heel-stick will check for is hypothyroidism (low thyroid hormone). Both conditions can cause mental retardation. They can be avoided if they are found and treated early. The baby also will be tested for hypoglycemia (low blood sugar), sickle cell anemia, and rare metabolic conditions. The tests the baby receives depends on which state you live in. You also can request that additional tests be done, but these tests may not be covered by your insurance.

➤ Give the baby a shot of vitamin K. A newborn's body can't make vitamin K on its own for a few days. Without it, blood won't clot. A vitamin K shot helps protect against a rare but severe bleeding disorder.

➤ Put a medicated ointment or liquid in the newborn's eyes. This guards against infection from germs that can get into the eyes during birth.

➤ Give the baby the first of three immunizations against hepatitis B. This virus can lead to severe illness and liver damage. Ask the doctor about the pros and cons of giving the vaccine to your newborn.

tests, he or she could have hearing loss that is not noticed. That can result in delayed speech or other speech problems.

There are two kinds of hearing tests for newborns. Both take 5 to 10 minutes. The tests are painless.

In one test, a tiny speaker and microphone are put in the baby's ear. The speaker makes soft clicking sounds. The ear's response to the sounds is measured by the microphone.

In the other test, soft earphones are placed over your baby's ears. Then three special sensors are attached to the baby's head. The earphones play soft clicks. The sensors measure brain-wave responses to the sounds.

If your baby does not pass the screening test for hearing, this does not always mean your baby has hearing loss. Some babies do not pass the screening test for other reasons. If the screening test shows there might be hearing loss, the doctor will refer your baby to a hearing specialist for further testing.

Circumcision

Whether to circumcise a baby boy is a matter of choice for parents. Circumcision means cutting away the **foreskin.** This is the layer of skin that covers the **glans**, the sensitive end of the penis. Circumcision is most often done by an ob-gyn or pediatrician soon after birth, before the baby leaves the hospital.

In most cases, there's no medical reason to circumcise a baby. It's not required by law or hospital policy. Some parents have their sons circumcised for religious or cultural reasons. Parents

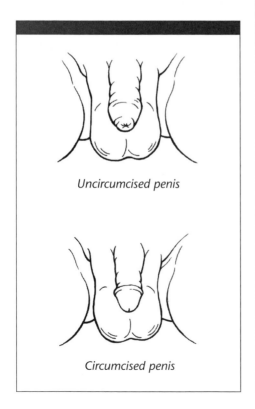

Uncircumcised penis

Circumcised penis

who want their sons circumcised must request it.

If you choose to have your baby circumcised, be sure that pain relief is provided. (See "Caring for Your Son's Penis" for more information on taking care of your baby after circumcision.)

Stocking Up for Baby

Many couples are so thrilled at the prospect of a new baby that they start shopping as soon as the pregnancy test result is positive. Friends and family, too, often shower parents-to-be with dozens of gifts.

Although cute clothes, toys, and high-tech baby gear sold today are appealing, a baby really doesn't need very much—at least at the start. You need basics such as clothes, diapers, a car seat, a baby carrier, and a place for your newborn to sleep. The other items can wait until later.

Baby Clothes

When choosing clothes for your new baby, be practical. If your newborn arrives in July, for instance, you won't need a thick blanket sleeper or bunting right away.

Don't buy many newborn outfits. A newborn grows so fast that these clothes may last just a few weeks. Buy baby clothes a little big. They'll last much longer this way. You can always roll up sleeves and hems. It's best to stick to a basic wardrobe.

How many of each item you need depends on how often you can do laundry. You may need to change your baby's outfit two or three times a day at first.

Baby Supplies

Whether you buy new baby gear, purchase it secondhand, or get hand-me-downs, be sure furniture and other supplies are clean, safe, and sturdy. Whether you are shopping for a crib or a car seat, it is important that your baby supplies meet current safety standards. Check with a consumer safety council for the latest guidelines.

Cribs

Cribs made since 1989 must meet strict safety standards. If you buy a new crib, be sure it has a Juvenile Products Manufacturers Association seal. If you use an older one, make sure it has certain safety features:

➤ Slats are no more than 2⅜ inches apart and none are missing or cracked (the baby's head or body could slip through).

➤ There are no cutouts or crossbars in the headboard or footboard (the baby's head could get trapped).

➤ There are no corner posts (the baby's clothing could get caught and strangle him or her).

➤ Latches are secure and can't be opened by a baby or a toddler.

➤ There are no rough edges, sharp points, or loose screws or bolts.

➤ The paint is lead-free and isn't chipping or peeling.

➤ There are at least 9 inches between the top of the side rail and the mattress when it's in the lowest position, and at least 26 inches when it's in the highest position.

No matter what kind of crib you pick, check for the following:

➤ The mattress is firm and fits snugly. No more than two fingers should fit between the mattress and the crib on all four sides.

➤ The mattress is waterproof. Don't use a plastic or rubber mattress cover—the baby could get trapped under it.

➤ The bumper pads fit snugly, go all the way around the crib, and are tied or strapped on tightly. Bumper ties should be no longer than 6 inches. Remove the bumper when your baby can pull up to stand.

Bassinets and Cradles

For the first few months a bassinet or cradle is a good option. You can use it as the only baby bed, or have one in addition to a crib. This can be helpful if your house has two floors. In addition, bassinets and cradles are easy to move from room to room. Be sure your bassinet or a cradle has the following features:

➤ The bottom is sturdy and the base is wide. This will prevent the cradle or bassinet from tipping over.

Baby Clothes and Supplies

These are basic clothes for your newborn:

___ Cotton undershirts or one-piece garments

___ Newborn gowns with drawstring bottoms

___ Footed stretch suits that snap at the crotch

___ Socks or booties

___ A sweater

___ Knit caps

___ A bunting (a "baby bag" with a zipper and a hood for cold weather)

Other supplies you should have on hand include:

___ Diapers (cloth or disposable)

___ Cloth diapers (to use as burp pads or to wipe up after your baby)

___ Receiving blankets

___ Baby washcloths and hooded towels

___ Bedding (fitted sheets and a light blanket)

___ A large diaper pail that closes tightly

___ A front carrier (so you can "wear" your baby when you go out for walks or even around the house)

___ A diaper bag

___ A rear-facing car safety seat

Many parents buy or borrow these items, although you can manage without them, too:

___ A changing table with safety straps

___ A plastic baby bathtub

___ A rocking chair or a glider to sit in while you feed or soothe your baby

___ A baby seat with a safety belt (this allows your baby to get a look at the world while you do dishes, pay bills, or take a shower)

___ A stroller with a reclining seat (a baby shouldn't be propped up in a stroller until he or she can sit up)

___ A baby swing

___ A baby monitor

___ A cool-air humidifier to moisten the air when your baby has a cold (steam vaporizers can cause burns)

➤ Folding legs lock firmly in place.

➤ The surfaces are smooth. Staples or other hardware that stick out could hurt the baby.

➤ The mattress is firm and fits snugly.

Be aware: older babies can tumble out of a bassinet or a cradle. Once your baby is sitting up, move him or her to a crib.

A Car Safety Seat

No single item will do as much to protect your baby as a car safety seat. In a crash, car safety seats do the following:

➤ Prevent injury 50% of the time

➤ Prevent death 71% of the time

➤ Reduce the need for hospitalization 67% of the time

The worst place for your baby to be in a car is in someone's arms. During a crash, a person can be thrown forward with enough force to crush the baby against the dashboard or windshield. Even if he or she is wearing a seat belt, the force of a crash can throw the baby from the car. If the seat belt also is wrapped around, the baby could be crushed between the belt and the person's body.

There are two kinds of car safety seats for babies. An infant seat is for babies who weigh up to 20–22 pounds. Most infant seats are made to pop out of a base. That way, you can carry the

seat by its handle or place it in a special stroller. An infant seat must be replaced when your baby hits 20–22 pounds. The other kind of car seat that is OK for newborns is a convertible seat. These seats aren't as portable as infant seats but can be used for infants and toddlers who weigh up to 40 pounds. If your baby is preterm or very small, ask the baby's doctor about the best seat to use.

It's illegal in all 50 states and the District of Columbia to drive a baby or a small child in a car without a safety seat. Most hospitals won't let you take your new baby home unless you have a car seat. Practice putting it in and out of the car to be sure you know how to install it when the time comes.

Your car owner's manual should have directions on how to install the seat. Newer cars use special anchors instead of the car seat belts to hold the infant seat in place.

The seat should be installed in a reclined, rear-facing position in the back seat of your car (the center of the back seat is best). In a head-on crash, the baby is pressed backwards into the safety seat, with less risk of harm. In a rear-end crash, the back seat acts as a buffer to hold the car seat tightly. (Once your baby weighs 20 pounds and is at least a year old, change from an infant safety seat to a front-facing toddler seat. Or, if you have a con-

Choosing and Using a Car Seat

➤ Don't confuse a plastic baby carrier with a safety seat. A regular baby carrier can shatter in a crash, even if a seat belt is placed around it.

➤ Look for a seat that's safe. The best seats have straps that hold the baby's body at each shoulder and hip and between the legs. This cuts down on the impact during a crash by spreading the force over more of the baby's body—much like a lap–shoulder belt does for an adult.

➤ Try before you buy. Before you buy a car seat, make sure it can be anchored in the back seat of your car. Choose a seat that's easy to use. While you are in the store, try locking and unlocking the buckle and changing the length of the straps.

➤ Send in the registration card that comes with the seat. That way, you'll be informed if the seat is recalled.

➤ Never use a rear-facing seat in the front seat of a car with a passenger-side airbag. In a crash, the airbag could inflate with enough force to harm or even kill your baby.

➤ If your baby's head flops forward, wedge a rolled towel under the car seat to level it out. Place rolled cloth diapers or blankets on both sides of your baby's head and shoulders to keep your newborn from falling to one side in the seat. You also can buy a special car-seat headrest for this.

➤ Dress your baby in clothes that let you put the safety straps between his or her legs.

➤ Never place a blanket between the baby and the harness straps, or underneath or behind the baby.

➤ Adjust the safety straps so they fit snugly. If the straps are loose, the baby could slip out or be thrown from the seat.

➤ Make sure the straps lie flat and aren't twisted.

➤ Fasten the seat's retainer clip at the level of your baby's armpits. This will keep the straps from slipping off of his or her shoulders.

For more details, contact National Highway Traffic and Safety Administration at 400 Seventh Street, SW, Washington, DC 20590, or visit the administration's website at www.nhtsa.dot.gov.

vertible seat, turn it around to face front.)

The seat should be strapped in as tightly as possible. Pressing down on the seat with your knee while you tighten the seat belt will help. Once the seat is installed, make sure that it doesn't move from side to side or forward and backward.

If you can't afford to buy a seat, you may be able to rent one. In addition, some communities and hospitals have programs for new parents to borrow a safety seat at no charge. Don't buy a used car seat. A used seat may look fine. If it's been in a crash, though, it won't work the way it should. You also won't know if the seat meets current safety standards or if it's been recalled. (A car seat rented from a reliable source is safe.) Check with your doctor, hospital, local baby stores, car dealers, or consumer safety council about child safety seats.

Taking Your Baby Home

In most cases, you and your baby can leave the hospital within a few days of delivery. At this early stage, you're both still recovering from birth and getting used to life together.

You more than likely found a doctor for your baby before he or she was born. If you haven't chosen a doctor yet, ask the hospital staff for leads. (See "Choosing Your Baby's Doctor" in Chapter 2).

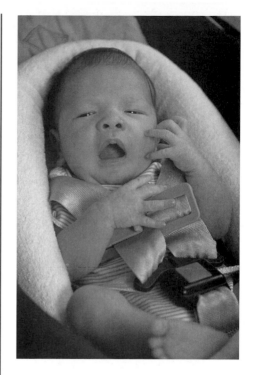

Be sure to set up a doctor's visit for your baby before you are discharged. The timing of this visit depends on how long your baby stays in the hospital, whether there are any special problems (such as jaundice or trouble breastfeeding), and what the doctor prefers. The first visit can be planned for a few days or a few weeks after delivery.

Don't be shy about asking the doctor questions. Doctors and nurses are used to lots of questions from new parents and welcome the chance to help. Some doctors' offices even have special call-in times for questions. Call right away if you're really worried about something.

Once you and your baby are settled in at home, don't try to do too much.

When To Call Your Baby's Doctor

Call the doctor if your newborn shows any of the following signs:

- Has trouble breathing (the baby has to work hard to get air in and out)
- Has skin that looks blue or very pale
- Has a seizure (shaking arms and legs)
- Has a fever higher than 100°F
- Doesn't want to wake up after sleeping for a few hours
- Doesn't seem as alert as normal when he or she wakes up
- Cries much more than normal and doesn't respond to comforting
- Moans as if in pain
- Acts very fussy
- Seems weak or cries more quietly than normal
- Has mucus, blood, or blood clots in his or her urine or stool
- Has diarrhea (a large, very watery bowel movement)

- Has fewer than six wet diapers a day
- Has dark or strong-smelling urine
- Has no stool for 48 hours
- Has stool that's not yellowish by day five if you are breastfeeding
- Vomits (not spits up) more than once a day
- Nurses poorly or doesn't want more than half a bottle for two feedings in a row
- Has very yellow skin or eyes
- Has bleeding or discharge from his or her eyes, nails, navel, or genitals
- Has diaper rash that doesn't go away or gets worse
- Has white patches in his or her mouth
- Just doesn't seem "right" to you

You may want to ask for extra help from your partner, relatives, or friends. If your employer doesn't offer paid maternity leave, find out if state or local agencies can give you help and support.

Newborns need time to get used to the outside world. Avoid loud noise, intense light, or lots of people. Instead, give yourself and your baby a couple of weeks of peace and quiet. Keep trips around town short. Limit visits from well-wishers. Use this time to rest, get to know your new baby, and settle into life as a family.

Remember, too, that each baby is unique. Some adapt well to their new surroundings. Others have a harder time at first.

Caring for Your Newborn

Newborn babies can function well in the outside world. Even so, they need lots of help to get nourishment and to stay clean, warm, safe, and healthy.

Keeping Your Baby Safe

New parents often worry about their baby's safety. Taking the following steps will keep your baby safe and help put your mind at ease:

➤ Lay your baby down to sleep on his or her back. This greatly lowers the risk of sudden infant death syndrome (SIDS). In the United States, nearly 5,000 babies younger than 1 year die from SIDS each year. No one knows for sure what causes SIDS. Experts think that putting babies down to sleep on their stomachs is the cause in some cases. (If your baby has health problems, talk to his or her doctor about the best sleeping position.)

➤ When you put your baby down to sleep, place him or her on a firm mattress. Don't let the baby sleep on a waterbed, sofa, sheepskin, or other soft surface. Remove pillows, quilts, comforters, toys, and stuffed animals from his or her crib. They can smother the baby. Babies should not sleep in the same bed as their parents. Dress your baby in a warm sleeper and do not use a blanket.

➤ Always use a car safety seat when your baby rides in a car, van, or truck. These are designed to protect babies and small children in a crash. (See "A Car Safety Seat.") Always use the safety straps that come in infant seats, strollers, and high chairs.

➤ Never leave your baby alone in a car. When it's hot outside, the temperature in parked cars can soar to more than 100 degrees in just a few minutes.

➤ Never leave your baby alone—even for a second—in the bathtub or on the changing table, bed, sofa, or anywhere he or she could fall or drown. Have all that you need within arm's reach. Keep a hand on your baby at all times. If you have to answer the phone or the doorbell, take your baby with you.

➤ Check your baby's toys and clothing for ribbons, buttons, or other small parts that could be pulled off and swallowed. Also, keep older children's toys, coins, and other small objects out of your baby's reach. These can lodge in the baby's throat and block the airway.

➤ Don't let anyone smoke around your baby. Infants and young children who are exposed to secondhand smoke have more colds and respiratory infections and are at higher risk of SIDS.

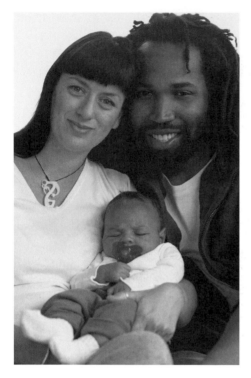

➤ Don't warm your baby's bottle in the microwave. This creates hot spots that can burn his or her mouth. Also, don't drink hot drinks or cook while you are holding your baby.

Feeding Your Baby

Breastfeeding is the best way to feed your new baby. Whether you choose to breastfeed or bottle feed your new baby, be sure to do it often (8–12 times every 24 hours). A newborn's stomach is about the size of his or her fist. Your baby can take in just a little breast milk or formula at a time. As a result, he or she needs to eat at least every few hours. (For how-tos on breastfeeding, see Chapter 10.)

If you are bottle feeding, the first thing you need to do is choose a formula. Formulas often are made with nonfat cow's milk and fat from soy, coconut, or corn. They also have vitamins, minerals, and other elements that closely mimic those found in breast milk. Most formulas have extra iron as well. Ask your doctor which type of formula he or she suggests. The Special Supplemental Food Program for Women, Infants, and Children provides formula for mothers who can't afford it.

Some babies are allergic to cow's milk or have trouble digesting it. If your baby reacts badly to formula, talk to his or her doctor about switching to a formula made with soy protein instead of milk.

Formula comes in powdered, condensed, or ready-to-serve form. Water must be added to powdered or condensed formula. If you buy either of these, follow the directions carefully. Formula that's too weak or too strong isn't good for your baby.

Next, choose the type of bottles you'll use. Baby bottles come in lots of designs. Bottles can be upright or angled. They either are made to use over and over or to hold special bags that are thrown away after each feeding.

No matter which type you choose, stock up on a supply of 4-ounce bottles for your newborn. Your baby won't be able to handle a feeding from a standard 8-ounce bottle until he or she is older.

Now, pick nipples for the bottles. Nipples can be standard, orthodontic, flat-tipped, or elongated.

For a baby who's fed only formula, a standard or orthodontic nipple may be fine. If you are combining breastfeeding and bottle feeding, though, a flat-tipped or elongated nipple may be the best choice. These nipples are made to prompt a type of sucking that's close to the sucking used to draw milk from the breast. This way, your baby is less likely to be confused about what he or she needs to do.

Before feeding your newborn, be sure the bottle and nipple have been cleaned well in hot, soapy water. Special bottle brushes help you scrub the hard-to-reach inside of your baby's bottles.

Give your newborn his or her first feeding within 6 hours of birth. Formula takes longer to digest than breast milk. That's why bottle-fed babies often can go for longer stretches (3–4 hours) between feedings. Still, follow your baby's cues, not the clock. If he or she seems hungry, offer a bottle.

When you're ready to start feeding, hold your baby in the crook of your arm. The baby's head and chest should be higher than his or her feet. Tilt the bottle so the nipple fills with formula. This will cut down on the amount of air your baby swallows and will help prevent gas.

Don't "prop" the bottle in your baby's mouth. This can lead to choking or ear infections because the formula pools at the back of the baby's throat.

Your newborn needs contact with you, too. Feeding provides a chance to relax and enjoy this time together.

Bathing Your Baby

You should keep your baby clean, but there's no need for a daily tub bath. Your newborn will get a good wash in the hospital after birth. Wait until your baby's umbilical stump has dried up and fallen off (7–10 days) before you give him or her another bath (see box).

In the meantime, sponge baths a few times a week will do. Here's how to keep your newborn's skin and scalp clean:

1. Undress your baby and wrap him or her in a towel.

2. Gently wipe your baby's eyes clean with a moist cotton ball.

3. Use a wet washcloth (no soap) to gently wipe your baby's face.

4. Uncover one part of your baby's body at a time to prevent him or her from getting cold.

5. Wipe each body part clean with a wet washcloth and a small amount of mild baby soap.

6. Pay close attention to the folds of skin in your baby's neck, arms, and legs.

7. Rinse and pat dry each area after you clean it.

Your Baby's First Tub Bath

Your baby's first real bath is a milestone. It can be a little scary, too. Don't worry—you'll get the hang of it in no time. A bath every few days (with spot cleanings in between) is more than enough to keep your baby clean. Here's how to tackle that first dip:

1. Gather your supplies. You'll need mild soap, baby shampoo, cotton balls, a washcloth, and a towel.

2. Use a sink lined with a foam pad or a special bathtub made for babies. Do not bathe your baby in the bathtub until he or she is old enough to sit up.

3. Fill the basin with 2 inches of water. Test the heat of the water with your wrist before putting your baby in. The water should be warm—not hot.

4. Start by wiping your baby's eyes and face clean with a wet cotton ball or washcloth.

5. Work your way down his or her body, ending up at the diaper area.

6. To keep your baby from getting chilled, wash his or her hair (or scalp) last and rinse with clean water.

7. If your baby seems to enjoy the bath, don't rush it. Let him or her relax, splash, and explore the water.

8. When the bath is over, wrap your baby snugly in a towel.

8. Wash the area normally covered by a diaper last.

Many mothers are nervous about bathing their newborns. If you have questions about how to do it, ask the nurses at the hospital to show you.

Caring for Your Baby's Umbilical Stump

In most cases, the stump of the umbilical cord dries up and falls off within 7–10 days of birth. The spot beneath the stump becomes your baby's belly button. Many parents wonder if the way the stump looks has anything to do with their baby's navel being turned in or out. It doesn't.

While the stump is drying out, keep the area clean and dry. This will speed healing and prevent infection. Expose the stump to air and protect it from urine and stool by folding down the top of your baby's diaper. Don't cover the stump with gauze or bandages.

Your doctor may suggest you use ointment or rubbing alcohol around the base of the stump for the first week or so. Call the doctor if the stump looks infected or the skin around it is red.

Diapering Your Baby

Most newborns empty their bladder and bowels within a day of birth. This may occur in the delivery room. Some babies wait more than 24 hours. If your baby takes more than 1–2 days to urinate or pass stool, his or her doctor will try to find out why. Most newborns urinate 6–18 times a day and pass stool as often as 7–8 times a day. It may be hard to tell if your baby is urinating (especially with super absorbent diapers). Placing a tissue in the diaper is a good test to check.

Choosing Diapers

You can use either cloth or disposable diapers. Each kind has pros and cons when it comes to cost and convenience. Here's a look at your options:

➤ *Disposable diapers.* Although they are the easiest to use, disposable diapers cost the most. Disposable diapers don't breathe as well as cloth diapers, so they can sometimes cause diaper rash. If you use disposables, try a number of brands until you find one you like. Avoid disposable diapers that shred when they are wet. Your baby could swallow loose pieces.

➤ *Cloth diapers that you buy and wash.* This is the cheapest option, but it takes the most time and energy. Cloth diapers come in two styles: flat and pre-folded. Flat diapers can be adjusted to fit your growing baby. They may be hard to find, though. Pre-folded diapers have the folds stitched in place so you don't have to fold them after laundering. No matter which type of cloth diaper you choose, start with at least three dozen of them. You'll also need at least three cotton diaper wraps. These hold the diaper in place and close with snaps or fasteners (so no diaper pins are needed). They also cut down on leaks and help keep clothes and bedding dry. They breathe better and are easier to use than rubber or plastic diaper covers, too.

➤ *Cloth diapers from a diaper service.* This is cheaper than using disposables. It's more costly than buying and washing your own diapers, though. Diaper services often pick up dirty diapers and drop off clean ones once or twice a week. They give you a choice of diaper sizes and often provide diaper wraps and a diaper pail for dirty diapers. Some parents use a diaper service for the first few months, when babies tend to go through the most diapers. Afterwards, they wash their own diapers or switch to disposables.

No matter which type you choose, change your baby's diaper each time he or she wets or soils it. This will help prevent diaper rash. You may go through nearly six dozen diapers a week at first. Have a good supply of clean ones on hand.

How to Diaper Your Baby

Before you change your baby's diaper, make sure you have the things you need within reach. Never leave your baby alone on a changing table or any other raised surface. He or she could roll or slide off.

Things you'll need:

➤ A clean diaper

➤ A diaper wrap (if you use cloth diapers)

➤ Alcohol-free diaper wipes or a washcloth and a basin filled with lukewarm water

➤ Diaper-rash ointment (if your baby has a rash)

➤ Cornstarch (for hot weather or if your baby has a rash)

What to do:

1. Remove the dirty diaper.

2. Have an extra cloth diaper handy in case your baby urinates when the diaper is off. Babies often do this. While you are changing your baby, place the extra diaper under the baby's bottom (for a girl) or on top of the penis.

3. Gently clean your baby's genitals and bottom. (If your baby's skin is irritated by baby wipes, use a wet washcloth instead.)

4. Be sure to wipe from front to back. This keeps bacteria from the baby's stool away from the urethra or vagina, where it can cause infection.

5. Pat the diaper area dry.

6. Apply diaper-rash ointment to irritated skin if your baby has a rash. If the rash is severe (has blisters or sores or does not go away in several days), talk to the baby's doctor.

7. Apply a light dusting of cornstarch if it's very hot out or if your baby has a rash. (Babies can inhale powder, which irritates the lungs. Don't use baby powder made with talc. Also, be careful not to shake out the powder near your baby's face. Never leave a container of powder within your baby's reach.)

8. Put on the new diaper as shown in the "Using Different Types of Diapers" box.

Dressing Your Baby

Although babies should be kept warm, there's no need to pile on layer after layer of clothing unless it's really cold. Your baby needs about the same amount of clothes as you do—plus one layer because he or she doesn't move around as much. Add a knit cap if it is cold when you and the baby go outside. Newborns can lose a lot of heat through their heads.

When it comes to choosing clothes, let the climate, the season, and the ease of dressing your baby be your guide.

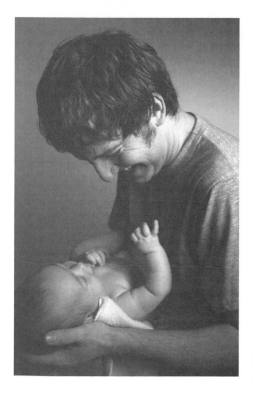

For the early weeks, footed one-piece baby suits are a good choice. They should be made with a soft material that breathes and doesn't irritate your baby's skin. Easy access to the diaper area also is vital. A zipper or snaps in the front are easier to deal with than closures in the back.

If it's chilly, layer an undershirt beneath the baby suit and a sweater or a bunting on top. If it's warm, a diaper and a one-piece garment may be all your baby needs.

Caring for Your Son's Penis

If your son was circumcised, a light dressing of gauze with petroleum jelly was placed over the head of your baby's penis after the procedure. This keeps it from rubbing against the diaper while it heals.

Keep the area clean. Wash your son's penis with soap and warm water each day. Change his diaper often so urine and stool don't irritate the tender tissue or cause infection. Dab the tip of your baby's penis with a little petroleum jelly to keep it from sticking to his diaper.

With one type of circumcision, a plastic ring is left on the penis. The ring will slip off on its own when the circumcision is fully healed. This takes about 7–10 days.

If you didn't have your son circumcised, you don't need to do anything special to care for his penis. Just wash the outside of the penis with soap and water when he takes his bath. Don't try to pull back your son's foreskin. The foreskin may not retract over the head of his penis until he's between 3 and 5 years old. Once this happens, you can teach your son how to clean under his foreskin.

Your New Family

The days and weeks after your baby arrives can be among the most challenging in your life. You may be tired and overwhelmed. Your baby may fuss a lot, be hungry around the clock, and have trouble settling into a regular sleep pattern.

Your biggest task during these early days with your baby is to learn how to read his or her signals. Chances are,

Using Different Types of Diapers

For both types of diapers, make sure it isn't too loose or too tight. The diaper should be snug but allow you to fit two fingers between the diaper and your baby's skin.

Disposable diaper:

1. Use one hand to grasp your baby's ankles and lift up his or her legs and bottom.

2. With the other hand, slide the back of the clean diaper under your baby's bottom. The top of the diaper should be level with your baby's belly button.

3. Lower your baby onto the diaper.

4. Bring the front of the diaper between your baby's legs and up over the genitals.

5. If your baby still has his or her umbilical stump, fold the top of the diaper down so the stump is exposed.

6. Unfasten the tabs on the back of the diaper. Stick them down on the front of the diaper.

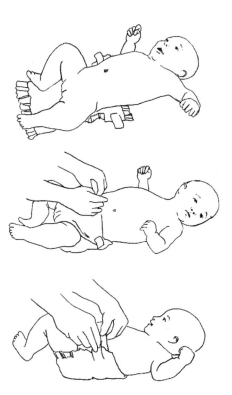

(continued)

Using Different Types of Diapers (continued)

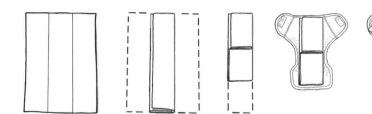

Cloth diaper:

1. Fold the diaper in thirds along its length.

2. Fold the bottom third of the diaper up.

3. Lay the folded diaper inside a diaper wrap.

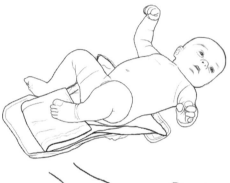

4. Fan out the top of the diaper.

5. Use one hand to grasp your baby's ankles and lift up his or her legs and bottom. With the other hand, slide the back of the diaper and the diaper wrap under your baby's bottom.

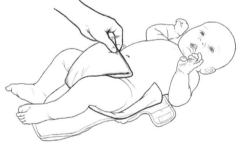

6. Lower your baby onto the diaper.

7. Bring the front of the diaper between your baby's legs and up over the genitals. (If your baby still has his or her umbilical stump, the top of the diaper and diaper wrap should be beneath the stump.)

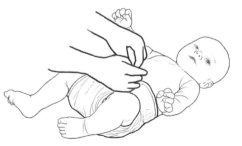

8. Bring the sides of the diaper toward the front, wrap snugly, and fasten them to the front.

these signals won't be the same as the ones used by your neighbor's baby, or a friend's baby, or even your last baby. Meet your baby's needs quickly and lovingly.

Give yourself time to master all the skills you'll need to take care of your baby, too. You become a mother the moment your baby is born. Mothering your child won't be second nature right away, though. Pretty soon, as you watch your baby grow, you'll wonder how you ever managed without him or her in your life.

CHAPTER 12

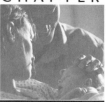

Postpartum Care

It may be hard to believe that childbirth is over and that this baby is really yours. You may be surprised by how anxious and stressed you feel. You may wonder whether you'll be a good mother. Tasks that you once did with ease seem harder. You are tired from birth and sleep deprived from caring for your new baby. You may feel a little down, despite having this precious new person in your life. If you know what's happening to your body and your emotions, you can better face the ups and downs of the first few months of being a mother.

Taking care of your physical and mental well-being is key. A good diet, exercise, and lots of rest boost your energy level and help your body get back to normal. Having people nearby for support helps ease you into your new role.

As you resume your daily life, you'll be faced with choices about going back to work, choosing child care, and plan-

ning your family. Don't feel you have to make all of these choices alone. Your doctor as well as your partner and other loved ones can help. Remind yourself that there are no "right" choices. Each mother must do what's best for her and her family.

Your Changing Body

While you were pregnant, your body worked round-the-clock for 40 weeks to help your baby grow. Now that your baby is here, there's more work to be done as your body recovers from pregnancy, labor, and delivery. It will take time for things to get back to normal.

Your Uterus

After delivery, your uterus is hard and round and can be felt behind your navel. It weighs about 2½ pounds. Six weeks later, it weighs only 2 ounces. You can no longer feel it when you press on your belly. The opening of your uterus—the cervix—also shrinks quickly.

Lochia

Once your baby is born, your body sheds the blood and tissue that lined your uterus. This vaginal discharge is called *lochia.*

For the first few days after delivery, lochia is heavy and bright red. It may have a few small clots. Soak up this discharge with sanitary pads—do not use tampons.

As time goes on, the flow gets lighter in volume and color. A week or so after birth, lochia often is pink or brown. Bright red discharge can come back, though. You may feel a gush of blood from your vagina during breastfeeding, when your uterus contracts. By 2 weeks postpartum, lochia often is light brown or yellow. After that, it slowly goes away. How long the discharge lasts differs for each woman. Some women have discharge for just a couple of weeks after their babies are born. Others have it for a month or more.

Return of Menstrual Periods

If you are not breastfeeding, your period may return about 6–8 weeks after giving birth. It could start even sooner.

If you are breastfeeding, your periods may not start again for months. Some nursing mothers don't have a period until their babies are fully weaned.

After birth, your ovaries may release an egg before you have your first

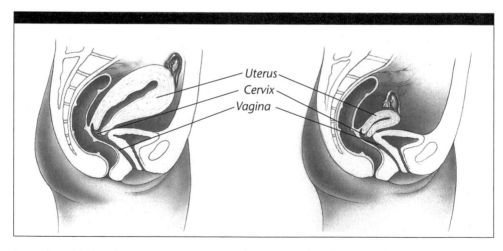

Uterus
Cervix
Vagina

Just after birth, the uterus measures about 7 inches long and weighs about 2½ pounds *(left)*. It can be felt just below the navel. In 6 weeks, it has returned to normal size *(right)*. The normal size is about 3 inches long, weighing about 2 ounces.

period. This means you can get pregnant before you even know you are fertile again. If you don't want another baby right way, start using birth control as soon as you resume having sex. (For details, see "Family Planning.")

Once menstruation returns, it may not be the same as before you were pregnant. Periods may be shorter or longer, for instance. Chances are, they'll slowly return to normal. Some women notice that menstrual cramps are less painful than they were before they got pregnant.

Your Abdomen

Right after delivery, you still look like you are pregnant. During pregnancy, the abdominal muscles stretched out little by little. They won't just snap back into place the minute your baby is born.

Give your body time to go back to normal. Exercise will help. Ask your doctor when it is safe to start exercising. Doing a few exercises at least three times per week will get you started. The box has some examples of postpartum exercises.

You may have backaches after delivery, too. Your stretched abdominal muscles don't help your back muscles support your weight. To prevent a sore back, practice good posture, support your back when you breastfeed, and try not to lift anything heavier than your baby for a while.

Postpartum Discomforts

When you imagined the days and weeks after your baby's birth, chances are you gave little thought to how your body would feel: sore. Most aches won't last. Following are some ways to relieve postpartum aches and pains.

Afterbirth Pains

Your uterus contracts and then relaxes as it shrinks back to its normal size. These cramps are sometimes called afterbirth pains. If you have given birth before or you are breastfeeding, they may be more painful. They'll go away in just a few days. In the meantime, take an over-the-counter pain reliever.

Painful Perineum

The perineum, the area between your vagina and rectum, stretches during delivery. You may have had an episiotomy, an incision to widen the vaginal opening during delivery. Or your perineum may have torn as your baby pushed through. Any of these causes may make this area feel a bit numb at first. Once the numbness wears off, it may feel swollen, bruised, and sore.

This tender tissue needs time to heal. During the weeks after birth, the perineal muscles will slowly start to regain some of their tone. You can help this process by doing Kegel exercises (see "Postpartum Exercises"). Start them

When To Call Your Doctor

Postpartum discomforts are normal. However, some can signal a health problem. Call your doctor if you have any of these symptoms:

➤ Fever more than 100.4°F (38°C)

➤ Nausea and vomiting

➤ Pain or burning during urination

➤ Bleeding that's heavier than a normal menstrual period or that increases

➤ Severe pain in your lower abdomen

➤ Pain, swelling, and tenderness in your legs

➤ Chest pain and cough or gasping for air

➤ Red streaks on your breasts or painful new lumps in your breasts

➤ Pain that doesn't go away or that gets worse from an episiotomy, perineal tear, or abdominal incision

➤ Redness or discharge from an episiotomy, tear, or incision

➤ Vaginal discharge that smells bad

➤ Feelings of hopelessness that last more than 10 days after delivery

soon after birth. Do them as often as you can, anytime and anywhere. To ease discomfort and speed healing:

➤ Ask for a cold pack right after delivery. Putting this on your perineum will cut down on swelling and help lessen soreness and stinging. During the days that follow, keep using cold packs.

➤ Apply chilled witch-hazel pads to the area.

➤ Ask your doctor about using a numbing spray or cream to ease pain.

➤ If it hurts to sit down, cushion the area with a pillow.

➤ Take sitz baths. Soaking in a few inches of warm water will bring relief.

➤ Use a water bottle you can squeeze to soothe the area with a stream of warm water after you urinate.

➤ Always wipe from front to back after you use the toilet. This will prevent a healing episiotomy or tear from getting infected with germs from your rectum.

Hemorrhoids and Vulvar Varicosities

If you had varicose veins in your vulva or hemorrhoids during pregnancy, they may get worse after delivery. These sore, swollen veins also can show up for the first time now because of the intense straining you did during labor.

For relief, try medicated sprays or ointments, dry heat (from a heat lamp or hairdryer turned on low), sitz baths, and cold witch hazel compresses. If hemorrhoids make bowel movements painful, be sure to eat a diet rich in fiber and drink plenty of fluids. A stool softener also may help. Ask your doctor before taking one. Try not to strain when you have a bowel movement. This can worsen hemorrhoids. In time, hemorrhoids and vulvar varicosities will get smaller or go away.

Bowel Problems

It may be hard to have bowel movements for a few days after delivery. There are lots of reasons for this: stretched abdominal muscles, sluggish bowels as a result of surgery or pain medication, and an empty stomach after not eating during labor. You also may be afraid to move your bowels because of pain from an episiotomy or hemorrhoids. Or, if you have stitches in your perineum, you may fear that having a bowel movement will open them. Don't worry about this—the stitches won't come out from moving your bowels.

If you have constipation and painful gas, try these tips to help the problem:

➤ Take short walks as soon as you can.

➤ Eat foods high in fiber and drink plenty of fluids.

➤ Ask your doctor about taking a stool softener.

You may find that the urge to have a bowel movement may not feel the way it used to. In some cases, you may not be able to control your bowel movements. Loss of normal control of the bowels is called fecal *incontinence*. It can be caused by the stretching and tearing of nerves near the rectum during birth. You may have gas when you do not mean to or did not expect it. If you have leakage of solid or liquid stool (feces), tell your doctor about your symptoms. Much can be done to help you regain control of your bowels.

Urinary Problems

In the first days after delivery, you may feel the urge to urinate but can't pass any urine. You may feel pain and burning when you urinate. That's because during birth, the baby's head put a lot of pressure on your bladder, your ure-

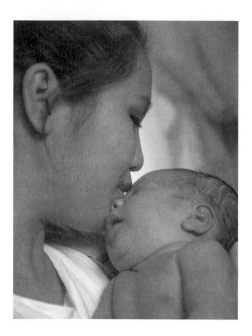

thra (the opening where urine comes out), and the muscles that control urine flow. This pressure can cause swelling and stretching that gets in the way of urination.

To lessen swelling or pain, try a warm sitz bath. When you are on the toilet, spray warm water over your genitals with a squeeze bottle. This can help trigger the flow of urine. Running the tap while you are in the bathroom may help, too. Be sure to drink plenty of fluids as well. This pain usually goes away within days of delivery.

Many new mothers have another problem: urinary incontinence. This means you can't stop the flow of urine—even when you are not trying to go to the bathroom.

With time, the tone of your pelvic muscles will return and the problem will go away in most cases. Kegel exercises also will help tighten these muscles (see "Postpartum Exercises"). If urinary problems persist more than a few weeks, let your doctor know. There are treatments he or she can offer.

Sweating

In the weeks after birth, many new mothers find themselves drenched with sweat. This happens most often at night. Don't worry about it. Your body is adjusting to changing hormones. To keep your sheets and pillow dry at night, you can sleep on a towel until the sweating eases.

Swollen Breasts

Your breasts fill with milk about 2–4 days after delivery. When this happens, they may feel very full, hard, and tender. The best relief for this engorgement is breastfeeding. Once you and your baby settle into a regular nursing pattern, the discomfort will go away. (Chapter 10 has details on easing engorgement.) Severe engorgement should not last more than about 36 hours. Until then, try the following:

➤ Wear a good-fitting support bra, sports bra, or chest binder.

➤ Apply ice packs to your breasts to reduce swelling.

➤ Don't express any milk. This sends a signal to your breasts to make more.

➤ Take pain medication if you need it.

Women who do not breastfeed may experience discomfort from engorgement for several days. When the breasts are not stimulated to produce more milk, this feeling will gradually subside.

Fatigue

You are going to be tired. You just finished a very hard task—childbirth. You also lost blood during delivery. Your new baby may be keeping you up all night, too.

Fatigue goes hand-in-hand with being a new mother. You can't really avoid it. You can take steps to ensure that you are rested during the days and weeks after giving birth:

➤ Ask for help. Your family and friends are more than likely eager to pitch in. Let them. Be specific when others want to know what they can do. Ask a friend to bring something for dinner, stop at the grocery store, start a load of laundry, or watch the baby or an older child for a couple of hours so you can take a nap.

➤ Sleep when your baby sleeps. Use your baby's nap time to rest—not to tackle household chores.

➤ Suggest quiet play. If you have an older child, set him or her up with a few puzzles, picture books, or other quiet activities so you and the baby can rest.

➤ Take it easy. Keep trips out of the house short.

➤ Only do what must be done. Some things will have to wait. It's important that you get the rest you need.

➤ Limit visitors. There will be plenty of time for people to meet your new baby when you are feeling rested. Until then, the last thing you need is a constant stream of well-wishers.

➤ Eat a healthy diet. It may be hard to find time to eat when you are caring for a new baby. Even so, it's vital that you do. Foods rich in protein and iron help fight fatigue.

If you feel really weak or the fatigue continues, talk to your doctor. Sometimes women have a change in thyroid function after pregnancy, especially if they had a thyroid problem before or during pregnancy or someone in their family has thyroid problems.

Postpartum Sadness

Many women have *postpartum blues* after delivery. This sadness also is called the "baby blues" or "maternity blues." Most often, it is mild. The blues should go away within a couple of weeks. In some cases, though, such feelings are intense and don't go away. This can signal a more serious condition called *postpartum depression*.

The Baby Blues

Many new mothers are surprised by how fragile, alone, and drained they feel after the birth of a child. Their feelings don't seem to match their expectations. They wonder, "What have I got to be depressed about?" Also, they fear that having these feelings means they are bad mothers. These emotions are normal. In fact, about 70–80 percent of new mothers get the baby blues.

About 2–3 days after birth, you may begin to feel anxious, sad, and upset. For no clear reason, you may feel angry with the new baby. These feelings are baffling and scary. They fade quickly, though. The baby blues tend to last from a few hours to a week or so. Most often, they go away without treatment.

When you feel blue, remind yourself that you have just taken on a huge job. Feeling sad, anxious, or even angry doesn't mean you are a failure as a mother. It also doesn't mean you are mentally ill. It simply means that your body is adjusting to the normal changes that follow the birth of a child.

Keep in mind, too, that things will soon start looking up again. Until then, do the following to help you conquer the blues:

➤ Talk to your partner or a good friend about how you feel.

➤ Get plenty of rest.

➤ Ask your partner, friends, and family for help.

➤ Take time for yourself.

➤ Get out of the house each day, even if it's only for a short while.

➤ Join a new mothers' group and share your feelings with the women you meet there.

Postpartum Depression

For some women, new motherhood brings with it more intense feelings. About 10 percent of new mothers have postpartum depression. This is marked by feelings of despair, severe anxiety, or hopelessness that get in the way of daily life. It can occur after any birth, not just the first.

Postpartum depression is more likely to occur in women who have had one or more of the following:

➤ Mood disorders before pregnancy

➤ Postpartum depression after a previous pregnancy

➤ Recent stress, such as losing a loved one, family illness, or moving to a new city

If you are prone to depression, seek professional help and enlist support from your loved ones before your baby arrives. Thyroid levels also may decrease after giving birth. Low thyroid levels can cause symptoms similar to depression. Your doctor may recommend that you have your thyroid levels checked to see if this is causing your symptoms of depression.

Treatment and counseling will help relieve postpartum depression. Talk to your doctor right away if you have any of these signs of depression:

➤ Baby blues that last for more than 2 weeks

➤ Strong feelings of depression or anger that come 1–2 months after birth

➤ Feelings of sadness, doubt, guilt, or helplessness that get worse each week and get in the way of day-to-day life

➤ Not being able to sleep, even when you are tired

➤ Sleeping most of the time, even when your baby is awake

➤ Eating much more or much less than normal

➤ Not finding pleasure in things that used to make you happy

➤ Intense concern and worry about the baby

➤ Lack of interest in or feelings for the baby or your family

➤ Panic attacks, such as being afraid to be left alone with the baby

➤ Thoughts of harming the baby or yourself

Return to Daily Living

Having a baby will change the way you live your daily life. Your relationship with your partner will be affected. Your old routines may no longer work. If you know this in advance and try to accept these changes rather than fight them,

you'll be a lot more relaxed as you start your life with the new baby.

Keep in mind, too, that a new baby touches the lives of the whole family. Each person has a role and should take part in the baby's care. There will be some tension as you all adjust to having a baby around. Talk about it. Share your feelings with your partner, your parents, and your children. Listen to their concerns, as well.

Talk to other new moms, too. Just hearing that your family isn't the only one feeling the effects of the birth of a baby can help you cope during this stressful time. The support of other mothers also can make you feel more comfortable in your new role.

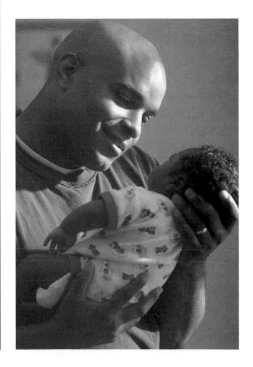

If the stress of parenting seems like too much to handle, get some help. Talk to your doctor or call a local crisis hot line. (These hot lines are listed in the community pages of the phone book.) All new parents reach the end of their rope from time to time. This is even more true if you don't have a lot of support or if your baby is fussy.

No matter what triggers them, never take out your emotions on your child. A baby can get injured easily, even if you don't intend to hurt him or her. Shaking a baby for just a few seconds, for instance, can do enough harm to cause life-long brain damage or even death.

If you ever fear that you are going to lose control and hurt your baby, hand him or her to your partner or another loved one and walk away. If you are alone, put your baby in a safe place, such as the crib. Then go into another room (if you can, one that's out of earshot of your baby's cries) until you calm down.

Once the episode has passed, ask yourself what you can do to prevent it from happening again. Tell your partner you need more help, for instance. Ask friends and relatives for help when you have been on baby duty for too long without a break. Find out what sort of community services—such as counseling, or financial help—are available to you.

You and Your Baby

First-time moms often think that knowing how to care for their newborns will come naturally. In fact, women have to learn mothering skills just as they learn other skills. Keep in mind during these early weeks that mastering baby care takes time, patience, and practice.

You also may feel bad about yourself if you don't have a "perfect" baby or don't measure up as the "perfect" mother. Rest assured—there's no such thing. First, babies have distinct characters right from birth. The fact is, some are just easier to care for than others. Also, it's very hard to juggle taking care of a new baby, running a household, caring for other children, and having a job.

Your Partner

Your partner, too, is going through a lot of changes right now. The needs and concerns of partners can be overlooked, with the focus on you and the baby. Partners are likely to get lots of advice about how to help the new mother, for instance. But getting used to a new baby can be just as hard for that other key person in the baby's life.

What if you are single and had the baby on your own, without the involvement of a life partner? In that case, don't try to shoulder the entire burden of raising a baby by yourself. There are many forms of family that help to enrich a child's life. Surrounding your-

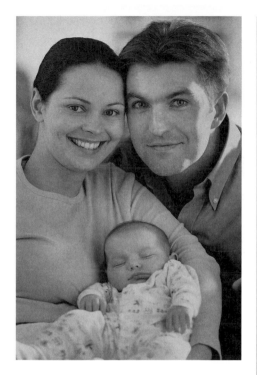

self with friends and family is good for you and good for your baby.

If you do have a spouse or significant other, that person may have mixed feelings about being a parent. Some plunge into family life with gusto. Others throw themselves into work to be a good provider for the new family. Still others, unsure about their new role, withdraw. They may even start spending more time away from home.

To enhance bonding with the baby, make sure your partner gets a chance to help. As a new mother, it may be hard to hand your baby to someone else. Most often, this is because of your own desire to do everything "right." Even so, not letting your partner or family mem-bers help sends the message that you doubt their ability.

Your partner needs to help with the baby now, or risk not learning and feeling more unsure as time goes by. To prevent this, be sure your partner has plenty of chances to hold, care for, and get to know the baby.

It's also vital for you and your partner to spend time alone. Many partners feel left out after a baby arrives. They even may be jealous of the baby for getting what seems to be all of your time, attention, and love.

Try to make time each day to spend together. Once you feel ready to leave the baby with a trusted sitter for an hour or two, make a "date" with each other. Go for a walk, see a movie, or go out to dinner.

Your Other Children

If you have other children, they can react to a new baby in many ways:

➤ They may feel let down that the baby isn't an instant playmate or that he or she is the "wrong" sex.

➤ No matter how well you prepare your children, they may be annoyed that all the baby does is eat, sleep, and cry.

➤ They may be jealous and insecure. As a result, they may try to get your attention by throwing temper tantrums, asking to nurse or be given a bottle, wetting their pants, changing their sleeping or eating patterns, or getting mad at you for paying so much attention to the baby.

➤ They may show anger toward the baby by hitting, biting, or throwing things.

When a new brother or sister comes home from the hospital, it's a perfect time for your partner and family to strengthen their relationship with your other children. Don't send your child to stay with someone else while you settle in at home. No matter how good your intentions, this may send your child the message that you no longer want him or her now that you have the baby. Instead, ask a relative or friend to stay with you and pay extra attention to the baby's brother or sister. Do the following after your baby is born:

➤ Give your child a new doll so he or she has a "baby," too.

➤ Spend time alone with him or her. Do this when the baby is sleeping or when your partner can take over on baby duty. Just 15 minutes per day spent talking, playing, reading, or simply snuggling with you helps remind your child how special he or she is.

➤ Listen to your child and respond to any questions, even if your hands are full with the baby.

➤ Ask your child to help you dress, bathe, feed, or burp the baby. Let a sibling amuse the baby by singing, talking, or making faces. A big brother or sister may want to keep his or her distance from the baby.

Single Mothers

If you are single, having a support network of friends and family is important. You may feel overwhelmed at times. The questions and concerns you have about your baby are not different from those of other mothers. These feelings are normal for all new mothers, single or not.

What is different for you is that you have sole responsibility for decisions that couples often make together. Build ties to be sure you have the help and support you need. Ask a family member or friend to stay with you when you first come home from the hospital. This is when you will be the most tired and often when the new baby is most demanding. You may need someone there during both days and nights for at least the first week—the first month is even better. If you don't have a family member or friend who can stay night and day, ask multiple people to help provide 24-hour coverage.

You may want to join a support group of single mothers. Such a group can give practical advice and also help you realize you are not alone. A single parents' group can deal with concerns you have as a new mother, such as breastfeeding, lack of sleep, and finding child care.

Your Baby's Grandparents

When a grandchild is born, some grandparents hold back. They may want to give new parents some space and not interfere. You may welcome this distance or be hurt by it. If you'd like your parents or in-laws to be more involved, invite them to see the baby. Call and ask how they dealt with a certain problem when they were new parents.

Other grandparents are eager to jump into their new role. They may visit often and give lots of advice. You may be thankful for this or see it as a nuisance. If you feel grandparents have overstayed their welcome, gently tell them that you need time alone as a family and set a date for their return home.

Your parents or in-laws may not approve of something you are doing— such as breastfeeding your baby, picking the baby up when he or she cries, or putting the baby down to sleep on his or her back. Remind them that parenting advice has changed a lot since they had their babies. Assure them you are doing what's best for the baby.

Getting Back in Shape

The demands of being a mother may have left you feeling too tired to exercise. The extra effort is worth it, though. Working out boosts your energy level and your sense of well-being. It also restores muscle strength and helps you get back in shape.

Most women can start working out as soon as they feel up to it (see the box on the following pages for some sample exercises). However, talk to your doctor about when you can get started. If you had a cesarean delivery, a hard birth, or problems after delivery, it may take a little longer to feel ready for exercise. For safety's sake, follow the same guidelines you did for a healthy lifestyle when you were pregnant (see Chapter 4).

If you stayed fit during pregnancy, you'll have a head start. Even so, don't attempt hard workouts right away. If you didn't do much exercise before, take it slowly now. Start with easy exercises and work up to harder ones.

Walking is a very good way to ease back into fitness. Take a brisk walk as

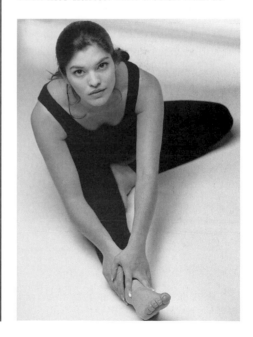

Postpartum Exercises

Leg Slides

This simple exercise tones abdominal and leg muscles. If you had a cesarean birth, it doesn't put much strain on your incision. Try to do leg slides a few times a day.

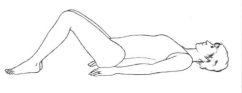

➤ Lie flat on your back and bend your knees slightly.

➤ Inhale and slide your right leg from a bent to a straight position.

➤ Exhale and bend it back again.

➤ Be sure to keep both feet on the floor and keep them relaxed.

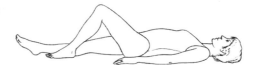

➤ Repeat with your left leg.

Head Lifts

Head lifts can progress to shoulder lifts and curl-ups. These all strengthen the abdominal muscles. When you can do 10 head lifts with ease, move on to shoulder lifts.

➤ Lie on your back with your arms along your sides.

➤ Keep your lower back flat on the floor.

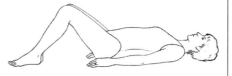

➤ Bend your knees so that your feet are flat on the floor.

➤ Inhale and relax your belly.

➤ Exhale slowly as you lift your head off the floor.

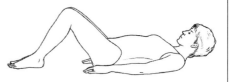

➤ Inhale as you lower your head again.

(continued)

Postpartum Exercises (continued)

Shoulder Lifts

Start this exercise the same way you would start head lifts. When you can do 10 shoulder lifts with ease, move on to curl-ups.

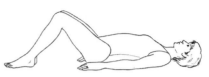

➤ Inhale and relax your belly.

➤ Exhale slowly and lift your head and shoulders off the floor. Reach with your arms so you don't use them for support. If this bothers your neck, place both hands behind your head.

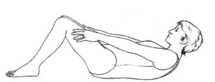

➤ Inhale as you lower your shoulders to the floor.

Curl-Ups

Start this exercise the same way you would start head lifts.

➤ Inhale and relax your belly.

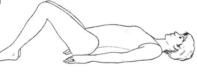

➤ Exhale. Reach with your arms and slowly raise your torso until it's halfway between your knees and the floor (about a 45° angle). If you need more support for your neck and head, place your hands behind your head.

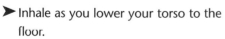

➤ Inhale as you lower your torso to the floor.

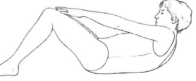

(continued)

Postpartum Exercises (continued)

Kneeling Pelvic Tilt

Tilting your pelvis back toward your spine helps strengthen your abdominal muscles.

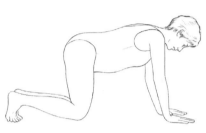

➤ Get on your hands and knees. Your back should be relaxed, not curved or arched.

➤ Inhale.

➤ Exhale and pull your buttocks forward, rotating the pubic bone upward.

➤ Hold for a count of three.

➤ Inhale and relax.

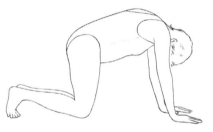

➤ Repeat five times. Add one or two repetitions a day if you can.

Kegel Exercises

Kegel exercises tone your pelvic-floor muscles. This, in turn, controls bladder leaks, helps the perineum heal, and tightens a vagina stretched from birth.

➤ Squeeze the muscles that you use to stop the flow of urine.

➤ Hold for up to 10 seconds, then release.

➤ Do this 10–20 times in a row at least three times a day.

often as you can—every day if possible. This will help prepare you for more intense exercise when you feel up to it. Walking is a great activity. It's easy to do, and you don't need anything except comfortable shoes.

Swimming is another great postpartum exercise. There also are exercise classes designed just for new mothers. To find one, check with local health and fitness clubs, community centers, and hospitals.

No matter what sort of exercise you do, design a program that meets your needs. You may want to strengthen your heart and lungs, tone your muscles, lose weight, or do all three.

Also try to choose a program you'll keep doing. Staying fit over the long haul is more important than getting into shape right after birth. Your doctor can suggest forms of exercise that will help you meet your fitness goals.

Nutrition and Diet

It's common to lose as many as 20 pounds in the month after delivery. It may be tempting to follow up this weight loss with a crash diet so you can squeeze back into your old clothes. Don't—dieting can deny your body vital nutrients and delay healing after birth. If you are nursing, strict dieting will deprive your baby of the calories and nutrients he or she needs. (For details, see "A Healthy Diet" in Chapter 10.)

Instead, try to be patient. Keep up the good eating habits you began in pregnancy. If you do, you'll be close to your normal weight within a few months. Combining healthy eating with exercise will help the process.

Going Back to Work

If, when, and how you go back to work after having a baby are personal choices. Paid maternity-leave policies vary from state to state and employer to employer.

The federal Family and Medical Leave Act (FMLA) guarantees women up to 12 weeks of unpaid leave after giving birth. (For more on the FMLA, see "Your Workplace Rights" in Chapter 4.)

Beyond your recovery from birth, there are other factors to take into account. You have to think about how much money you make and how long your family can do without it. You have to look at the costs of and options for child care, too. If you are breastfeeding, you should give yourself time to establish a good nursing relationship with your baby. You also will want to decide about going on with breastfeeding when you go back to work. (For details, see "Work" in Chapter 10.)

No matter what you choose to do about work, try to discuss it with your boss before the baby is born. Be careful to build in some leeway for yourself. In other words, be sure your employer knows you can't predict for sure what will happen. You can't know how you'll feel about work until after your baby is born. For instance, some women plan to scale back on work or even put their careers on hold for a few years. Then they find that they miss the excitement and self-esteem they get from their jobs. Other women plan to go back to work full-time shortly after giving birth. Once their babies arrive, though, they are less sure about being both a mother and a full-time worker.

Working mothers have a number of options these days. A growing number

Finding Good Child Care

Follow this step-by-step guide to find the right care for your baby:

1. *Gather the facts.* Make a list of childcare providers, family childcare homes, and childcare centers in your area. Then find out the following:

   Where is it located?_____

   Does the provider care for infants? _____

   What hours are available?_____

   Is it open year-round?_____

   What's the policy on sick children?_____

   What's the cost for care?_____

2. *Check it out.* If you are thinking about family home or center care, visit more than once. Make an appointment the first time. If you like what you see during this visit, drop in the next time. (If drop-in visits aren't allowed, keep looking.) Find out:

   Is the facility clean, safe, well-equipped, and child-friendly?_____

   Are there enough care providers (one adult per three to four infants, four to five toddlers, or six to nine preschoolers)?_____

   Are the caregivers attentive and loving?_____

   How is discipline handled?_____

   Do the children seem happy and well cared for?_____

   What's a normal day like?_____

   What's served at meal and snack times?_____

3. *Set up an interview.* Schedule a chat with a family childcare provider, nanny, or center director. Have your baby with you and note how the caregiver responds to him or her. Ask the following:

   What experience and training do the care providers have? _____
   _____

   Have they cared for infants before? _____

(continued)

Finding Good Child Care (continued)

Why did they go into this line of work? _____

How long do they plan to stay in it? _____

What do they like most—and least—about caring for children? _____
_____

What's their philosophy on caring for and disciplining children? _____
_____

For an individual caregiver, why did she leave her last job? _____
_____

For a center, what's the staff turnover rate?_____

Do babies at a center have one main caregiver or do a number of caregivers take care of the babies? _____

Do the care providers have training in first-aid and CPR?_____

Are they willing to give your child prescribed medications?_____

What plans are in place in case of a medical emergency?_____

If you are nursing, how do they feel about handling pumped breast milk?
_____

Is the home or center licensed, or is the caregiver certified?_____

4. *Check credentials.* Never leave your baby with someone until you have checked out his or her background. Ask for the following:

   ➤The document showing that the home or center is licensed or registered or that the caregiver is certified; call the licensing agency to ask about any complaints

   ➤Written policies on philosophy, procedures, or discipline

   ➤References from other parents who have used the caregiver, home, or center; call at least three other parents

5. *Try it out.* Once you have chosen a caregiver, do a few "practice" runs before you go back to work. This way, if anything strikes you as being "off," you still have time to keep looking. It also will help you and your baby get used to the setup before your maternity leave ends.

of employers let new mothers work part-time, work from home 1 or 2 days a week, job share, condense their work weeks, or work flexible hours. Also, some companies offer onsite childcare. This is a real bonus for new mothers—they can bring their babies to work with them and visit them during breaks and lunch hours.

There are three basic options to finding good child care: 1) your baby can be cared for in your home, 2) in a caregiver's home, or 3) in a child care center. If you want to hire someone to care for your baby in your home, contact agencies that focus on child care placements. Keep in mind that this type of care is very costly. To cut costs, some parents share a caregiver with another family. The caregiver in these "share-care" setups is paid to watch two babies in one family's home.

A less costly option is having a relative or a licensed provider care for your baby in their home. In most cases, these caregivers watch more than one child.

Child care centers are yet another option. This type of setting may take care of many groups of children of all different ages. Some accept babies as young as 6 weeks and some do not take infants until they are out of diapers, so check ahead of time.

No matter which option you'd like to pursue, be sure to start your search early even while you are still pregnant. Ask around: your pediatrician, friends, neighbors, and coworkers are all good sources of information on child care. Also check with parents' centers and your local child care resource and referral agency (listed in the phone book). The box on the previous pages also has tips on how to find good child care.

Sex After Birth

Your doctor will tell you when you can resume having sex. It likely will be a month or so after delivery. After giving birth, you may find that you don't have much interest in sex. There are many reasons for this:

➤ *Fatigue.* Once you get your baby to sleep, all you or your partner may want to do is sleep, too.

➤ *Stress.* Coping with your baby's demands can leave you with little desire for sex.

➤ *Fear of pain.* Your breasts may be tender and your perineum may be sore. If you are breastfeeding, low estrogen levels may make your vagina dry. This can make sex uncomfortable.

➤ *Lack of desire.* Hormone levels decrease after birth. As a result, so does your desire for sex.

➤ *Lack of opportunity.* Sex takes energy, time, and focus. When you are a new parent, these all tend to be in short supply.

Even if you want to have sex, wait until the healing process is complete to avoid hurting fragile tissues. It is fine to resume sex as soon as you feel comfortable. Most often, this takes at least 4 weeks. Make sure your partner understands this, too. Do the following when you feel ready to start having sex again:

➤ Spend private time with your partner. Talk about yourself and each other instead of the baby or the household.

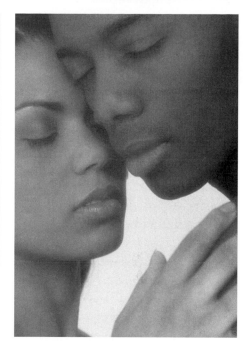

➤ Get in the mood. Find a time for sex when you are not rushed. Wait until the baby is sound asleep or you can drop him or her off with a friend or a relative for a couple of hours.

➤ Proceed slowly and gently. Start with a soothing massage. Try foreplay. Be sure to tell your partner what does— and doesn't—feel good.

➤ Use a lubricant. Your vagina may be less moist than normal, especially while breastfeeding. A water-soluble cream or jelly will help. If the problem persists, see your doctor.

➤ Try different positions. You may find that side-lying or kneeling on top of your partner gives you more control and freedom of movement, for instance. This can help you relax and can aid arousal.

➤ Try other approaches. There are numerous ways to give and receive sexual pleasure. If sex isn't comfort-able yet, try mutual masturbation or oral sex.

➤ Talk about it. If you have concerns about sexual problems, discuss them with your partner. This will help both of you avoid frustration and hurt feelings.

Family Planning

If you and your partner are ready to start having sex again, it is vital to start thinking about post-delivery birth control. Birth control can allow your body to heal before having another baby and allow you to plan your family.

Even if you want your children to be close in age, it's best to wait at least 18 months before getting pregnant again.

It is believed that babies conceived less than 6 months (or more than 10 years) after you give birth have a higher risk of preterm birth, low birth weight, and small size. Babies born soon after their siblings may have these problems because the mother's body has not had time to replace nutritional stores. Postpartum stress also is a factor. It is unclear why the longer time between pregnancies may affect fetal health. Of course, each family has different needs and desires when it comes to child spacing. Discuss the issue with your partner and your doctor.

If you are not breastfeeding, you can be fertile within weeks of giving birth. If you are breastfeeding, it can be hard to tell when fertility returns. Keep in mind, too, that if you used fertility drugs to conceive your first baby, it doesn't mean you can't get pregnant without them.

To be on the safe side, choose a form of birth control before you have sex for the first time, even if you are breastfeeding. Breastfeeding is only a temporary method of birth control and is effective only under certain conditions (see Chapter 10 for more details). Today, there's a wide array of birth control methods for both women and men. Each has pros and cons. Before choosing one, talk about it with your partner and your doctor. That way, you are more likely to choose birth control that best meets your needs. Some questions to ask:

➤ How well does the method work?

➤ How safe is it for your body (and, if you are nursing, for your baby)?

➤ How easy is it to use?

➤ How convenient is it (will you need to plan in advance or put sex on hold for a few minutes to use a certain method)?

➤ Will it prevent sexually transmitted diseases (STDs) as well as pregnancy?

➤ What are the side effects?

➤ How much does it cost?

➤ Is it permanent?

Any method of birth control can do a good job of preventing pregnancy if it's used the right way and used all the time. You may find that one form of birth control suits your needs at a given time better than others.

That's why you shouldn't just start using your old birth control method after your baby is born. Certain types of birth control may interfere with breastfeeding. (For details on using birth control during breastfeeding, see "Birth Control" in Chapter 10.) Birth control pills, hormone injections every 3 months, and the *intrauterine device (IUD)* are among the most effective methods. They also leave you the option of having more children later.

Used the right way, these methods give you constant protection from pregnancy. You don't have to do anything special when you want to have sex. Surgical sterilization also offers constant protection. However, you must be sure you don't want any more children.

Hormones

Hormonal birth control works by preventing ovulation. When there's no egg to fertilize, you can't get pregnant. You still have your period each month with some types of hormonal birth control. There are four main types of hormonal contraception:

1. *Birth control pills.* **Oral contraceptives** are the most common method of hormonal birth control. Taken as directed, the pill also is one of the most effective forms of birth control. Combination pills contain man-made estrogen and progesterone. If you are breastfeeding, estrogen can cut down on your milk supply. As a result, combination pills should not be used until milk flow is steady. This occurs about 3 months after delivery. Until then, use other methods that do not contain estrogen. Minipills

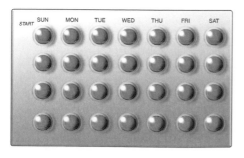

contain progestin only. They are a better choice if you are breastfeeding because there is no estrogen to affect the milk supply. The dose of progestin is even lower than that found in low-dose birth control pills. Unlike other birth control pills, each pack consists of 28 tablets of active hormone. Minipills can be used by some women who cannot take estrogen.

2. *Injections.* This is another easy method to use. Each injection provides birth control for 3 months. You need four injections per year. As long as your injections are up-to-date, you don't have to do anything else to prevent pregnancy. Injections without estrogen may be used if you are breastfeeding.

3. *Skin patch.* A contraceptive patch is small—about 1¾ square inches—and sticks to your skin. It releases estrogen and progestin through your skin. You put a new patch on every week for 3 weeks each month. During the fourth week, you have your period.

4. *Vaginal ring.* This is a flexible, plastic ring that you place in your upper vagina. It releases both estrogen and progestin. You insert the ring and leave it in for 21 days, then take it out for 7 days. During the week it is out, you have your period.

Intrauterine Device

The IUD is a small plastic device that contains copper or hormones. It's inserted into the uterus by a doctor. The copper or hormones in the IUD prevent an egg from being fertilized or prevent a fertilized egg from implanting in the uterus.

Both types of IUDs are T-shaped, but they work in different ways. The hormonal IUD releases a small amount of progesterone into the uterus. The copper IUD releases a small amount of copper in the uterus. A hormonal IUD must be replaced each year. A copper IUD can stay in place for up to 10 years. It also may be used while a woman is breastfeeding. Both types of IUDs can be removed if you want to get pregnant or switch to another form of birth control.

The IUD is simple to use. You don't need to do anything else to prevent pregnancy once it's in place. It's also very effective. However, the IUD may not be the best choice for women who have more than one sex partner.

Barrier Methods

Barrier methods include a spermicide, diaphragm, cervical cap, sponge, and male and female condom. They work by keeping sperm from getting to the egg.

➤ *Spermicides.* These are chemicals that kill sperm. They are contained in various forms: creams, jellies, foams, and vaginal inserts and suppositories. Before sex, you place the substance containing the spermicide in your vagina, close to the cervix.

➤ *The diaphragm.* This is a round rubber dome that you insert before sex. It fits inside your vagina and covers your cervix. If you used a diaphragm before, you must be refitted after giving birth.

➤ *The cervical cap.* This is a small rubber cup that fits over your cervix. It stays in place with suction. If you used a cervical cap before, you must be refitted after giving birth to your baby.

➤ *The male condom* This is a thin sheath worn over a man's penis. It is made of latex (or, less often, animal membrane). Latex condoms also help prevent STDs.

➤ *The female condom.* This is a plastic pouch that lines the vagina. It is held in place by a closed inner ring at the cervix and an open outer ring at the entrance of the vagina. Female condoms may help prevent STDs.

➤ *The Lea's Shield.* This dome-shaped, silicon device with a loop for removal fits inside the vagina and covers the cervix. It does not prevent STDs.

If you choose a barrier method, be sure to use it each time you have sex. To further reduce your chances of getting pregnant, use spermicide with a diaphragm, cervical cap, or condoms.

Natural Family Planning

Natural family planning also is called "periodic abstinence" or "the rhythm method." It involves not having sex during the days of the month that you are most fertile.

To prevent pregnancy, you must know when you ovulate. You can predict ovulation by watching for changes in your body temperature or cervical mucus or by charting your menstrual cycle. For best results, it's a good idea to combine all three of these methods. Ovulation predictor kits also are available. Menstrual cycles often aren't regular after childbirth and during breastfeeding. Thus, natural family planning may not work well for new mothers.

Sterilization

Sterilization is an option if both you and your partner are sure you want this baby to be your last. Sterilization is more than 99% effective, and, in most cases, it's permanent. Talk to your doctor about it well ahead of time if you think you want to be sterilized after giving birth to your baby. It usually is done within 1–2 days of birth.

Sterilization is done by surgery. General or local anesthesia is used. As with any surgery, sterilization has some risks. Serious complications, such as infection or bleeding, occur in about 1 in 1,000 women who have the operation. Most of the time, these problems can be treated and corrected.

Female sterilization is called tubal ligation. It is commonly known as "getting your tubes tied." It does not affect either partner's ability to have or enjoy sex. It closes the fallopian tubes and stops the egg from going from the ovary

Female Sterilization

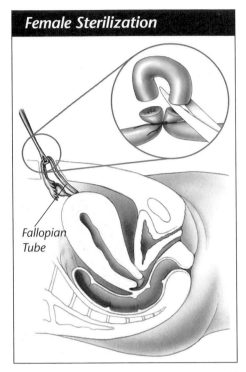

Fallopian Tube

During postpartum sterilization, a small vertical or horizontal cut is made near the navel, and each fallopian tube is pulled through the incision. A section of the tube is closed off, and the section between the ties is removed.

to the uterus. It also blocks sperm from reaching an egg. In a tubal ligation, fallopian tubes are cut, cauterized (burned), or blocked with bands or clips. Tubal ligation won't affect your periods or your pleasure of sex.

Male sterilization is called **vasectomy**. It involves cutting or tying the vas deferens (tubes through which sperm travel). This means no sperm is released when a man ejaculates. Vasectomy does not affect a man's ability to get erections or have orgasms.

Both types of sterilization can be done at any time. In most cases, the surgery is done so the patient can go home the same day. Some women choose to get sterilized right after their babies are born, while they are still in the hospital. The surgery is easier then because the uterus is still enlarged and pushes the fallopian tubes up in the abdomen. The doctor can grasp them easily through a small cut near the navel. The tubes are then tied or cut. If you want to be sterilized after giving birth to your baby, talk to your doctor about it well ahead of time. In some cases, it can be done a few minutes after the birth, with the same anesthesia used for the delivery.

Male Sterilization

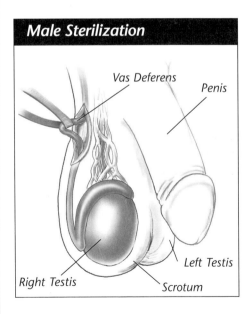

Vas Deferens

Penis

Right Testis

Left Testis

Scrotum

During a vasectomy, one or two small cuts are made in the skin of the scrotum. Each vas is pulled through the opening until it forms a loop. A small section is cut out of the loop and removed.

You should be certain that you won't change your mind about having more children later. Although there is surgery to reverse sterilization, it doesn't always work. Also, the operation to reverse sterilization is major surgery. Most insurance plans won't cover it.

Emergency Contraception

What if you and your partner have sex before you have settled on a birth control method? Or, in the rush to make use of your baby's half-hour nap, you forget contraception one time? Talk to your doctor right away about emergency contraception. This is even more vital if your period has returned or you are not breastfeeding and you don't want to become pregnant.

Emergency contraception is a high dose of birth control pills taken within 72 hours of sex. It is followed by a second dose 12 hours later. This lowers the odds of getting pregnant by about 75 percent. Your doctor also can insert an IUD after unprotected sex to help prevent pregnancy.

These methods work by preventing ovulation, blocking fertilization, or keeping a fertilized egg from implanting in the uterus. There are two types of emergency contraceptive pills. One type is combined oral contraceptives—birth control pills that contain the hormones estrogen and progestin. The other type uses only one of the hormones—progestin. Your doctor may prescribe a combination of regular birth control pills or a package with two pills.

After taking emergency birth control pills, you may feel sick to your stomach for 1 or 2 days. Your belly also may feel bloated and your breasts may feel tender. Your next period may be earlier or later than you expect. If you don't get your period within 3 weeks, take a home pregnancy test.

Your Follow-up Visit

Arrange a visit to see your doctor 4–6 weeks after your baby's birth. (If you had a cesarean birth, the doctor may want to see you about 2 weeks after surgery to check the incision.) The goal of this checkup is to make sure that your body has recovered from pregnancy and birth and that you are not having any problems.

During the visit, the doctor will check your weight, blood pressure, breasts, and abdomen. He or she also will do a pelvic exam to make sure a tear or episiotomy has healed and that your vagina, cervix, and uterus have returned to their normal state.

Use this time to bring up any questions or concerns you have about the healing process, breastfeeding, birth control, weight loss, sex, or your emotions. To help you remember everything to talk about, jot down any questions you have and bring them with you to this visit.

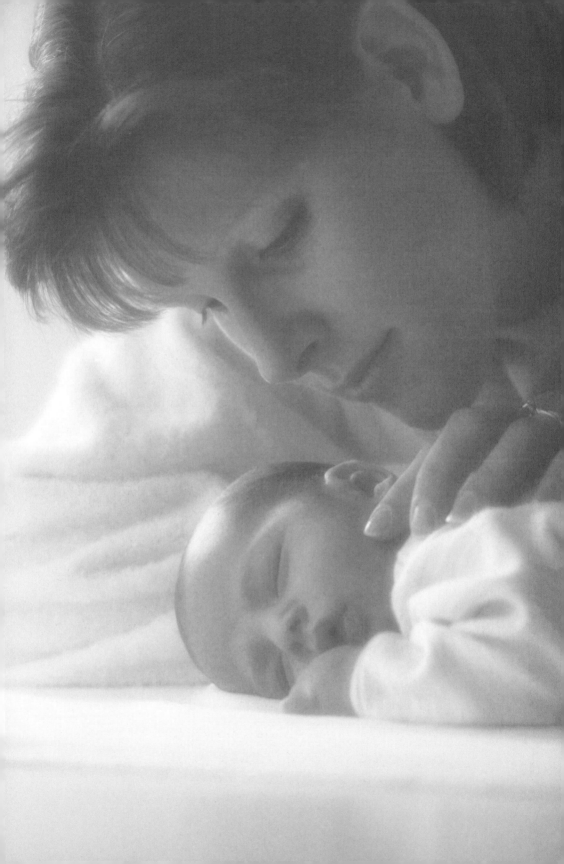

Special Care

Most of the time, pregnancy goes the way it should: the mother is healthy, the fetus grows normally, and the childbirth is a happy and trouble-free event. Sometimes, however, problems can arise that require special attention.

A mother or father may pass an inherited disorder to the baby. A baby may not develop the way it should. A woman may have a health condition—or develop one during pregnancy—that puts her and her baby at risk. Complications can arise as a result of the pregnancy itself.

In some of these cases, close monitoring and treatment can help prevent problems or make them less severe. That is why getting early and regular prenatal care is so vital to having a healthy baby.

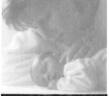

CHAPTER **13**

Genetic Disorders
and **Birth Defects**

Almost every mother-to-be worries about her baby having a problem. Most of the time, this worry is needless. Almost all children in the United States are born healthy. Out of 100 newborns, only two or three have major birth defects. Birth defects may affect the baby's health, or his or her ability to function. Some can be prevented, and many can be treated or corrected with medication or surgery.

Some birth defects are passed from parent to child. Just as a baby gets hair and eye color from his or her parents, the baby can inherit certain diseases or conditions. Other birth defects result from being exposed to harmful things during pregnancy. Sometimes, a mixture of inheritance and exposure during pregnancy is the cause. In many cases, the reason for a defect isn't known.

Many birth defects can be seen right away. A defect that's present at birth—

no matter when it is diagnosed—is called a ***congenital disorder***. A congenital disorder may or may not be inherited. There are many types of birth defects, and they can range from mild to severe. Some can be detected in advance, and others occur without warning. There are no tests to detect many disorders.

Many babies with birth defects are born to couples with no known risk factors. However, the chance of having a baby with a birth defect is greater when the parents have certain risk factors. Before pregnancy or during prenatal care, some tests are offered to check the parents' risks for having a baby with certain defects. The results of these tests, along with genetic counseling, will let parents know about their risk of having a baby with a problem.

Being tested is a personal choice. Some couples choose not to be tested for birth defects. Others find that testing and counseling can help them make decisions and consider options.

Chromosomes and Genes

Genetics is the branch of science that deals with how traits are passed from parent to child through *genes*, which are in *chromosomes*. A man's sperm and a woman's egg each have 23 chromosomes. All other cells in the body have 46. When an egg and a sperm join, the 23 chromosomes from the mother's egg and the 23 chromosomes from the father's sperm pair up. The fertilized egg then becomes a cell with 46 chromosomes. This cell multiplies to create the baby.

Whether a baby is a boy or girl is determined by a pair of chromosomes called the sex chromosomes. The baby gets one from the mother's egg and one from the father's sperm. The egg always has an X chromosome. The sperm can have either an X or a Y chromosome. Thus, the baby always gets an X chromosome from the mother, and either an X or Y from the father. A combination of XY sex chromosomes creates a male. An XX combination creates a female. So, it is the sex chromosome in the father's sperm that determines the sex of the child.

Each chromosome contains many genes. When the chromosomes pair up to create a baby, the genes also pair up. Each gene pair controls a certain characteristic, called a "trait," such as height or hair color. Some traits are controlled by a single gene pair. Other traits—including skin color, hair color, and height—are the result of many pairs of genes working together.

Some genes are dominant and some are recessive. In a gene pair, the dominant gene overrides the recessive gene. For a recessive trait to show up in the baby, both genes in a pair must be recessive. Disorders, like other traits, can be created by recessive and dominant genes.

Genetic Disorders

Genetic defects fall into 1 of 3 categories: 1) inherited (single gene), 2) chromosomal (many genes), and 3) multifactorial (combination of genes and environment). Aspects of some of the most common genetic disorders are listed at the end of the chapter. Some of these disorders can be detected before or during pregnancy.

Inherited Disorders

An inherited disorder is caused by a gene that is passed from parent to child. These disorders can be dominant, recessive, or X-linked.

Dominant Disorders

A dominant disorder is caused by just one gene from either parent. Some dominant disorders are common and not serious. Others are rare, but can be life-threatening. If one parent has the gene, each child of the couple has a 1-in-2 (50%) chance of inheriting the disorder. Two examples of dominant disorders are Huntington's disease and *polydactyly.*

Recessive Disorders

For recessive disorders, both parents must have the gene before the problem will occur in their child. Everybody carries a few abnormal recessive genes. Most of the time, these don't cause a problem. That is because the normal genes override the abnormal genes. A person who has a recessive gene for a certain disorder is a *carrier* for that disorder. Although that person may show no signs of the disorder, it can be passed on to his or her children.

If both parents are carriers of the same recessive disorder, each of the children has a 1-in-4 (25%) chance of having the disorder. If one parent has the disorder and the other doesn't (and isn't a carrier), the children will be carriers. Bloom syndrome, Tay-Sachs disease, *cystic fibrosis*, and sickle-cell disease are examples of recessive disorders that are more common in certain ethnic groups. For each disorder, both parents must have the gene for the baby to be born with the disorder.

X-Linked Disorders

Disorders that are caused by genes on the X chromosome are called "X-linked" or "sex-linked" disorders. In most X-linked disorders, the abnormal gene is recessive. When an X-linked disorder is caused by a recessive gene, a woman can carry the gene but usually does not have that disorder. That's because she has two sex chromosomes (XX) (see "Chromosomes and Genes"). If she is a carrier, one of her X chromosomes has the recessive disorder, but her other X chromosome has the normal gene, which overrides the abnormal gene. So she is either not affected or has only a slight effect from the disorder.

A male baby inherits an X chromosome from his mother and a Y chromosome from his father. If he inherits the X chromosome with the disorder, he gets the disorder. That's because he doesn't have another X chromosome with a normal gene to cancel out the one with the disorder.

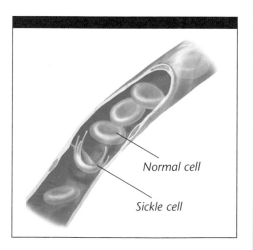

Normal cell

Sickle cell

The red blood cells of a person with sickle cell disease are shaped like a crescent (or a "sickle"). Normal red blood cells are circular.

If a women is a carrier for an X-linked disorder and the father of the baby doesn't have the disorder, there is a 1-in-2 (50%) chance a son will have the disorder and a daughter will be a carrier. Very rarely, a daughter has an X-linked recessive disorder. In this case, her father has the disease and her mother is a carrier, and the daughter receives the abnormal gene from both parents. Genetic testing sometimes can show if a woman is a carrier of an X-linked disorder or if the fetus is affected. Examples of X-linked disorders are hemophilia and *fragile X syndrome.*

Chromosomal Disorders

A chromosomal disorder, such as **Down syndrome**, can be caused by a missing, damaged, or extra chromosome. Chromosomal problems are rarely inherited. Instead, they usually are caused by an error that occurs when the egg and sperm are joining. Extra, missing, or incomplete chromosomes often cause severe health problems. Most children with chromosomal disorders have physical defects and some have mental defects. Two examples of chromosomal disorders are Down syndrome and trisomy 18.

The risk of having a child with a chromosomal disorder increases as a woman ages (see Table 13–1). For instance, a 35-year-old woman has a 1-in-192 (less than 1%) chance of having a baby with a chromosomal disorder. The chance increases to 1 in 66 (about 1.5%) in a woman 40 years old.

Table 13–1. How Common Are Chromosomal Disorders?

Chromosomal disorders occur when there are too few or too many chromosomes. The table shows your risk of having a baby with Down syndrome or any chromosomal disorder. Your risk is based on your age.

Mother's Age	Risk of Down Syndrome	Risk of Any Chromosomal Disorder
20	1/1,667	1/526
25	1/1,250	1/476
30	1/952	1/385
35	1/378	1/192
36	1/289	1/156
37	1/224	1/127
38	1/173	1/102
39	1/136	1/83
40	1/106	1/66
41	1/82	1/53
42	1/63	1/42
43	1/49	1/33
44	1/38	1/26
45	1/30	1/21

Modified from Hook EB, Cross PK, Schreinemachers DM. Chromosomal abnormality rates at amniocentesis and in live-born infants. JAMA 1983;249:2034–2038 (ages 33–49), copyright 1983, American Medical Association; Hook EB. Rates of chromosome abnormalities at different maternal ages. Reprinted with permission from the American College of Obstetricians and Gynecologists (Obstetrics and Gynecology 1981;58:282–285).

Multifactorial Disorders

Multifactorial disorders are disorders that are thought to come from a mix of genetic and environmental factors. The actual cause is unknown. Some of these disorders can be detected during pregnancy. They often can be treated with surgery. Examples of multifactorial disorders are *cleft palate*, clubfoot, abdominal wall defects, and neural tube defects. These are defects that result when the coverings over the spinal cord or brain do not close properly. Neural tube defects include *spina bifida* and *anencephaly*.

Birth Defects

Birth defects are caused by an error in the way the bone, brain, skin, or tissue developed. They may affect how the body looks, works, or both. Heart defects are the most common type of birth defect. About 1 in 125 babies is born with a heart defect. Many birth defects are mild, but some can be severe and even cause death. Babies with birth defects may need surgery or other medical treatments.

There are many different types of birth defects. They can be genetic or inherited or caused by the fetus being exposed to a harmful agent. For instance, some birth defects can occur if the woman gets certain infections, drinks alcohol, or takes certain medications during pregnancy. Birth defects also can be caused by exposure to toxic substances such as mercury or lead. In some cases, they are caused by a combination of things. For about 70% of babies born with birth defects, the cause is not known. See Chapter 17 for details about infections during pregnancy. Chapter 5 covers birth defects that can be caused by drugs, alcohol, or poor nutrition.

Some birth defects can be prevented and others can be found during pregnancy. Most birth defects occur during the first 3 months of pregnancy, but some do not appear until later in life. Prenatal tests can be done to detect certain birth defects. Some are offered based on risk factors, and others are offered to all women.

Are You at Risk?

Many babies with birth defects are born to couples with no risk factors. However, the risk of birth defects is higher when certain factors are present:

➤ Age 35 years or older when the baby is due

➤ Family or personal history of birth defects

➤ Previous child with a birth defect

➤ Use of certain medicines around the time of conception

➤ Diabetes before pregnancy

When you have your pre-pregnancy checkup or start prenatal care, your doctor may give you a list of questions to find risk factors. Your answers to these questions will help your doctor advise you on your risk of having a baby with a genetic defect.

Risk Factors for Genetic Disorders

Answer the following questions about risk factors. If you answer "yes" to any of them, you may be at increased risk for having a baby with a genetic disorder:

___ Will you be age 35 years or older when your baby is due?

___ Will the baby's father be age 50 years or older when your baby is due?

___ If you or the baby's father are of Mediterranean or Asian descent, do either of you or anyone in your families have thalassemia?

___ Is there a family history of neural tube defects?

___ Have you or the baby's father ever had a child with a neural tube defect?

___ Is there a family history of congenital heart defects?

___ Is there a family history of Down syndrome?

___ Have you or the baby's father ever had a child with Down syndrome?

___ If you or the baby's father are of Eastern European Jewish, French Canadian, or Cajun descent, is there a family history of Tay–Sachs disease?

___ If you or your partner are of Eastern European Jewish descent, is there a family history of Canavan disease or any other genetic disorders?

___ If you or your partner are African American, is there a family history of sickle cell disease or sickle cell trait?

___ Is there a family history of hemophilia?

___ Is there a family history of muscular dystrophy?

___ Is there a family history of cystic fibrosis?

___ Is there a family history of Huntington's disease?

___ Does anyone in your family or the family of the baby's father have cystic fibrosis?

___ Is anyone in your family or the baby's father's family mentally retarded?

___ If so, was that person tested for fragile X syndrome?

___ Do you, the baby's father, anyone in your families, or any of your children have any other genetic diseases, chromosomal disorders, or birth defects?

___ Do you have a metabolic disorder such as diabetes or phenylketonuria?

___ Do you have a history of pregnancy issues (miscarriage or stillbirth)?

If you are in a high-risk group, you may be offered carrier testing, which can be done before, after, or during pregnancy. You also may have tests during pregnancy to detect your risk of a problem or to diagnose it. Some tests for birth defects are offered to all pregnant women. Others may be offered if your medical history, family history, or physical exam raises concerns about your baby's health.

Carrier Testing

Carrier testing of both parents will detect if either parent is a carrier of a certain genetic defect. All women may be informed about carrier screening for cystic fibrosis. Other screening tests can be done if your family history, ethnic origin, or other factors increase your risk of being a carrier. Unfortunately, there are no carrier screening tests for most inherited birth defects.

For the test, a sample of blood or saliva is studied in a lab to detect a defective gene for a certain inherited disorder. Your doctor or genetic counselor will help you understand the chances of the defect being passed on to your baby. If the carrier screening is done before you are pregnant, you can use the results to decide if you want to get pregnant. If the screening is done after you are pregnant, for some disorders, the baby can then be tested for the defect.

Screening Tests

Screening tests are offered to all pregnant women, even when there are no symptoms or known risk factors. However, a screening test only shows there is an increased risk that a defect will occur. Based on the results of the screening test, further tests may be done to check the baby's health. Some of the common problems found through screening tests include neural tube defects, abdominal wall defects, heart defects, Down syndrome, and trisomy 18.

A test result could be positive (showing there is a risk of a problem) even though the baby is healthy. Likewise, a birth defect can occur even if the test results do not show a problem. Most tests focus on a certain problem, and not all disorders can be found by testing. A genetic counselor can explain the test results and what they mean.

Maternal Serum Screening

Tests of maternal serum (blood) are done during pregnancy to detect a higher-than-normal risk of having a baby with certain birth defects. With *maternal serum screening*, several tests often are performed together. This is known as the "multiple marker screening." These tests measure the level of the following three or four substances in woman's blood:

1. *Estriol.* Estriol is a hormone made by the woman, placenta, and the baby.

2. *Human chorionic gonadotropin (hCG).* This is a hormone made by the placenta.

3. ***Alpha-fetoprotein (AFP).*** Alpha-fetoprotein is a substance made by the baby, a small amount of which crosses the placenta and enters the mother's blood.

4. *Inhibin-A.* This is a hormone produced by the placenta.

With maternal serum screening, a sample of blood is tested. This usually is done between 15 and 20 weeks of pregnancy. The timing of the test is important because certain levels can only provide an accurate reading at a specific point in pregnancy. For instance, a high AFP level can simply mean a woman is further along in pregnancy than she thought or that she is carrying more than one baby.

Tests results can be combined to determine the risk of certain disorders (Table 13–2). The test results show if there is an increased risk for neural tube defects, Down syndrome, trisomy 18, or abdominal wall defects. If the results are not in the normal range, further testing may be needed.

An abnormal result, while alarming, only signals a possible problem. In most cases the baby is healthy even if there is an abnormal blood test result. In some cases, abnormal levels can be explained with an ultrasound exam.

Combined Screening

A screening test that combines the results of a special ultrasound test and blood (serum) tests is called "combined screening." It can be done between 10 and 14 weeks of pregnancy to detect signs of Down syndrome, trisomy 18, and heart defects. This type of screening is fairly new and is not done everywhere.

The ultrasound test is called ***nuchal translucency screening***. This test uses ultrasound to measure the thickness on the back of the neck of the fetus. A thickening may be a sign of Down syndrome.

The serum test measures the level of two substances in the mother's blood:

Table 13–2. Maternal Serum Screening Test Results

Birth defect	Level of Substance in Maternal Serum			
	Estriol	hCG	Inhibin-A	AFP
Neural tube defect or abdominal wall defect	Normal	Normal	Normal	High
Down syndrome	Low	High	High	Low
Trisomy 18	Low	Low	Normal	Low

Abbreviations: hCG, human chorionic gonadotropin; AFP, alpha-fetoprotein pregnancy-associated plasma protein-A (PAPP-A) and free-beta human chorionic gonadotropin (hCG). The combined results of the nuchal translucency screening and the serum screening levels show if the fetus might have a defect. If the results show there is an increased risk of a birth defect, further testing can be done.

If the nuchal translucency test shows increased thickness, but the combined screening does not show a risk of a Down syndrome or trisomy 18, there could be a heart defect. To check on this, a detailed exam of the fetal heart can be done.

Diagnostic Tests

If a screening test or other factors raise concerns about the baby, further tests often are done to diagnose certain birth defects. Diagnostic tests include a detailed ultrasound exam, amniocentesis, and chorionic villus sampling.

Detailed Ultrasound Exam

A detailed ultrasound exam may be done if there is a family history showing risks for birth defects. It also may be done if there is an abnormal result from a screening test. The results of the ultrasound exam can help explain abnormal results and provide more information. This type of exam may need to be done in a special center equipped to perform them. (See Chapter 3 for more information about ultrasound.)

A detailed ultrasound exam can show some birth defects. If heart problems are suspected in the fetus, a fetal echocardiogram also may be done to examine the baby's heart in more detail. In some cases, other diagnostic tests are needed to provide more information.

Amniocentesis

Most often, *amniocentesis* is performed at 15–20 weeks of pregnancy. To perform the procedure, a doctor guides a thin needle through the abdomen and uterus. A small sample of amniotic fluid is withdrawn and sent to a lab.

In the lab, cells that have been shed from the baby are grown in a special culture. This can take up to 3 weeks. Next, the chromosomes in these cells are studied under a microscope. This shows if there is an extra chromosome (as in Down syndrome). It also can show if there are other chromosomal defects. Testing the AFP level in the amniotic fluid can help determine if the fetus has a neural tube defect.

If there is a risk for a certain disorder such as cystic fibrosis or muscular dystrophy the fetal cells can be studied to see if the baby will have these conditions. However, such testing is done only if a genetic history or carrier screening test suggests a risk for the single gene disorder.

Complications from amniocentesis are rare. Side effects may include cramping, vaginal bleeding, and leaking

Amniocentesis

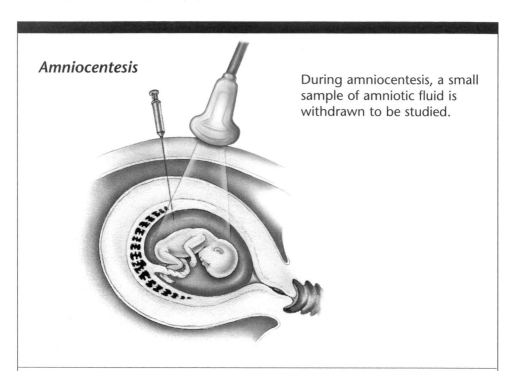

During amniocentesis, a small sample of amniotic fluid is withdrawn to be studied.

Chorionic Villus Sampling

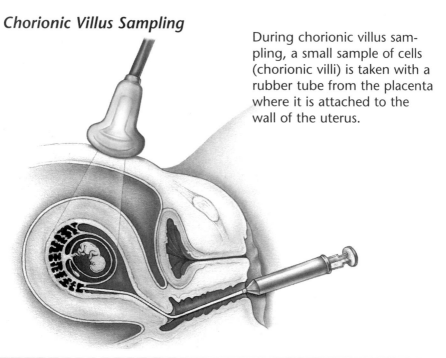

During chorionic villus sampling, a small sample of cells (chorionic villi) is taken with a rubber tube from the placenta where it is attached to the wall of the uterus.

of amniotic fluid. Very rarely, the fetus is injured. There is a slight chance of miscarriage (about 0.5%) as a result of amniocentesis.

Chorionic Villus Sampling

Chorionic villus sampling (CVS) detects some of the same chromosomal problems that amniocentesis does. It can be performed earlier than amniocentesis—often at 10–12 weeks of pregnancy.

To perform CVS, a doctor guides either a small tube through the vagina and cervix or a thin needle through the abdomen and uterine wall. The doctor then takes a small sample of chorionic villi from the placenta. Chorionic villi (the plural of villus) are tiny, finger-like projections of placental tissue. Villi come from the same fertilized egg as the fetus. This means they have the same genetic makeup.

The villi are sent to a lab, where they are grown in a culture. This can take up to 3 weeks. Chromosomes from the villi then are studied under a microscope to check for chromosomal or other defects.

Chorionic villus sampling carries some risks. There is a small chance (about 1%), for instance, that the test will cause miscarriage.

Fetal Blood Sampling

Cordocentesis, also called fetal blood sampling, is used to test for chromosomal defects and other abnormalities. At 18 weeks of pregnancy or later, blood is taken from a vein in the umbilical cord. Fetal blood sampling usually is used when the results of amniocentesis, chorionic villus sampling, or ultrasound are unclear. As with amniocentesis, possible effects from this procedure are infection, cramping, and bleeding. The miscarriage rate after cordocentesis is about 1–2%.

Genetic Counseling

Genetic counseling can help a couple assess their risk of having a baby with a genetic disorder, decide whether to be tested, and consider their options. A genetic counselor has special training in genetics. He or she can offer expert advice on types of genetic disorders and how they affect babies born with them.

The genetic counselor will ask a couple for a detailed family history. If a family member has a problem, the counselor may ask to see that person's medical records. He or she also may refer the woman or her partner for physical exams, blood tests, or prenatal tests. Using all the information gathered, the counselor will try to figure out the baby's risk of having a problem. The counselor then will explain and discuss the options.

Whether to have genetic testing is up to a woman and her partner. Some people would rather not know if they are at risk for having a child with a problem.

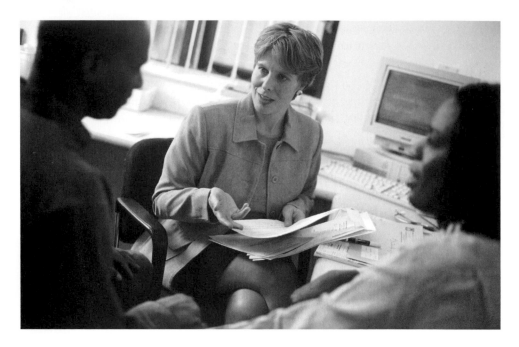

Even so, there are benefits to finding out:

➤ If a woman is tested before trying to conceive, the results can help her decide whether to become pregnant. If she learns that she has a strong chance of having a child with a birth defect, she can explore other options for starting a family, such as adopting a child, or being artificially inseminated with sperm from a donor. She also may choose to have a donated egg fertilized by her partner's sperm and implanted in her uterus. Using a technique called preimplantation genetic diagnosis, the embryo can be tested before it is implanted in the uterus so that only unaffected embryos will be transferred.

➤ The test results can provide information that will help other family members. Siblings and other relatives who may want to have children of their own someday can benefit from the knowledge that the family has the gene for a certain disorder.

➤ Testing can help a woman prepare for the birth of a child with special needs. She can learn about the effects of the disorder, line up special medical care for her baby, and seek out others for support.

➤ Testing for birth defects during pregnancy can help a woman decide whether to continue her pregnancy. If she finds out her baby has a severe problem, she has the option to end the pregnancy, depending on how far along she is in the pregnancy.

Most often the test results will reveal that the baby is normal. If test results show that the baby may have a birth defect, learn the facts and talk about your feelings with your partner, your doctor, and others with whom you can share your thoughts. You may have to make some hard choices in a short time.

There is no "right" choice in these cases. The decision is based on the values unique to each person. The choice that's right for one woman may not be right for another. Counseling may help sort out the issues.

Some choose to end a pregnancy. Others may choose to continue it even if the baby will have a problem. The months before the birth can be used to plan for the baby's future. That way, he or she will have the best care right from the start and the best chance to lead a full and happy life.

Facing the issues of genetic disorders creates many questions and challenges for couples who will need to consider choices and make decisions. Information about the risks of specific genetic disorders and options for testing and treatment are outlined on the following pages (Table 13–3).

Table 13–3. Genetic Disorders

Disorder	Description	Risk Factors
Dominant Disorders		
Huntington's disease	This is a nerve disorder that causes loss of control of movements and mental function. Symptoms usually start between the ages of 35 and 50 years, but they can begin any time from childhood to old age.	Family history of the disease
Polydactyly	This is a disorder in which a baby is born with extra fingers or toes.	Family history of the disorder; African American descent
Recessive Disorders		
Bloom syndrome	With this disorder, a child may have growth problems during pregnancy and after birth. There also is a risk of skin problems, learning problems, and mental retardation.	European Jewish descent (Ashkenazi Jews)
Familial dysautonomia	This disorder can affect digestion, breathing, tearing, and the regulation of blood pressure and body temperature. Taste and the perception of pain, heat, and cold also may be affected.	European Jewish descent (Ashkenazi Jews)
Fanconi anemia group C	This disorder mainly is a blood disease, but, in some cases, there are physical defects as well.	European Jewish descent (Ashkenazi Jews)
Mucolipidosis IV	This disorder can cause mental retardation, physical problems, breathing problems, and other problems.	European Jewish descent (Ashkenazi Jews)

Risk of Occurring	Test Available?	Treatment
About 1 in 100,000 people	If there is a family history of the disease, genetic testing can tell if the parents or the baby have the gene and will later develop the disease.	There is no cure, and death often follows about 15 years after the onset of symptoms.
About 1 in 125,000 people	No	It's easily corrected with surgery.
About 1 in 40,000 babies with Ashkenazi Jewish ancestry is born with Bloom syndrome. The chance of being a carrier is 1 in 100.	Carrier testing can find out if the parents are carriers. Amniocentesis and chorionic villus sampling are used to detect Bloom syndrome in a fetus.	There is no current treatment.
About 1 in 3,600 babies with Ashkenazi Jewish ancestry is born with this disorder. About 1 in 32 Ashkenazi Jews are carriers.	Carrier testing can find out if the parents are carriers. Amniocentesis and chorionic villus sampling are used to detect familial dysautonomia in a fetus.	There is no cure, but there are some treatments that can improve the length and quality of life.
About 1 in 32,000 babies with Ashkenazi Jewish ancestry is born with this disorder. About 1 in 89 Ashkenazi Jews are carriers.	Carrier testing can find out if the parents are carriers. Amniocentesis and chorionic villus sampling are used to detect Fanconi anemia group C in a fetus.	Some children have been treated with bone marrow transplants.
About 1 in 62,500 babies with Ashkenazi Jewish ancestry is born with this disorder. About 1 in 127 Ashkenazi Jews are carriers.	Carrier testing can find out if the parents are carriers. Amniocentesis and chorionic villus sampling are used to detect mucolipidosis IV in a fetus.	There is no current treatment.

(continued)

Table 13–3. Genetic Disorders (continued)

Disorder	Description	Risk Factors
Recessive Disorders (continued)		
Niemann–Pick disease type A	Children with this disorder have problems with eating. There also is a loss of early motor skills. Most children with this disorder do not live past 2–3 years of age.	European Jewish descent (Ashkenazi Jews)
Sickle cell anemia	This is a blood disorder in which the red blood cells have a crescent, or "sickle," shape rather than the normal doughnut shape. Because of their odd shape, these cells get caught in the blood vessels. This prevents oxygen from reaching organs and tissues, which causes pain. Also, the body destroys sickle cells faster than it can make normal cells to replace them. Anemia often results.	African-American descent
Tay–Sachs disease	This is a disease in which harmful amounts of a fatty substance called ganglioside GM2 collects in the nerve cells in the brain. Tay–Sachs disease causes severe mental retardation, blindness, and seizures. Symptoms first occur at about 6 months of age.	European Jewish descent (Ashkenazi Jews) and French Canadian descent
Gaucher's disease	This is a disease in which an enzyme needed to break down a certain kind of fat is lacking. This causes the fat to build up, mostly in the liver, spleen, and bone marrow, which causes pain, fatigue, jaundice, bone damage, anemia, and even death.	European Jewish descent (Ashkenazi Jews)

Risk of Occurring	Test Available?	Treatment
About 1 in 32,000 babies with Ashkenazi Jewish ancestry is born with this disorder. About 1 in 90 Ashkenazi Jews are carriers.	Carrier testing can find out if the parents are carriers. Amniocentesis and chorionic villus sampling are used to detect Niemann–Pick disease type A in a fetus.	There is no current treatment.
About 1 in 600 African American babies and 1 in 1,000–1,400 Hispanic–American babies are born with this disorder. About 1 in 12 African Americans is a carrier.	Carrier testing can find out if the parents are carriers. Amniocentesis and chorionic villus sampling are used to detect sickle cell anemia in a fetus.	There is no current treatment.
About 1 in 3,000 babies with Ashkenazi Jewish ancestry is born with Tay–Sachs disease. The chance of being a carrier is 1 in 30 for Ashkenazi Jews and French Canadians and 1 in 300 for other people.	Carrier testing can find out if the parents are carriers. Amniocentesis and chorionic villus sampling are used to detect Tay–Sachs disease in a fetus.	There is no current treatment. Most children with Tay–Sachs disease do not live past 5 years of age.
About 1 in 900 babies with Ashkenazi Jewish ancestry is born with Gaucher's disease. About 1 in 15 Ashkenazi Jews are carriers.	Carrier testing can find out if the parents are carriers. Amniocentesis and chorionic villus sampling are used to detect Gaucher's disease in a fetus.	Enzyme replacement therapy is available for those more severely affected.

(continued)

Table 13–3. Genetic Disorders (continued)

Disorder	Description	Risk Factors
Recessive Disorders (continued)		
Canavan disease	This is a rare disorder that causes the brain to degenerate. Death usually occurs before 4 years of age, although some children may survive into their teens and twenties.	Canavan disease can occur in any ethnic group, but it is more frequent among Ashkenazi Jews from eastern Poland, Lithuania, and western Russia and among Saudi Arabians.
Cystic fibrosis	This disorder causes problems with digestion and breathing. Symptoms appear in childhood—sometimes right after birth. Some people have milder symptoms than others. Over time the symptoms tend to become worse and are harder to treat.	Caucasian people of Northern European descent
Thalassemia (also called "Cooley's anemia")	This disorder causes anemia. There are different types of thalassemia. Some are more severe than others.	Depending on the type of disorder, it is more likely to occur in people of Mediterranean (especially Greek or Italian) descent, Middle Eastern descent, African descent, or Asian descent
X-Linked Disorders		
Hemophilia	Males with hemophilia lack a substance in the blood that helps it clot. When they are injured, they are at risk for bleeding to death.	Male

Risk of Occurring	Test Available?	Treatment
About 1 in 6,400 babies with Ashkenazi Jewish ancestry is born with Canavan disease. About 1 in 40 Ashkenazi Jews are carriers.	Carrier testing can find out if the parents are carriers. Amniocentesis and chorionic villus sampling are used to detect Canavan disease in a fetus.	There is no current treatment.
The chance of being a carrier is 1 in 29 for whites, 1 in 46 for people of Hispanic background, 1 in 65 for African Americans, and 1 in 90 for Asian Americans. About 1 in 2,500 babies with Ashkenazi Jewish ancestry is born with cystic fibrosis. About 1 in 29 Ashkenazi Jews are carriers.	Carrier testing can find out if the parents are carriers. Amniocentesis and chorionic villus sampling are used to detect cystic fibrosis in a fetus.	There are treatments but no cure. People with cystic fibrosis usually have a shortened life span. Some die in childhood. Others live into their 40s or even longer.
As high as 1 in 20 (if member of risk group)	Carrier testing can find out if the parents are carriers. Amniocentesis and chorionic villus sampling are used to detect thalassemia in a fetus.	The more severe types can lead to fetal death or a need for blood transfusions for a person's entire life.
About 1 in 10,000 males has this disorder. Females can be carriers of this disease.	Carrier testing can find out if the parents are carriers. Amniocentesis and chorionic villus sampling are used to detect hemophilia in a fetus.	There is no current treatment.

(continued)

Table 13–3. Genetic Disorders *(continued)*

Disorder	Description	Risk Factors
X-Linked Disorders (continued)		
Duchenne muscular dystrophy	This is the most common severe form of muscular dystrophy. Signs of muscle weakness begin at about 2 years of age. As the arm and leg muscles weaken, a boy will have trouble standing and walking. By 12 years of age, he may be confined to a wheelchair.	Male
Fragile X syndrome	This genetic disorder is the most common cause of inherited mental retardation. People with fragile X syndrome have varying degrees of mental retardation or learning disabilities and behavioral and emotional problems. Boys with the disorder have a long, triangular face and ears that stick out. Women can be carriers of the fragile X gene but not have any symptoms.	Male
Chromosomal Disorders		
Down syndrome	A person with Down syndrome has an extra chromosome—three number 21 chromosomes instead of two. This is called trisomy 21. Down syndrome causes mental retardation. Most people with Down syndrome have IQs in the mild to moderate range of mental retardation. Some are more severely retarded. Down syndrome also can cause heart defects, hearing loss, and vision disorders.	The risk of having a baby with Down syndrome increases as a woman ages.

Risk of Occurring	Test Available?	Treatment
About 1 in 3,500 male births	Carrier testing can find out if the parents are carriers. Amniocentesis and chorionic villus sampling are used to detect Duchenne muscular dystrophy in a fetus.	There is no current treatment. Death usually occurs in the late teens or early 20s.
This disorders affects 1 in 1,200 male births and 1 in 2,500 female births. In the United States, about 1 in 250 women carries the fragile X gene.	Prenatal tests can show if the baby has the fragile X gene. However, the test cannot always tell whether a baby will be mentally retarded. Almost all boys who have the full mutation have mental retardation or serious learning disabilities, but only about one third to one half of affected girls do.	There is no current treatment.
About 1 in 800 babies is born with Down syndrome in the United States.	Maternal serum screening tests; nuchal translucency test; chorionic villus sampling; amniocentesis	There is no current treatment.

(continued)

Table 13–3. Genetic Disorders (continued)

Disorder	Description	Risk Factors
Chromosomal Disorders (continued)		
Trisomy 18	This is a problem caused by having three number 18 chromosomes. The fetus has serious problems with growth and development. After birth, there may be physical problems such as an open spine or heart defect. Most infants with trisomy 18 die within the first year of life.	Previous child with trisomy 18
XXY (sometimes called "Klinefelter's syndrome" or "47XXY")	This disorder occurs when a boy has an extra X chromosome. He has two X chromosomes and one Y chromosome, for a total of 47 chromosomes. XXY males often are sterile and have a rounded body type and enlarged breasts. Even though they are not mentally retarded, they often learn to talk later than other children and may have difficulty learning to read and write.	Male
Turner's syndrome	This disorder occurs when a girl is born with just one X chromosome. These girls tend to be short—usually not more than 5 feet tall. Girls with Turner's syndrome usually start puberty late and are almost always infertile. Some have other health problems, including kidney or heart defects, high blood pressure, diabetes mellitus, thyroid disease, and arthritis.	Female
Multifactorial Disorders		
Anencephaly	A type of neural tube defect that occurs when the brain and head don't form the way they should.	None

Risk of Occurring	Test Available?	Treatment
About 1 in 8,000 births are affected by this disorder.	Maternal serum screening tests; nuchal translucency test; chorionic villus sampling; amniocentesis	There is no current treatment.
About 1 in 500–1,000 male births is affected by this disorder.	Maternal serum screening tests	There is no current treatment.
About 1 of every 2,500 female births is affected by this disorder.	Chorionic villus sampling; amniocentesis	Treatment with growth and sex hormones can help increase height.
One in 1,000 live births is affected by this disorder.	Ultrasound and maternal serum screening tests	There is no current treatment. Babies with this disorder often are stillborn. If not, they usually die within a few hours or days after birth.

(continued)

Table 13–3. Genetic Disorders (continued)

Disorder	Description	Risk Factors
Multifactorial Disorders (continued)		
Spina bifida	With this type of neural tube defect, affected babies have varying degrees of paralysis and bladder and bowel problems. The effects depend on where the defect is located. When the defect is low in the spine, problems often are mild. If the defect is higher in the spine, it can cause leg paralysis, loss of feeling, lack of bladder and bowel control, hydrocephalus (extra spinal fluid in the brain), mental retardation, and even death.	None
Omphalocele	In this defect, the muscle and skin that cover the wall of the abdomen are missing. As a result, the organs in the abdomen are covered by only a membrane. The amount of missing tissue varies from little to most of the abdominal wall.	None
Gastroschisis	Gastroschisis is a small opening in the abdominal wall, next to the baby's navel. With this disorder, part of the stomach and the intestines stick out through this hole.	None
Congenital heart disease	This is heart disease that is present at birth. The severity of the disease depends on the type of heart defect and whether other problems also occur. Chromosomal disorders cause about 30–40% of cases of congenital heart disease.	If a parent has a congenital heart defect, his or her children are at increased risk for having a heart defect.

Risk of Occurring	Test Available?	Treatment
This disorder occurs in about 1 in every 2,000 live births in the United States.	Spina bifida often can be detected before birth with maternal serum screening tests.	Surgery
This disorder occurs in about 1 in 5,000 births.	An omphalocele often can be detected by ultrasound and maternal serum screening tests. Amnio-centesis also may be suggested.	There is no current treatment.
This disorders occurs in about 1 in 10,000 births. The rate is higher in babies born to teenaged mothers.	The disorder usually can be found by a prenatal ultrasound exam. If it is found, the fetus will need to be monitored regularly by ultrasound for the rest of the pregnancy.	In most cases, the opening can be repaired by surgery after birth.
This disorder occurs in about 1 in 125 births.	Congenital heart disease may be found during a routine ultrasound exam, but only about 1 in 10 cases is detected this way.	There are treatments available, but currently no cure.

(continued)

Table 13–3. Genetic Disorders (continued)

Disorder	Description	Risk Factors
Multifactorial Disorders (continued)		
Cleft lip and cleft palate	A cleft lip is a gap in the upper lip. A cleft palate is a gap or hole in the roof of the mouth. Cleft lip and cleft palate are among the most common congenital defects.	In most cases of cleft lip and cleft palate, the cause is not known. But cleft lip also can be caused by a chromosomal disorder or inherited as a dominant trait.
Clubfoot	With clubfoot, a baby is born with one or both feet twisted at the ankle. Clubfoot is caused by a combination of heredity and other factors that may affect prenatal growth. These include infection, drugs, and disease.	Boys are more likely than girls to have a more severe form of clubfoot.
Pyloric stenosis	In pyloric stenosis, the opening between the stomach and the intestine is blocked. Symptoms often show up 2–8 weeks after birth. It can cause vomiting that doesn't go away, constipation, and failure to gain weight.	None
Cerebral palsy	This disorder affects control of movement and posture. Cerebral palsy may be congenital, or the damage to the brain may happen around the time the baby is born. Symptoms range from mild to severe.	Sometimes certain infections in the early months of pregnancy and a variety of genetic disorders can cause the problem, but often the cause is unknown.

Risk of Occurring	Test Available?	Treatment
One of these disorders occurs in about 1 in 1,000 births	An ultrasound exam sometimes can detect the problem during pregnancy, but it is often difficult to get an image of the defect.	After birth, surgery can correct the defect.
This disorder occurs in about 1 in 1,000 births	An ultrasound exam sometimes can detect the problem during pregnancy.	It is not painful, and it doesn't bother the baby until he or she starts to stand and walk. If the problem is slight, special exercises often will correct it. For more severe cases, a baby may need to wear splints or casts for up to a year or have surgery.
This disorder occurs in about about 1 in 500–1,000 babies, mostly males.	An ultrasound exam sometimes can detect the problem during pregnancy.	This defect is easily treated with surgery.
This disorder occurs in about 2–3 in 1,000 babies.	No. Cerebral palsy usually is not diagnosed until the child is 2–3 years old.	Currently no cure is available, but many children with cerebral palsy have other problems that require treatment, such as mental retardation, learning disabilities, seizures, and problems with seeing, hearing, or speech.

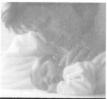

CHAPTER **14**

Managing Medical Problems

Pregnancy puts many new demands on your body. It can affect a health problem that you already have. Some conditions can affect the baby. It's best if any health problems you have are under control before you become pregnant. This increases the chances that your baby will be born healthy.

Doctors keep close tabs on medical problems and their effect on pregnancy. If you have a medical problem, during pregnancy you may need to have extra tests, see the doctor more often, or have special treatment. You may need to monitor your condition from home and check in often with the doctor or stay in the hospital while you are pregnant.

Most women with medical problems have healthy babies. It takes special care and extra effort. A team of doctors may work together to make sure that both you and your baby receive the special care needed.

High Blood Pressure

Blood pressure is vital for the body's circulatory system—the heart, arteries, and veins—to function. It is created in part by the steady beating of the heart. Each time the heart contracts, or squeezes, it pumps blood into the arteries. The arteries carry the blood to the body's organs. The veins return it to the heart.

Small arteries, called arterioles, also affect blood pressure. These blood vessels are lined with a layer of muscle. When the blood pressure is normal, this muscle is relaxed and the arterioles are dilated (open) so that blood can flow through them easily. However, if a signal is sent to increase the blood pressure, the muscle layer tightens and the arterioles narrow. This makes it harder for the blood to flow. The pressure then increases in the arteries.

A blood pressure reading has two numbers. Each number is separated by a slash: 110/80, for instance. (You may hear this referred to as "110 over 80.") The first number is the pressure in the arteries when the heart contracts. This is called the **systolic blood pressure.** The second number is the pressure in the arteries when the heart relaxes between contractions. This is the **diastolic blood pressure.**

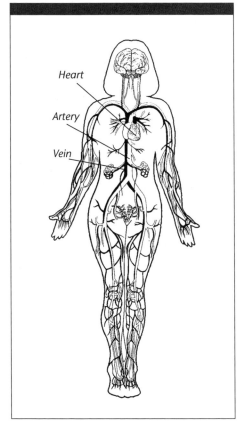

The heart pumps blood rich in oxygen through the arteries (light blood vessels) to the body. Veins (dark blood vessels) carry blood back to the heart.

Blood pressure changes from person to person. It changes often during the day. It can increase if a person is excited or exercises. Most often, it decreases when a person is resting. These short-term changes in blood pressure are normal. It is only when a person's blood pressure stays high for some time that it may signal a problem.

In most pregnant women, readings less than 120/80 are normal. If a pregnant woman's systolic pressure is 140 or her diastolic pressure is 90 on several readings, it is too high.

Because of the normal ups and downs in blood pressure, if a woman has one high reading, another reading may be taken again later to see if it is at a normal level. Normal blood pressure can be an average of a number of readings taken at rest.

In a healthy pregnancy, the baby receives all of the nutrients and oxygen needed for normal growth from the mother. This happens when the correct amount of the woman's blood flows through the placenta and the nutrients and oxygen pass through the umbilical cord to the baby.

High blood pressure can cause problems during pregnancy. When a woman has high blood pressure in pregnancy, it may affect the growth of the baby.

Chronic Hypertension

When high blood pressure has been present for some time before pregnancy,

Your Blood Pressure Reading

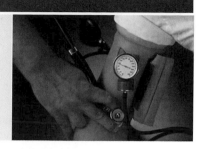

$$\frac{110}{80} = \frac{\text{systolic}}{\text{diastolic}} = \frac{\text{pressure in arteries when heart contracts}}{\text{pressure in arteries when heart relaxes}}$$

it is known as chronic, or essential, hypertension. This condition remains during pregnancy and after the birth of the baby. It is vital that chronic hypertension be controlled because it can lead to health problems such as heart failure or stroke.

During pregnancy, chronic hypertension also may affect the growth of the baby. Many women with chronic hypertension can stop taking medication during pregnancy because their blood pressure returns to normal. Other women need to continue treatment during their pregnancies. Talk to your doctor about the best treatment for you. In some cases, a woman may need to switch to a different medication that still helps control her blood pressure but is safer to use during pregnancy.

Gestational Hypertension

When high blood pressure first occurs during the second half of pregnancy, it is known as *gestational hypertension.* This type of high blood pressure goes away soon after the baby is born. A woman with this condition may need to see the doctor more often to have her blood pressure checked. When gestational hypertension occurs with other findings it is called preeclampsia. Gestational hypertension may lead to preeclampsia.

Preeclampsia

Preeclampsia is a serious medical condition affecting all organs of the body. For example, preeclampsia causes stress on the kidneys, which results in increased amounts of protein in the woman's urine. Other signs of preeclampsia may include:

➤ Headaches

➤ Visual problems

➤ Rapid weight gain

➤ Swelling (edema) of the hands and face

Doctors do not know why some women get preeclampsia. They do know that some women are at a higher risk

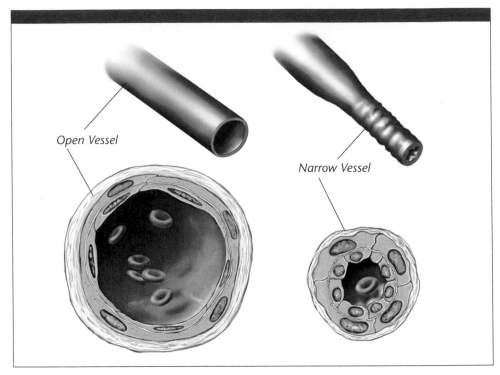

Open Vessel

Narrow Vessel

When your blood pressure is normal, blood vessels are open so that blood can flow easily through them. When your pressure is high, though, the vessels are narrow. This makes it harder for the blood to flow.

than others. The risk of developing preeclampsia is increased in certain women who:

➤ Are pregnant for the first time

➤ Have had preeclampsia in a previous pregnancy

➤ Have a history of chronic hypertension

➤ Are 35 years of age or older

➤ Are carrying more than one baby

➤ Have certain medical conditions such as **diabetes** or kidney disease

➤ Are obese

➤ Are African American

➤ Have certain immune disorders, such as lupus

A woman with preeclampsia may need to stay in the hospital so that she and her baby can be monitored. In some cases, her baby may be delivered early. When preeclampsia becomes severe, the woman's organs can be damaged, including the kidneys, liver, brain, heart, and eyes. In some cases, seizures will occur. This is call eclampsia.

Severe preeclampsia may require early delivery, even if the baby is not fully grown. If a baby is born prematurely, it may have complications. Preeclampsia is a very serious illness for both the woman and baby and can, in rare cases, cause the death of both.

Special Care

If a woman knows she has high blood pressure before pregnancy, there are steps she and her doctor can take to reduce the chance of severe effects to herself or her baby (see box). For this reason, the best thing a woman can do is to see her doctor before pregnancy and get regular prenatal care.

At each prenatal visit, weight, blood pressure, and a urine sample (to check for protein) are taken. This helps detect any changes that might have occurred. Once the doctor is aware that a woman's blood pressure is high, she may be checked more often.

What You Can Do If You Have High Blood Pressure

If you have chronic high blood pressure, follow these steps to help make your pregnancy safer:

Before pregnancy

➤ Work with your doctor to lower your blood pressure.

➤ Lose weight through diet and exercise, if needed.

➤ Take blood pressure medication as prescribed.

➤ Ask your doctor if your blood pressure medication is safe to use during pregnancy.

➤ Stop smoking

During pregnancy

➤ See your doctor regularly, starting as soon as you can, so that changes in your blood pressure and weight can be found as soon as they occur.

➤ If you have high blood pressure, kidney disease, or any other risk factors, be sure to tell your doctor early in pregnancy.

➤ If you develop any of the warning signs of preeclampsia, tell your doctor right away.

➤ Check your blood pressure and weight at home, if your doctor suggests you do so.

When blood pressure increases slightly in early or midpregnancy, bed rest may help reduce the pressure. Bed rest may be at home or in the hospital. If the blood pressure does not increase to dangerous levels, pregnancy may be allowed to continue until labor begins naturally.

If preeclampsia develops, the only real cure is having the baby. The decision to deliver the baby depends on the risks to the mother and whether the risk to the baby is greater in the woman's uterus or in a special nursery. Labor may occur naturally or be induced (brought on). Sometimes a cesarean birth is needed depending on the health of the mother and baby.

Before deciding to deliver the baby early, the doctor may wait to see if the situation improves. During labor, medication may be given to help prevent seizures or lower blood pressure.

Diabetes

Diabetes occurs when the body has trouble making or using insulin. Insulin is a hormone that converts the glucose in food into energy. Glucose is a sugar that is the body's main source of fuel. If there isn't enough insulin, or if the insulin doesn't convert enough glucose into fuel, the level of glucose in the blood becomes too high. Good control of the levels of blood glucose decreases the risks to the mother and baby.

Some women have diabetes before they become pregnant; others develop the disease only during pregnancy. In either case, insulin and other medications may be needed to control glucose levels.

Diabetes Before Pregnancy

About 1 woman in 100 has diabetes before she gets pregnant. If you have diabetes, it's best that the disease be brought under control before you are pregnant. During pregnancy, your health should be closely monitored and blood glucose levels kept in check. With planning, control, and expert care, the chances of having a healthy baby are very good.

Diabetes can't be cured. It can only be controlled. Women who have diabetes should get early care to help lower the risk of problems. Diabetes increases your risk of the following conditions:

➤ *Miscarriage.* The risk of pregnancy loss is even greater if the condition isn't under control.

➤ *Birth defects.* Heart defects, kidney defects, and spinal problems are more common in babies whose mothers have diabetes. The rate of such birth defects is even higher if the disease isn't well managed.

➤ ***Hydramnios*** (too much amniotic fluid). Hydramnios may make it hard for the mother to breathe—fluid in the uterus constricts the lungs. It also can lead to preterm labor and birth.

➤ *Macrosomia.* An overly large baby can make it hard to give birth vaginally. If the doctor suspects that the baby has grown too large, cesarean birth may be considered.

➤ *Stillbirth.* Although stillbirth is rare, mothers with diabetes are more likely to lose their babies than women without the disease.

➤ *Respiratory distress syndrome.* Diabetes may cause the baby's lungs to mature more slowly. Respiratory distress syndrome can occur when the baby's lungs aren't fully developed. This can affect his or her breathing after birth.

➤ *Preeclampsia.* (See "Preeclampsia" for more information.)

Gestational Diabetes

Diabetes that occurs during pregnancy is called gestational diabetes. It usually goes away after the baby is born. More than half of the women who have gestational diabetes get diabetes later in life.

Some women who develop gestational diabetes have no known risk factors. But certain things make it more likely:

➤ Being older than age 30 years

➤ Being overweight (See BMI chart in Chapter 5)

➤ Having one or more family members with diabetes

➤ Being a member of an ethnic group with a high rate of diabetes (Hispanic, Native American, Asian, African American)

➤ Having had gestational diabetes in the previous pregnancy or having had a very large baby

Your doctor may do a screening test for diabetes if you have several of these risk factors. A glucose screening test is often given at 24–28 weeks of pregnancy or earlier based on risk factors. For the test, the patient drinks a special sugar mixture. An hour later, a blood sample is drawn and sent to a lab. There, a technician measures the level of sugar in the blood.

If a glucose screening test shows the level is high, a glucose tolerance test is given. This test is similar to glucose screening. However, it lasts longer—about 3 hours—and requires four blood samples. The test is done while fasting on an empty stomach. The 3-hour test gives the doctor more precise information on the diagnosis so the disease can be treated.

With mild gestational diabetes, blood glucose levels often can be controlled with a special diet and exercise. If the problem is more severe, medication, in addition to a special diet may be needed. The level of glucose in the blood should be tested each day.

If diabetes isn't controlled, the extra sugar in the blood increases the risk of having a baby with macrosomia. Babies with macrosomia are overly large. They weigh 10 pounds or more. They may be too big to fit safely through the birth canal.

Overly large babies often have health problems:

➤ Low glucose levels

➤ Low blood calcium and magnesium levels

➤ Too many red blood cells

➤ Jaundice

➤ Breathing problems

To see how the baby is doing, the doctor may order special tests. Ultrasound may be used to assess the baby's weight. Amniocentesis can show if the baby's lungs are mature enough to handle an early delivery, if it is needed.

A few months after birth, the glucose tolerance test may be repeated. If test results are normal, health can be maintained with a balanced program of diet and exercise. This may decrease the chances of problems in future pregnancies and help reduce the risk of diabetes later in life.

Controlling Diabetes

Women who have diabetes should keep a close check on the following areas to keep glucose levels under control:

➤ *Diet.* The amount of calories needed depends on weight. Even if diabetes

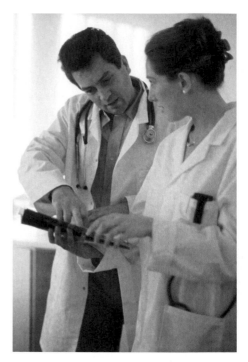

is well controlled, a new diet may be needed during pregnancy. Most often, the diet consists of special meals and snacks spread over the course of the day. A bedtime snack helps keep blood glucose at the right level during the night. The diet may need to be adjusted as delivery nears. A change may be needed to help decrease glucose levels or better meet the growing baby's needs.

➤ *Exercise.* Exercise decreases the amount of insulin needed to keep blood glucose at normal levels. The type and amount of exercise needed depends on a woman's health and fitness level and how far along she is in pregnancy.

➤ *Medications.* Treatment may be given as insulin in shots or hypoglycemic agents in pills depending on a number of factors. These medications will help blood glucose stay at a normal level. It doesn't cross the placenta, so it doesn't affect the fetus directly. How much and how often medication is needed depend on a number of factors. It's likely the need for medication will increase during pregnancy and level off near the end. This means the dosage will have to be adjusted from time to time.

➤ *Blood glucose levels.* To find out how much medication is needed, blood glucose levels must be checked at home each day. The levels may need to be checked several times a day. There are various ways to do this at home.

Special Care

Women who have diabetes need special medical care during pregnancy. If you have diabetes you may need to do the following:

➤ See the doctor more often.

➤ See a doctor who has special training in diabetes care.

➤ Work with a dietitian to develop meal plans.

➤ Stay in the hospital if treatment at home isn't working.

➤ Have certain tests that will help spot any problems that arise.

One test can show the average blood sugar control during the previous 2–3 months. This test measures a substance in the blood called hemoglobin A_{1C}. In the blood, glucose binds to hemoglobin. The amount of glucose bound to hemoglobin is the hemoglobin A_{1C}. When the hemoglobin A_{1C} level increases, it means glucose levels have been poorly controlled for a number of weeks.

Tests also may be needed to tell how the baby is doing. Tests such as ultrasound, amniocentesis, and fetal monitoring allow the doctor to track the baby's health (see Chapter 13 for details on these tests). When it's time for the baby to be born, most women are able to have a vaginal birth.

Heart Disease

Heart disease affects about 1–4% of pregnant women. Heart problems include congenital defects (defects that are present at birth), rheumatic heart disease, previous heart surgery, and a previous heart attack.

Women who have heart disease should talk to their doctors before trying to conceive. The risk of problems during pregnancy depends on the type of defect and how severe it is. The care of a maternal–fetal specialist or a cardiologist (an expert in heart disease) also may be needed. They can provide details on how a heart problem may affect pregnancy and how pregnancy may affect the heart. Sometimes steps can be taken before pregnancy to correct a condition.

Pregnancy brings about major changes in the circulatory system. The amount of blood volume increases by 40–50%. This increase makes the heart work harder. Taking it easy will help offset the extra demands on the heart.

Labor and delivery also put added stress on the heart. Labor contractions increase the heart's workload. Pain medication will help reduce this problem.

Even though labor contractions put stress on the heart, vaginal delivery is safer than cesarean birth in most cases. The doctor may use forceps or vacuum extraction to decrease the amount of pushing and shorten labor time.

Heart disease can increase the risk of early delivery or a small baby. Also, women who have congenital heart disease have a 4–5% chance of having a baby with a birth defect.

Lung Disorders

It is common to feel short of breath during pregnancy. This does not mean the baby is not getting enough oxygen. (For hints on dealing with this symptom, see "Shortness of Breath" in Chapter 7.) However, some lung disorders can cause problems:

➤ *Asthma.* This lung disease causes wheezing and trouble with breath-

ing. Asthma can deprive the baby of oxygen if it's not treated. Most asthma medicine is safe to use during pregnancy. A woman with asthma should not stop using an inhaler or taking prescribed pills when she gets pregnant without first talking to her doctor. With many cases of severe asthma, the attacks will continue during pregnancy. Regular medical care is vital so the baby's health can be monitored and the asthma can be controlled.

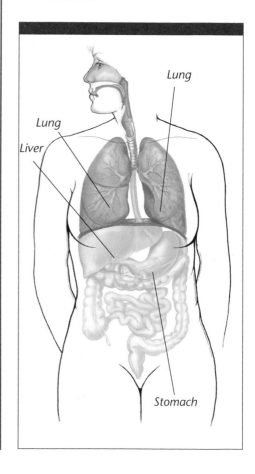

➤ *Pneumonia.* This lung infection may be more severe in pregnancy than it is at other times. It can cause both the woman and the baby to get less oxygen. If a doctor suspects pneumonia, he or she may order a chest X-ray to find out for sure. This type of X-ray isn't thought to be harmful during pregnancy, but the woman should tell the X-ray technician that she is pregnant. To be on the safe side, a lead apron will be draped over the belly to shield the fetus from radiation. Antibiotics are needed to treat pneumonia. In some cases, a stay in the hospital may be needed until the infection clears up.

Kidney Disease

Kidneys that have been scarred from an illness or don't function the way they should could affect pregnancy. Kidney disease in pregnancy may cause hypertension, preterm birth, and stillbirth.

Kidney disease often can be diagnosed from medical history, physical exam, and blood and urine tests. Protein in the urine can be a sign of kidney disease, for instance. This is another reason a urine sample may be obtained at each prenatal visit.

Seizure Disorders

Epilepsy and certain other disorders cause seizures (convulsions). A seizure can consist of a few muscle twitches, or it can be a major attack that causes a blackout and loss of bladder or bowel control.

Most women with seizure disorders have healthy babies, but problems can occur. Birth defects happen two to three times more often if the mother has a seizure disorder than in pregnancies where the mother does not. Cleft lip, cleft palate, and heart defects are the most common problems in babies born to women with seizure disorders. No one is certain why these problems occur. Some of the medications used to treat the condition may be the cause.

If you have a seizure disorder and get pregnant, do not stop taking your **anticonvulsant** medication without talking to your doctor first. In some cases, seizures may be more harmful than the medication used to control or prevent them.

The amount of medication needed often changes during pregnancy. The doctor will monitor drug levels and adjust the dosage as needed. With good control of drug levels, there should be little change in the number or strength of seizures.

Medications that treat seizure disorders can use up stores of folic acid. This is a vital nutrient during pregnancy. Neural tube defects are linked with not getting enough folic acid (see "Genetic Disorders and Birth Defects" in Chapter 13). Taking folic acid supplements will decrease the risk of having a baby with a neural tube defect.

Obesity

Obesity during pregnancy can cause problems for both the mother and the baby. Obesity is defined as having a body mass index of more than 29 (see the BMI chart in Chapter 6). Obesity is a major health problem. More than 30% of adult women are obese.

Obese pregnant women are at risk for many serious health problems. They are 10 times more likely to have high blood pressure during pregnancy (see "High Blood Pressure"). They also have an increased risk of having gestational diabetes (see "Gestational Diabetes") and are more likely to have a cesarean birth. The rate of complications from cesarean delivery is increased for obese women. Diabetes or high blood pressure increase the chance of needing a cesarean delivery. The baby also has an increased risk of being born with birth defects, especially neural tube defects.

Obese women who are planning to get pregnant, should lose weight first. Talk to your doctor about your plans for having a baby. Your doctor can help you work out a healthy plan to lose weight before you become pregnant.

Obese pregnant women should not try to lose weight. For such women, a healthy weight gain during pregnancy is no more than 15 pounds (see "Weight Gain in Pregnancy" in Chapter 6).

Autoimmune Disorders

With autoimmune disorders, the immune system attacks the body's own tissues. As a result, organs such as the thyroid or other parts of the body can be injured.

Many autoimmune diseases have symptoms that overlap with other illnesses. This makes them hard to detect. Most of these disorders are chronic. Often, they have no cure because the cause isn't always known. Symptoms may go away for a time and then flare up with little warning and for no clear reason.

The effect of an autoimmune disorder on pregnancy depends on the type of disorder and how severe it is. Women who have these disorders need special care during pregnancy.

Systemic Lupus Erythematosus

Systemic lupus erythematosus (SLE) is an autoimmune disease, often referred to simply as "lupus." It can affect the whole body, including the skin, joints, kidneys, and nervous system. Some women with SLE have a rash on their faces. Others get a more severe condition that causes their kidneys to fail and affects the nervous system, heart, and blood.

SLE tends to strike women during their childbearing years. Having SLE increases the risk of miscarriage, preterm birth, fetal growth problems, and stillbirth. It also can affect the fetal heart rate and damage the baby's heart.

About 20–30% of pregnant women with SLE will have gestational hypertension (see "High Blood Pressure"). If you have SLE, you will need to see your doctor more often during pregnancy.

For about one third of women who have SLE and become pregnant, the disease gets worse during pregnancy. Symptoms also can flare up after delivery. If a woman's kidneys aren't affected by SLE and she goes 6 months without symptoms before getting pregnant, she is less likely to have problems during pregnancy. SLE may be treated with medications called *corticosteroids* or other medications that can be used during pregnancy.

Rheumatoid Arthritis

Rheumatoid arthritis is an autoimmune disease that affects the joints. It causes pain, soreness, heat, and swelling in small- and medium-sized joints. It also can cause stiffness in the morning and a general feeling of fatigue and discomfort.

Rheumatoid arthritis can flare up and then lessen for a time, or it can get worse and damage the joints. During pregnancy, rheumatoid arthritis greatly improves for many women.

Rheumatoid arthritis often is treated with anti-inflammatory medications such as aspirin and acetaminophen.

Other drugs may be prescribed along with rest and physical therapy. Certain drugs sometimes used to treat rheumatoid arthritis should be avoided during pregnancy. These include methotrexate and cyclophosphamide.

Antiphospholipid Syndrome

Antiphospholipid syndrome is a condition caused when the body produces high levels of the antiphospholipid antibody. Antibodies are proteins that are made in response to a stimulus. For instance, in some cases, they are helpful in protecting the body against disease. Sometimes antibodies can be harmful.

During pregnancy, the disorder can cause preeclampsia, blood clots, and stroke. It also is associated with miscarriage, slow fetal growth, and fetal death. It often can be treated successfully during pregnancy. Antiphospholipid syndrome often is treated with a blood thinner and low-dose aspirin.

Multiple Sclerosis

Multiple sclerosis (MS) is a disease that affects the central nervous system. Symptoms of MS vary from person to person. They include extreme fatigue, vision problems, loss of balance and muscle control, tremors, and stiffness.

Symptoms also change from time to time in the same person. A person can have relapses or flare-ups when symptoms get worse and also can have periods with no symptoms.

Pregnancy is not at risk with MS. The baby grows normally. Also, pregnancy does not make MS worse. The best therapy is to follow a healthy lifestyle of good nutrition, exercise, rest, and prenatal care.

During birth, sometimes weakness from MS can keep a woman from pushing hard enough. If this is the case, the doctor may use forceps or suction to help the baby through the birth canal.

Thyroid Disease

The thyroid is a gland in the neck that controls key body functions. Certain disorders cause the thyroid to release too much or too little thyroid hormone. Hypothyroidism means the thyroid isn't as active as it should be. Hyperthyroidism means the thyroid is too active. Either can harm you or your baby during pregnancy (see box).

Treatment with medication and close monitoring by your doctor can decrease the risk of problems. Your doctor will check the levels of thyroid hormone in your body at regular intervals during your pregnancy to be sure they are at healthy levels. The chance of problems during pregnancy is greatest when thyroid disease is not treated and controlled.

Many medications used to treat thyroid disease in pregnancy are safe for a fetus. However, radioactive iodine, which is sometimes used to treat hyperthyroidism, should not be taken during pregnancy. It may injure the thyroid

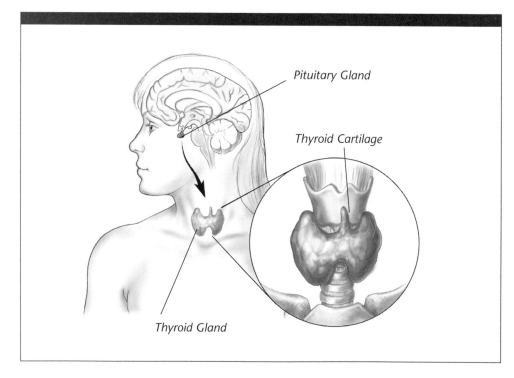

Pituitary Gland

Thyroid Cartilage

Thyroid Gland

Risks of Thyroid Disease During Pregnancy

Risks of Hypothyroidism

Baby

➤ Smaller than normal

➤ Preterm birth (born before 37 weeks of pregnancy)

➤ Decreased mental ability (if untreated or uncontrolled)

Mother

➤ Preeclampsia—A condition of pregnancy in which there is high blood pressure, swelling due to fluid retention, and abnormal kidney function

➤ Placental abruption—A condition in which the placenta has begun to separate from the inner wall of the uterus before the baby is born.

Risks of Hyperthyroidism

Baby

➤ Smaller than normal

➤ Preterm birth

➤ Possible death

➤ Hyperthyroidism that requires treatment with medications for a short time after birth

Mother

➤ An irregular heartbeat or heart failure

➤ Thyroid storm (severe hyperthyroidism)

gland of the fetus. This may cause the baby to have hypothyroidism.

Some women may not have thyroid problems during pregnancy but develop problems after birth. This is called postpartum thyroiditis. This often is a short-term problem, and hormone levels quickly return to normal. Sometimes this condition can lead to long-term hypothyroidism, which will require treatment.

If you have a history or symptoms of thyroid disease and are thinking of becoming pregnant or are pregnant already, talk to your doctor. Testing the

function of the thyroid gland is not a routine part of prenatal care.

Physical Disability

For women who are physically disabled, pregnancy and being a parent pose special challenges. That doesn't mean they can't—or shouldn't—become mothers.

It's a good idea for women with disabilities and their partners to meet with the doctor before getting pregnant. This will help reduce the odds of medical problems during pregnancy.

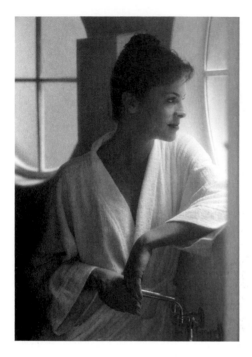

Special care also will be needed after pregnancy begins. The doctor may work closely with the primary care doctor or other specialists. He or she also may suggest occupational or physical therapy to help you better cope with the stresses pregnancy puts on the body.

Before the baby arrives, special equipment may have to be installed or modified at home to help in caring for the baby. Leaving the hospital may require postpartum home care for mother and baby.

Mental Illness

As many as 1 in 6 pregnant women have mental health problems. The fol-lowing mental health problems can affect a woman before and during pregnancy:

➤ Mood disorders, such as severe depression and bipolar disorder

➤ Schizophrenia

➤ Anxiety disorders, such as obsessive–compulsive disorder and phobia

➤ Personality disorders

Some mental illnesses may have a genetic factor. A woman who has a mental illness may want to see a genetic counselor to find out the chances of passing it on to her baby.

Mental illness can affect pregnancy in a number of ways. If you have a mental illness or had one in the past, be sure to tell your doctor about it. The doctor can arrange for counseling or community agencies to provide social or mental health services.

Being pregnant can cause mental illness to worsen. Or, pregnancy may cause emotional problems to reoccur. This may be a result of hormonal changes or stress.

For some women, depression can occur during a pregnancy or after delivery, even if she has no history of it. More than 1 in 10 mothers-to-be have depression that doesn't go away. If you have symptoms of depression or any other mental illness, it is important to get treatment (see box). Ask for support from your partner and loved ones and seek counseling if you need it.

If a mental illness is not treated, a woman may do things that could harm her baby. For example, she could have trouble eating well, getting enough rest, or taking care of herself in other ways. She also may be less likely to get regular prenatal care.

The doctor needs to know about any medications that are taken to control a mental or emotional disorder. Some medications can harm a growing baby. Other drugs are thought to be safe during pregnancy (for instance, antidepressants), and with some the effect on the baby simply isn't known.

A doctor and mental health provider can advise a woman on whether to stop taking medication that has been prescribed. In many cases, the benefit of keeping a mental condition under control outweighs any possible risks from the drug used to treat it.

Mental health care is vital after the baby is born. Some women have a mental health problem after delivery. Women with mental health problems are 20 times more likely to be admitted to a hospital for a psychiatric illness in the month after giving birth than they are in the 2 years that led up to it. They

Signs of Depression

The signs of depression can seem like the normal ups and downs of pregnancy. That can make it hard to spot depression during pregnancy. A blue mood now and then is normal. You should tell your doctor if you are sad most of the time for at least 2 weeks or have any symptoms of depression:

➤ Depressed mood most of the day, nearly every day

➤ Loss of interest in work or other activities

➤ Feeling guilty, hopeless, or worthless

➤ Thinking about death or suicide

➤ Sleeping more than normal or lying awake at night

➤ Loss of appetite or losing weight (or eating much more than normal and gaining weight)

➤ Feeling very tired or without energy

➤ Having trouble paying attention and making decisions

➤ Having aches and pains that don't get better with treatment also are more likely to have postpartum depression. (For more information, see "Postpartum Depression" in Chapter 12.)

The first weeks after a newborn arrives can be stressful for any new mother. During the early weeks, help and support is important to make a woman feel comfortable as she adjusts to being a mother.

What You Can Do

If you have a medical condition, with proper care, you have a good chance of having a healthy pregnancy and baby. If you learn for the first time during pregnancy that you have an illness, it can come as a shock. In addition to learning about pregnancy and birth, you must learn how to care for a medical condition. A doctor can help you adjust and work out a treatment plan.

Remember that many women with medical problems have healthy babies. Work with your doctors to monitor your health and take steps that may be needed to make sure you and your baby have the best outcome possible.

CHAPTER 15

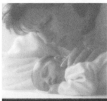

Complications During Pregnancy

Although pregnancy and childbirth are natural events, problems can arise despite the best of care. Some problems require prompt treatment or special care to do the best for you and your baby. Certain factors can increase a woman's risk of problems. In some cases, these risks can be detected in advance. In even the most healthy and fit women, things can go wrong with no warning.

If you have a high-risk pregnancy, your doctor and health care team will watch your progress closely. They will adjust your prenatal care as needed and give you special care through labor and delivery. If you suspect or find any problems, such as the ones described here, contact your doctor.

Miscarriage

A miscarriage occurs when the pregnancy ends before 20 weeks of gestation. Miscarriage sometimes is called "spontaneous abortion." It occurs in about 15–20% of all pregnancies, often during the first 3 months. Bleeding is the most common sign that a miscarriage might occur. Another sign is cramping pain in the lower abdomen. This pain often comes and goes and is stronger than that of menstrual cramps.

The cause of miscarriage often is not known. When it is known, it can include the following problems:

➤ *Chromosomes.* More than 75% of miscarriages in the first 13 weeks of pregnancy are caused by problems with the chromosomes of the baby. Many times these problems occur by chance; however, sometimes these problems are related to the woman's age. Rarely, it can be caused by a genetic problem (see Chapter 13).

➤ *Illness in the mother.* Problems such as heart disease or uncontrolled diabetes can be linked to repeated mis-

Warning Signs of Miscarriage

Call your doctor if you have any of the following symptoms:

➤ Spotting or bleeding with or without pain

➤ Heavy or constant bleeding with abdominal pain or cramping

➤ A gush of fluid from your vagina but no pain or bleeding (you may need an exam to see if your membranes have broken)

If you have heavy bleeding and think you have passed fetal tissue, place it in a clean jar and take it to the doctor to be checked. Your doctor will want to examine you to see if your cervix has dilated.

carriage. Treating the illness before pregnancy can help decrease the risk.

➤ *Hormone imbalance.* The woman's body may not be making the amount of the hormone progesterone needed for pregnancy to continue.

➤ *Immune system disorders.* The woman's body may be making antibodies that are not needed or too many antibodies.

➤ *Uterine problems.* Some women are born with a uterus that is not shaped properly. Other uterine problems that may be linked to miscarriages are **fibroids** (benign growths in the uterus). These problems can be treated with surgery.

Women who have more than one miscarriage may be referred to a doctor with special skill in this area. A complete physical exam and blood tests will be done to try to find out if there is a problem. Some of these procedures also may be done:

➤ Hysterosalpingography. An X-ray of the uterus and fallopian tubes is taken after the organs are injected with a small amount of fluid.

➤ Hysteroscopy. A thin, telescope-like device called a hysteroscope is guided through the vagina and cervix to view the inside of the uterus.

➤ Laparoscopy. A slender device called a laparoscope is inserted through a small incision made near the navel. The device shines light inside so the doctor can view the pelvic organs.

➤ Ultrasound. Sound waves are used to view the internal organs.

➤ Sonohysterography. A saline solution is injected into the uterus to expand the walls of the uterus. An ultrasound probe is inserted into the vagina to examine the uterine structures and lining.

The feelings of loss after a miscarriage can be intense. Women often find themselves searching for reasons and may blame themselves. Emotional healing is as important as physical healing. (See Chapter 16 for more information about grieving and coping with loss.)

Vaginal Bleeding

Vaginal bleeding in pregnancy can have many causes. Exams and tests, such as ultrasound, may be needed. A repeat pregnancy test or ultrasound exam may help find out if any of these situations apply:

➤ The pregnancy is ectopic (located outside the uterus).

➤ Miscarriage has occurred or is about to occur.

➤ The pregnancy is normal.

In many cases, the bleeding stops on its own and the baby is carried to term with no problems.

Sometimes bleeding can become serious and require prompt treatment. You should report any bleeding to your doctor. He or she can decide the proper course of action based on your symptoms and stage of pregnancy.

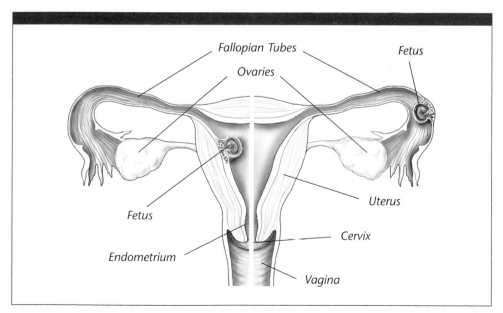

Normal pregnancy (*left*) occurs in the uterus. An ectopic pregnancy (*right*) may occur in the fallopian tube.

Early pregnancy

At the start of pregnancy, some women may have light bleeding (spotting or staining). This is called implantation bleeding and can happen when the fertilized egg becomes attached to the lining of the uterus. Some women may confuse this bleeding with a menstrual period. When there is doubt, a lab test can confirm you are pregnant.

Many women who have bleeding have little or no cramping. In more than half of the women who bleed in early pregnancy, the bleeding stops and the pregnancy goes on to term. At other times, the bleeding and cramping become more heavy and strong, ending in miscarriage.

Late Pregnancy

The cause of bleeding during the second half of pregnancy may be something minor. Bleeding might occur if the cervix becomes inflamed, for instance. However, some bleeding can be severe and may pose a threat to you or the baby. Contact your doctor or nurse right away if you have any bleeding in late pregnancy. You may need to go to the hospital for special care.

Heavy vaginal bleeding often suggests a problem with the placenta. The most common problems are placental abruption and placenta previa. With placental abruption, the placenta separates from the wall of the uterus before or during birth. This often causes

Placental Problems

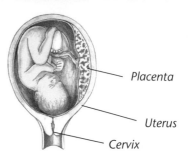

In a normal pregnancy, the placenta is attached to the uterine wall away from the cervix.

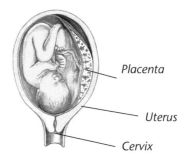

Placental abruption is when the placenta becomes detached from the uterine wall.

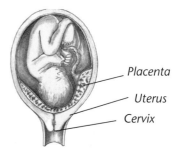

Placenta previa is when the placenta lies low in the uterus and blocks the cervix.

vaginal bleeding and constant, severe pain in the abdomen. The baby may get less oxygen, which could be harmful.

With placenta previa, the placenta lies low in the uterus and covers part or all of the cervix. This blocks the baby's exit from the uterus. Women who have placenta previa and are bleeding require prompt care and may need to stay in the hospital.

Both placental abruption and placenta previa may be severe enough to require that the baby be delivered early. Some women with placenta previa will need to have cesarean delivery.

Blood Group Incompatibility

Each person's blood is one of four major types: A, B, AB, or O. Blood types are determined by the types of antigens on the blood cells. Antigens are proteins on the surface of blood cells that can cause a response from the immune system.

Type A blood has only A antigens, type B has only B antigens, type AB has both A and B antigens, and type O has neither A nor B antigens. There are other antigens that can make blood types even more specific. One of the most common is the Rh factor.

As part of your prenatal care, you will have blood tests to find out your blood type. If your blood lacks the Rh antigen, it is called Rh negative. If it has the antigen, it is called Rh positive. More than 85% of people in the world have Rh-positive blood.

If the mother is Rh negative and the baby's father is Rh positive, the baby can inherit the Rh factor from the father. This makes the baby Rh positive, too. Problems can arise when the baby's blood has the Rh antigen and the mother's blood does not.

If a small amount of the baby's blood mixes with the mother's blood, her body may respond as if it were allergic. It then makes antibodies to the Rh antigens in the baby's blood. This means she has become sensitized. Antibodies then can attack the baby's blood. The antibodies will break down red blood cells of the baby and cause anemia. This can lead to severe illness or even death in the baby or newborn.

If the baby has an Rh type blood opposite the mother's, the first pregnancy poses little risk. It takes time for antibodies to build up after being exposed to the antigens. Once antibodies are formed, they do not go away. Thus, they would be a problem in later pregnancies. The best course is to keep from being sensitized and forming antibodies in the first place.

If the mother is Rh negative and blood tests show that she has not become sensitized, her doctor will prescribe *Rh immune globulin (RhIg)* shots to prevent antibodies to the Rh antigens from forming. RhIg shots are

Sensitization and Rh Immune Globulin

Sensitization can occur any time fetal blood mixes with the mother's blood. This can happen during pregnancy or after an abortion, miscarriage, ectopic pregnancy, or amniocentesis. After any of these events, an Rh-negative woman often is given RhIg to prevent sensitization. The effects of RhIg seem to last only about 12 weeks. For this reason, it is given again any time blood from the baby and mother might mix.

It is safe for pregnant women to receive RhIg. The only known side effects are soreness from the injection or a slight fever. There is no risk of infection with human immunodeficiency virus (HIV) with RhIg shots.

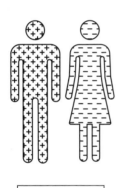 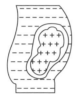 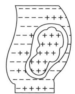 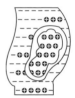

- Rh-negative
+ Rh-positive
⊕ Antibodies

First pregnancy: An Rh-negative woman may have an Rh-positive baby.

Cells from Rh-positive baby enter the mother's bloodstream. Woman may become sensitized—antibodies form to fight Rh-positive cells.

Second pregnancy: In the next Rh-positive pregnancy, antibodies attack fetal blood cells.

given at about 28 weeks of pregnancy and again right after the birth (if the baby is Rh positive) to prevent harm to the next child. RhIg also is given if the mother had a miscarriage or certain procedures, such as amniocentesis, during pregnancy.

If the mother has become sensitized already, the baby is at risk. The levels of antibodies in mother's blood are checked during pregnancy. If they become high, tests may be done to check the health of the baby.

The baby may be anemic and need a blood transfusion. After 18 weeks of pregnancy, a transfusion can be given while the baby is still in the uterus. If the baby is old enough, early birth may be an option. The baby most likely will be taken care of in a special-care nursery.

Breech

It is normal for a baby move about until 34 weeks of pregnancy. Around that time, most babies move so their heads are down near the birth canal. This is called a **vertex presentation** (the vertex is the top of the head). If this does not happen, the baby's buttocks, or buttocks and feet, will be in place to come out first during birth. This is called breech presentation. It occurs in about 1 of 25 full-term births.

The causes of breech presentation are not fully known. It is more likely for some women if:

➤ She has had more than one pregnancy.

➤ There is more than one baby in the uterus.

➤ The delivery is early.

➤ The uterus has too much or too little amniotic fluid.

➤ The uterus is an abnormal shape or has growths, such as fibroids.

➤ Placenta previa occurs.

Birth defects are slightly more common in breech babies. A birth defect may be the reason the baby has not moved into the vertex position before birth.

Sometimes, the baby can be turned into a head-down position by **external version**, also known as "version." Version may be an option for some women. Version can be done at 36 weeks of pregnancy. Version does not involve surgery, but there is some discomfort. Medication may be given first to relax the uterus. The doctor will do an ultrasound exam to check the condition and the placement of the baby, the location of the placenta, and the amount of amniotic fluid in the uterus. Ultrasound also is used during the procedure to check on the progress of the turn.

With version, the doctor places his or her hands at certain key points on your lower abdomen. The doctor then pushes to turn the baby. The baby slowly turns as if it were doing a somersault. Before, during, and after version, your baby's heartbeat will be checked closely.

More than half of the tries at version succeed in turning the baby. However, some babies will shift back into a breech position. If that happens, your doctor may try version again.

Although problems seldom occur with version, there is some risk for the following:

➤ Rupture of membranes

➤ Problems with the baby's heart rate

➤ Beginning of labor

➤ Placental abruption

If any problems arise, efforts to turn the baby will be stopped right away. Your doctor may then advise cesarean delivery. If the baby is still in the breech position by the due date, a cesarean

Breech Birth

In a vertex delivery, the baby's head emerges first and usually stretches the cervix enough to allow the rest of the body to pass through the birth canal.

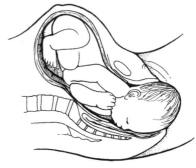

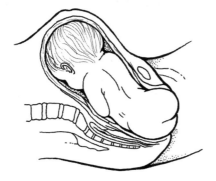

In a breech birth, where the lower body is delivered first, there may be less room for the head to be guided out.

delivery may be the best option. Although cesarean delivery has some risks, it may pose less risk than a vaginal delivery for a breech baby.

A baby in the breech position is harder to deliver than a baby in the normal, head-down position. Vaginal delivery of a breech baby carries more risks than vaginal delivery of a baby in the normal position. This is because at the time of birth, the baby's head is the largest and firmest part of its body. When the baby is in the normal, head-down position, the baby's head emerges first. In most cases, the rest can be

guided out through the birth canal. In a breech birth, though, the baby's head emerges last. It may be harder to ease it through the birth canal. During a vaginal delivery, there also is an increased risk of a prolapsed cord. This is when the umbilical cord slips through the cervix and comes into the birth canal before the baby. This can stop the flow of blood through the cord.

Breech babies are more difficult to deliver even by cesarean birth. Also, cesarean delivery won't solve all of the problems, such as birth defects, that are linked to breech presentation. If labor is advanced and delivery is near or if a woman is having twins, it may not be possible to plan a cesarean delivery of a baby in the breech position.

Multiple Pregnancy

When a woman is carrying more than one baby it is called a multiple pregnancy. Multiple pregnancies have become more common in the last two decades. They now make up about 3% of all pregnancies. One of the reasons for the increase in multiple pregnancies is that more women are using fertility treatments to help them get pregnant. With this treatment, multiple eggs are produced and fertilized.

The following factors can increase the chances of a multiple pregnancy:

➤ Family history of multiple pregnancy.

➤ Fertility drugs or other treatments.

➤ Age older than 35 years.

The most common kind of multiple pregnancy is twins, when the uterus contains two fetuses. Twins are born once in about every 32 births in the United States. There are two types of twins. Either two separate eggs are fertilized, causing *fraternal twins*, or a single egg divides into two fetuses, known as *identical twins*. Identical twins are somewhat rare. They occur less than once in every 100 births.

Even more rare is a pregnancy with three or more babies. Three or more babies can be formed by more than one egg being fertilized, a single fertilized egg splitting, or both methods combined. The birth of triplets (three babies) or more babies occurs once in about every 540 births in the United States. However, triplets occur naturally in only 1 of about 3,000 births. The other births of multiple babies occur as the result of fertility treatments.

Most multiple pregnancies are found before delivery. If the doctor suspects a multiple pregnancy, an ultrasound exam may be done to confirm it. Ultrasound also is used to check the growth of the babies. There are some signs of multiple pregnancy:

➤ Extreme bouts of nausea and vomiting in the first trimester.

➤ More fetal movement than in previous pregnancies.

➤ The uterus grows more quickly or is larger than expected.

➤ More than one heartbeat can be heard.

The risk of problems during pregnancy increases with the number of babies. That is, there is a higher risk of problems with twins than with a single fetus, a higher risk with triplets than with twins, and so on.

Women who are carrying more than one baby, may need special care during pregnancy, labor, and delivery. During pregnancy, you need to eat about 500 more calories per day about a total of

How Are Twins Formed?

You may wonder why sometimes twins look so much alike and at other times don't seem to look alike at all. It has to do with how twins are formed.

Fraternal Twins

Most twins are fraternal. Each grows from a separate egg and sperm. As a rule, a woman's ovaries release one egg each month to be fertilized. Sometimes two or more eggs are released and both become fertilized. This creates fraternal twins. (Sometimes these twins will be described as dizygotic, meaning two zygotes or two fertilized eggs.)

Each fraternal twin has its own placenta and amniotic sac. Because each twin grows from the union of a different egg and a different sperm, these twins are similar only in the same way any brothers and sisters are. The twins can be both boys, both girls, or one of each.

Identical Twins

Sometimes, for unknown reasons, one fertilized egg splits early in pregnancy and grows into two or more fetuses. Two fetuses formed this way are identical (or monozygotic) twins. They share a placenta. Often each has its own amniotic sac.

Because identical twins share the same genetic material at the start, they are the same sex and have the same blood type, hair color, and eye color. These twins can look so much alike that even their mothers may have difficulty telling them apart.

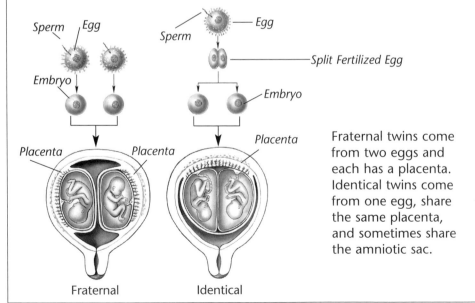

Fraternal twins come from two eggs and each has a placenta. Identical twins come from one egg, share the same placenta, and sometimes share the amniotic sac.

2,700 calories per day for twins. Extra vitamins and minerals can be taken to meet these needs.

Certain complications are more likely with a multiple pregnancy:

➤ High blood pressure or anemia

➤ Preterm labor (see "Preterm Birth")

➤ Premature rupture of membranes (see "Early Rupture of Membranes")

➤ Fetal growth problems

With twins, one or both may need to be born by cesarean birth. How they are born depends on their position, weight, and health. If both are in the head-down position, they may be born vaginally. The heart rates of each twin will be monitored during labor. In pregnancies with three or more babies, cesarean delivery usually is performed. Twins and triplets often are delivered before 37 weeks of gestation. A pediatrician or neonatologist—a doctor who is an expert in the care of newborns—will examine the babies after birth.

Preterm Birth

Pregnancy typically lasts about 40 weeks. Babies born before 37 weeks are *preterm*, and usually are not fully grown. This occurs in about 12% of babies born in the United States each year. The earlier the baby is born, the greater the risk of a problem. Preterm birth accounts for 75% of newborn deaths that are not related to birth defects. Preterm babies may have problems right away that need special care in the hospital, and they may have long-term problems, including learning and behavioral problems and trouble with vision, hearing, and breathing.

Preterm labor can happen to anyone, without warning. Some of the following factors have been linked to preterm labor:

➤ Past pregnancies with preterm labor or birth

➤ Special problems in this pregnancy

➤ Multiple pregnancy

➤ Abdominal surgery during pregnancy

➤ Infection in the mother

➤ Bleeding in mid-pregnancy

➤ Weight of the mother less than 110 pounds

➤ Previous pregnancy loss in second trimester

➤ Placenta previa

➤ Premature rupture of membranes ("water breaks" too soon)

➤ High blood pressure

➤ Chronic illness in the woman

➤ Too much fluid in the amniotic sac

➤ Birth defects in the baby

Defects in the uterus, such as an incompetent cervix, also have been linked to preterm labor. A cervix is called incompetent when it opens before the full term of pregnancy. The causes of this are not certain. An ultrasound exam may be done to measure the length of the cervix.

For some women with an incompetent cervix, a procedure called *cerclage* may be done. Cerclage is a procedure that "stitches" the cervix closed. The stitch usually is taken out at the 37th week of pregnancy.

Signs of Preterm Labor

Preterm birth can result if labor starts before the end of the 37th week. If preterm labor is found early, attempts may be made to postpone birth to give your baby extra time to grow and mature. Even a few more days in the womb may mean a healthier baby. The box lists signs of preterm labor.

Sometimes the signs that preterm labor may be starting are fairly easy to detect. For instance, you can monitor yourself to see if you are having contractions. Lie down on your side and gently feel the entire surface of your lower abdomen with your fingertips. Feel for a firm tightening over the surface of your uterus. Often this tightening is not painful. If you feel these contractions, keep track of them for an hour. Note when each one starts and ends. If you have contractions that occur four times every 20 minutes or if

you have contractions eight times an hour that last for more than an hour, call your doctor right away. You may be in preterm labor.

The only way to know whether a woman is truly in preterm labor is to check her cervix. In labor, the cervix thins out (effaces) and opens up (dilates) so the baby can enter the birth canal.

Fetal monitoring also can be done to check the heartbeat of the baby and contractions of the uterus. Ultrasound may be used to estimate the size and age of the baby and to check the cervix.

Sometimes contractions have begun, but the membranes have not ruptured and the cervix has not dilated. If this happens between weeks 24 and 35 of pregnancy, the doctor may measure the amount of a substance called *fibronectin* in the vaginal discharge. If the amount of fibronectin is normal, preterm birth is unlikely within the next 2 weeks.

If preterm birth seems likely, a decision must be made whether to deliver the baby. A key factor is if the baby's lungs are mature enough to function outside the uterus. Amniocentesis may be used to check your baby's lungs. If the lungs are not mature, they are not coated with enough of a substance called *surfactant*. Without this coating, the baby may have trouble breathing. This is called respiratory distress syndrome. It is the most common cause of death in preterm babies.

Signs of Preterm Labor

Call your doctor or nurse right away if you notice any of these signs:

➤ Change in vaginal discharge (becomes watery, mucus-like, or bloody)

➤ Increase in amount of vaginal discharge

➤ Pelvic or lower-abdominal pressure

➤ Constant, low, dull backache

➤ Mild abdominal cramps, with or without diarrhea

➤ Regular or frequent contractions or uterine tightening, often painless (four times every 20 minutes or 8 times an hour for more than one hour)

➤ Ruptured membranes (your water breaks—whether a gush or a trickle)

If it looks as though the baby may come, a medication called a corticosteroid is given. This will increase the amount of surfactant in the baby's lungs. It helps the baby's lungs mature, reduces bleeding problems, and increases the baby's chance to live. Corticosteroids are most likely to work when preterm labor begins between 24 and 34 weeks of pregnancy.

Preventing Preterm Birth

In the earliest stages of labor if there is no sign that the mother or the baby are in danger from infection, bleeding, or other problems, attempts can be made to try to stop labor. This will allow the baby more time to grow and mature.

Medications may be used to stop or slow preterm labor. These medications are called *tocolytics.* They may delay birth for 2–7 days. Sometimes a tocolytic is given to allow the corticosteroid to help the baby's lungs. Also, a delay can allow time for transfer to a hospital with special care for premature babies.

As with all medications, tocolytics can have side effects. Each woman responds in her own way. Side effects can include the following:

➤ Fast pulse

➤ Chest pressure or pain

➤ Feeling dizzy

➤ Headache

➤Feeling of warmth

➤Feeling shaky or nervous

Women at risk for preterm labor, may be asked to limit their activities. Some women may need to stay in the hospital for a while. The advice of your doctor depends on the findings of the exam and other tests.

Progesterone may help prevent preterm birth in some women who have had a previous preterm birth. More research is needed to find out if progesterone can prevent preterm birth in women with other risk factors, such as carrying multiple babies.

Your Preterm Baby

Sometimes preterm labor may be too advanced to be stopped. In some cases, the baby is better off being born—even if the birth is early. Reasons can include infection, high blood pressure, bleeding, or other signs that the baby is having problems.

Preterm labor and delivery involve risks that require special care. You or your baby may be moved to a hospital

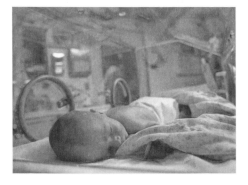

that can provide this expert care. The baby may need to stay in the hospital after you are discharged.

Preterm babies look different from term babies. They may be red and skinny because they have little fat under their skin and their blood vessels are close to the surface. The earlier a baby is born, the less developed he or she is. This can lead to breathing problems (such as respiratory distress syndrome), feeding problems, or an increased risk of infection. Survival rates are best for babies after 24 weeks. After 32 weeks the baby is less likely to have long-term problems.

Early Rupture of Membranes

In most cases, when "the water breaks" (rupture of the membranes that hold the amniotic fluid), it is followed by other signs of labor. Sometimes, though, the membranes break before labor begins. This is called ***premature rupture of membranes.***

Call your doctor if you have a discharge of fluid from your vagina. The doctor will want to see you to evaluate if your membranes have ruptured. Sometimes you may have a discharge for other reasons. Diagnosis of rupture of the membranes depends on your medical history, physical exam, and lab tests. It is confirmed when there is amniotic fluid in the vagina. Other tests, such as ultrasound, can be done when the diagnosis is not clear.

Although some fluid is lost when the membranes rupture, the baby will produce more fluid. This may cause more leaking from the uterus.

One of every 10 women has premature rupture of membranes. The reasons are not clear. Some causes may be infection or bleeding.

With premature rupture of membranes, other problems can occur:

➤ Infection of the amniotic fluid, the baby, or the mother

➤ Umbilical cord problems

➤ Placental abruption

If these problems occur, the doctor will decide to induce labor. If premature rupture of membranes occurs before the baby is ready to be born (before 37 weeks of pregnancy), this is called preterm premature rupture of membranes. If this happens, usually efforts are made to delay birth until the baby is more developed.

Most women with premature rupture of membranes need to stay in the hospital. That is because an infection can occur suddenly, and the baby also is at risk for umbilical cord compression.

Rest, fluids, and medications may be used to manage preterm premature rupture of membranes. Antibiotics or corticosteroids may be given depending on the stage of pregnancy. Antibiotics can lower the risk of infection and respiratory distress syndrome. Corticosteroids are used to help the baby's lungs mature and to reduce the risk of respiratory distress syndrome.

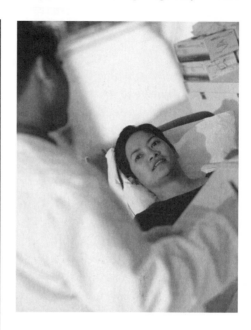

Postterm Pregnancy

Most women (80%) give birth between 38 and 42 weeks of pregnancy. These pregnancies are called term pregnancies. Up to 10% of normal pregnancies are not delivered by 42 weeks. These are called postterm pregnancies.

Knowing the gestational age of the baby is key in knowing if a pregnancy is postterm. It can be hard, though, to pinpoint the age of the baby. A woman may not be sure when her last period was, for instance. For this reason, more than one method may be used to cross-check the age of the baby (see "Due Date" in Chapter 2).

Only a small number of pregnancies that go past 42 weeks have problems. In fact, about 95% of postterm babies are born without problems. As pregnancy moves past 42 weeks, the baby has a higher risk of the following conditions:

➤ *Dysmaturity syndrome.* The baby is malnourished and born with a long and lean body, an alert look on the face, lots of hair, long fingernails, and thin, wrinkled skin.

➤ *Macrosomia.* The baby grows larger than normal, which can pose problems during and after birth.

➤ *Meconium aspiration.* The baby inhales meconium (greenish waste that is emptied from the baby's bowels into the amniotic fluid). This blocks the airways, causing the baby to gasp for air. It requires treatment right away.

A number of tests can be used to check the well-being of the baby. Tests often are started between 40 and 42 weeks of pregnancy. Some tests are done in the doctor's office. Others are done in the hospital. (Chapter 3 gives details about testing for fetal well-being.)

If the baby seems to be active and healthy and the amount of amniotic fluid appears normal, monitoring may be done at set times until labor starts on its own. At 42 weeks of pregnancy, labor is induced to avoid problems of postterm birth. Some women wonder why the doctor doesn't simply bring on labor before 42 weeks of pregnancy. First, there is a chance that the due date is off. Often, neither the mother nor her doctor can be sure that the baby is fully mature and ready to be born. Second, in

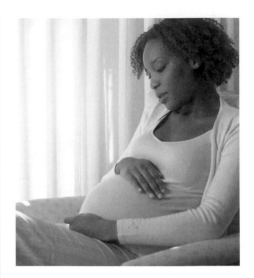

some women, the cervix is not ready for labor to start.

If the cervix is not ready, a number of agents can be used to help dilate the cervix. These are called "cervical-ripening" agents. If the baby seems to be having problems, labor may need to be induced. This can be done in a number of ways. (For more details on cervical ripening and inducing labor, see "Helping Labor Along" in Chapter 8.)

If problems arise, the baby may be delivered by cesarean birth. After birth, a postterm baby may need special care.

Special Care

If your pregnancy involves certain complications, your doctor will monitor your health until you give birth. In most cases, you will give birth to a healthy child. You should follow your doctor's advice and take steps to keep yourself healthy.

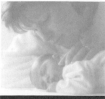

CHAPTER **16**

Pregnancy Loss

Most babies are born healthy. Even with the best of care, however, things can go wrong. If you lose a baby, you may feel shock, anger, guilt, sorrow, and pain. If your baby is alive but has a severe physical or mental problem, you also may have feelings of grief and loss. These feelings are normal. There are ways to work through the normal grieving process to help you and your loved ones cope with the loss.

Most women get emotionally attached to their babies long before the actual birth. This process is called bonding. The bond grows stronger throughout pregnancy. As the weeks and months of your pregnancy go by, you may imagine how the baby will look and what he or she will be like. Around 16–20 weeks of pregnancy, when you first feel your baby move, the bond may become much more intense. The father also develops a strong tie to

his unborn child. He may have many of the same feelings you do.

Losing your baby can bring intense sadness and shock. In almost all cases, you did not expect it to happen. The loss of a baby at any stage—during pregnancy or after birth—is tragic.

Miscarriage

Miscarriage, also known as early pregnancy loss, can occur in any pregnancy. Early pregnancy loss can cause pain and disappointment. How intense your feelings are does not always relate to the time in pregnancy when the loss occurs. A miscarriage can bring the same sorrow as a stillbirth.

In addition to grief, you may have feelings of guilt or a sense of failure. The truth is you may never know the reason for the miscarriage. But it is not your fault. There is no evidence that

Dealing With Loss

Consider some of these activities to help you after a pregnancy loss:

➤ Talk about the baby with family and close friends.

➤ Read books and articles about dealing with loss or that offer comfort.

➤ Express yourself by writing in a journal or by writing letters to the baby and others.

➤ Stay physically active—take a daily walk, for instance.

➤ Tell friends and family what they can do for you, whether cooking a meal, running errands, or just spending time with you.

➤ Join a support group, either in person or online.

➤ Find a grief counselor; the hospital may be able to refer you to someone.

➤ Get enough sleep every night.

➤ Eat healthy, well-balanced foods.

➤ Don't drink alcohol or take drugs.

working, exercising, or having sex increase the risk of miscarriage, for instance. Also, miscarriage usually is not something that can be prevented. Some women have repeated miscarriages, which can make it even more difficult to handle.

A miscarriage can be devastating, and there is no right or wrong way to grieve. Takes steps to help yourself cope with your feelings.

Stillbirth and Neonatal Death

The death of a baby in the womb after week 20 of pregnancy is called a still-birth. This happens in about 1 in 200 pregnancies. Most of these deaths occur before labor begins.

Usually, the first sign of a problem is that your baby has stopped moving. Ultrasound then is used to see if the baby is alive. If your baby dies in the womb, your doctor will talk with you about the best options for delivery. Often, the best thing may be to induce labor. This decision depends on your health and the stage of your pregnancy.

After birth, the baby and placenta are examined to help find the cause of death. In as many as one third of the cases, the reason for stillbirth is unknown.

When a baby dies within 28 days of birth, it is referred to as neonatal death. This event can make you feel overwhelmed and angry. You want to know why this happened to your baby.

Neonatal death most often occurs because a baby had birth defects or was born early. There also may be complications during labor and delivery that can cause death. These include problems with the placenta, the umbilical cord, infection, and lack of oxygen.

Having a baby that is stillborn or dies soon after birth is a profoundly painful event. You will need to heal both physically and emotionally.

Grieving

Grief is a normal, natural response to the loss of your baby. Working through grief and mourning your loss are healing processes that help you adapt and move ahead with your life.

The goal is not to "get over" the loss of your baby. That will never happen. But you can learn to move on.

The Stages of Grief

Grieving includes a wide range of feelings. Just as each pregnancy is unique, ways to react to a pregnancy loss also are unique. The process you follow will be affected by your experiences with death, the culture you were raised in, your role in the family, and what you think others expect of you.

The grieving process that follows the death of a loved one may last 2 years or more. It goes through certain stages that can overlap and repeat. Each person who goes through the grieving process will heal in his or her own way. However, the process often seems to follow a common pattern in many people and consists of shock, numbness, and disbelief; searching and yearning; anger or rage; depression and loneliness; and acceptance.

Shock, numbness, and disbelief

When faced with news of their baby's death, parents often think "This is not really happening" or "This can't be true." You may deny that the loss has occurred. You may have trouble grasping the news or feel nothing at all. Even though you and your partner may be together physically, you may each feel a very private sense of being alone or empty.

Searching and yearning

These feelings tend to overlap with your initial shock and get stronger over time. You may start looking for a reason for your baby's death—who or what caused him or her to die? It is common during this stage to feel very guilty. You may think that somehow you brought about your baby's death and blame yourself for things you did or did not do. You may have dreams about the baby and yearn for what might have been. You may even think you are going crazy.

Anger or rage

"What did I do to deserve this?" and "How could this happen to me?" are common feelings after losing a baby. In this stage of grief you may find yourself questioning your religious beliefs. You may direct your anger at your partner, the doctor, the hospital staff, or even other women whose babies were born healthy. If you or your partner feel angry toward each other, it may be hard for you to comfort each other. It's good to accept your anger, express it, and try to get it out of your system. Anger becomes unhealthy if you turn it inward and direct it toward yourself.

Depression and loneliness

In this stage, the reality sinks in that you have lost your baby. You may feel tired and run down, sad, out of sorts, and helpless. You may have trouble getting back into your normal routine. The support from friends and family that you received during the early weeks of your loss may be gone, even though you still need comfort and kindness. Your relationships with people may be strained because others do not understand your feelings. Slowly you will start to get back on your feet and work through your loss.

Acceptance

In this final stage of grieving, you come to terms with what has happened. Your baby's death no longer rules your thoughts. You start to have renewed energy. Although you will never forget your baby, you begin to think of him or her less often and with less pain. You pick up your normal daily routine and social life. You laugh with friends and make plans for the future. You may feel ready to start planning your next pregnancy.

Other Signs of Grieving

As you grieve, you may have other feelings or symptoms that are natural and normal. The following symptoms are likely to occur in the first months after your loss:

➤ Aches and pains in the breasts and arms

➤ A tight feeling in the chest and throat

➤ Heart flutters

➤ Headaches

➤ Trouble sleeping

➤ Nightmares

➤ Loss of appetite

➤ Tiredness and easy fatigue

➤ Loss of memory and trouble concentrating

➤ Pictures of the baby in your mind

Grieving mothers often feel as if their bodies have failed them. At first you may want to ignore your health or work or how you look. These feelings may be worse if your body is sore or slow to heal from the baby's birth.

Although you may not be concerned about your own health, you need to take special care of yourself. If at any time you have concerns about what's going on in your body or mind, talk to someone who makes you feel comfortable and will listen. Allow yourself time to heal, both physically and emotionally.

You and Your Partner

Your relationship with your partner may be affected by the stress of the loss of your child. You may have trouble getting your thoughts and feelings across to each other. One or both of you may feel hostile toward the other. You may find it hard to have sex again or do other things together that you used to enjoy. This is normal. Try to be patient with each other. Let your partner know what your needs are and what you are feeling. Take time to be tender, caring, and close. Make an extra effort to be open and honest.

Throughout the grieving process, your partner may not respond in the same way as you do. Your partner may feel differently from you and may be able to move on before you are. Your partner may not be ready to talk about the loss when you are. Each person should be allowed to grieve in his or her own way. Try to understand and respond to your partner's needs as well as your own.

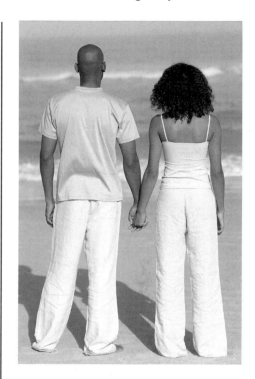

Making Decisions

When you lose a baby, you must make certain decisions—even if you don't feel like facing anything. You also may choose to take certain actions, such as naming the baby or holding a memorial service, that help you through the healing process.

Saying Goodbye

You may or may not want to see your baby when it is born. Although this may sound scary or morbid at first, other bereaved parents suggest that seeing your baby may be very helpful to you. It may help you realize your loss more fully and make it easier to let go of him or her. It can create a personal memory of your baby that you can carry with you. Most parents find that the truth is far kinder and gentler than they had imagined.

Choosing a Name

Naming the baby helps give him or her an identity. A name allows you, your friends, and your family to refer to a specific child, not just "the baby you lost." You may want to use the name you first chose or pick another one.

Mementos

Many parents treasure mementos of their baby. You may want to ask the nurse to give you a lock of hair, a handprint or footprint, an ID bracelet, or a crib card from your baby.

Photos also can help create a memory of your baby. Even if you don't think you will want pictures of your baby, think about having them taken anyway so that you will have them if you change your mind later.

Autopsy

Your doctor may ask to do an *autopsy*—an exam of your baby's organs—or other tests to help find the cause of death. Although the doctor may not be able to tell the exact reason why your baby died, an autopsy may help answer questions about what happened. The information the autopsy provides may be useful for your family in planning future pregnancies.

Many parents are relieved to know the cause of death or to learn that no special problems were found. An autopsy does not delay burial and does not prevent having an open casket at a funeral. The costs may not be covered by insurance.

Funeral or Memorial Service

You may choose to have a religious or memorial service. For many parents, it is a great comfort to have family and friends acknowledge the life and death of their baby and to express their sorrow at a special service.

You will need to decide what will be done with your baby's body. You may wish to contact a funeral home for burial or cremation. Some parents find comfort in having a grave site they can visit. Check with your hospital to see what your options are.

Going Home

It's hard to leave the hospital with empty arms and face an empty nursery. Once you arrive home, it also may be hard to deal with family and friends. Most people will not be aware of the effect your loss has on you or how best to support you as you grieve. Although they do not mean to hurt you, people often cannot understand the pain involved in losing a baby.

They care for you and want to comfort you. However, they may say things that cause you pain, such as "You're young, you can try again," "Be grateful for your other children," "Some things happen for the best," "Be brave," or "You'll get over it." Some people may avoid you. They may avoid talking about the baby because they feel awkward.

During this time you should put your own needs first. Let people know what you want from them and how you are feeling. You don't need to force yourself to be brave just to please others.

To ease the pain of telling other people what has happened, you can send out announcements of the baby's birth and death. People you know casually who see that you are no longer pregnant may not be aware of your loss. They may ask questions. Prepare a simple sentence you can use in response.

If you have other children at home, tell them that the baby has died. Trying to shield children from death doesn't work. They can sense your sadness, anger, and fear. When telling young children about what happened to the baby, avoid placing blame. Make sure they understand that the baby's death is not their fault. Children often feel angry and jealous toward a new baby. The news of the baby's death may make them wonder if their thoughts and feelings somehow caused it.

Children sometimes fear that they or their parents also may be in danger of dying. You need to assure them that nothing they did caused the baby's death and that there is no danger to them or you. Children's responses to

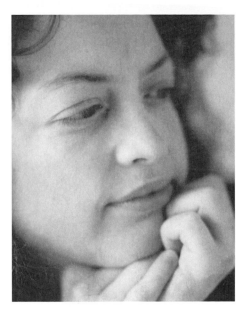

death vary. It depends on their ages and personalities. Let them know you can see they are upset over the baby's death and that you feel the same way. Be sure to include your children in any funeral or memorial service.

Once you've returned home, take off the time you had planned after the baby's birth if you can. Going back to the pressures of work and seeing coworkers can be hard if you are not up for it. Sometimes you have no choice but to go back to your job or resume a full life right away.

Don't be surprised if feelings of grief come back on your due date or on anniversaries of your baby's birth or death. This is called an "anniversary reaction" or "shadow grief." You may dread these days and suffer through them, while family and friends seem to have forgotten. It helps to be aware of

Support Systems

Getting in touch with one of the resources listed here may help you cope with your loss. These organizations offer support, friendship, and understanding. They offer services on the Internet and some have local support groups that you can join.

CLIMB: Center for Loss in Multiple Birth, Inc.
PO Box 91377
Anchorage AK 99509-1377
907-222-5321
E-mail: climb@pobox.alaska.net
www.climb-support.org

The Compassionate Friends
PO Box 3696
Oak Brook, IL 60522-3696
877-969-0010 or 630-990-0010
Fax: 630-990-0246
E-mail: nationaloffice@compassion
  atefriends.org
www.compassionatefriends.org

First Candle/SIDS Alliance
1314 Bedford Avenue, Suite 210
Baltimore, MD 21208-6605
800-221-7437 or 410-653-8226
Fax: 410-653-8709
E-mail: info@firstcandle.org
www.sidsalliance.org

International Stillbirth Alliance
1427 Potter Road
Park Ridge, IL 60068
E-mail: info@stillbirthalliance.org
www.stillbirthalliance.org

RESOLVE/The National Infertility Association
1310 Broadway
Somerville, MA 02144
617-623-1156 or 888-623-0744
E-mail: info@resolve.org
www.resolve.org

SHARE: Pregnancy and Infant Loss Support, Inc.
St. Joseph's Health Center
300 First Capitol Drive
St. Charles, MO 63301-2893
800-821-6819 or 636-947-6164
Fax: 636-947-7486
E-mail:
share@nationalshareoffice.com
www.nationalshareoffice.com

these feelings and to let others know how you feel. Often, parents find that doing something special to mark the date—such as making a visit to the grave site or giving money to a charity in the baby's name—is helpful.

Seeking Support

As you grieve, you will feel defenseless at times. The pain of your baby's death can remind you of painful experiences from the past, such as other losses and deaths, infertility, or family problems. Often, the pain from these past experiences can return and get in the way of the healing process.

Find a network of people who can support you right after the baby's death and in the months that follow. Know you are not alone. A number of people have the knowledge and skills to help you. Your doctor or nurse may be able to direct you to support systems in your community. These can include childbirth educators, self-help groups, social workers, and clergy. Some of these resources may be more helpful than others. You will need to find the one that fits your needs.

Many grieving parents find it helpful to get involved with groups of parents who have gone through the same loss. Members of such support groups respect your feelings, understand your stresses and fears, and have a good sense of the kindness you need.

Professional counseling also can help to relieve your pain, guilt, and depression. Talking with a trained counselor can help you understand and accept what has happened. You may wish to get counseling for yourself only, for you and your partner, or for your entire family. These are some reasons for seeking help:

➤ You feel "stuck" in a phase of the grief process so that you cannot work through certain problems.

➤ You have severe physical or emotional problems that keep you from functioning. These include not feeling able to return to work, losing interest in your health and looks, having trouble sleeping, or staying in bed all day. (For more information on depression see Chapter 12.)

Another Pregnancy?

Before thinking about getting pregnant again, allow time for you and your partner to work through your feelings. After losing a baby, some couples feel a need to have another baby right away. They think it will fill the empty feeling or take away the pain. A new baby cannot replace the baby that was lost. If you have another baby too soon after your loss, you may find it hard to think of the new child as a separate and special person.

Should you choose to have another pregnancy, keep in mind that the chances of losing another baby are very small in most cases. Even so, you may be anxious and worried during your next pregnancy. Talk with your doctor or nurse about the baby's death. Find out the chances that it could happen again and what you can do to reduce these risks. Your doctor may suggest certain tests before or during your pregnancy to find problems as early as possible. (Chapter 18 has more details related to planning your next pregnancy.)

The Future

The pain of losing your baby will never vanish completely, but it will not always be the main focus in your life and thoughts. At some point you will be able to talk and think about the baby more easily and with less pain. One day you'll find yourself doing more of the things you used to do—like enjoy favorite activities, renew friendships, and look forward to the future.

CHAPTER 17

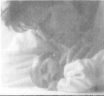

Infections During Pregnancy

Infections are caused by tiny organisms that invade the body and then spread. These organisms can be bacteria or viruses. The body draws on its immune system to fight back and try to kill the invaders. While this fight is going on, symptoms of the infection, such as a rash, pain, fever, and swelling, may occur. You also form antibodies in your blood.

Antibodies are special proteins that form in the blood to combat infection when it strikes. They are a key part of the immune system. Tests can show if they are present. If antibodies to a disease are present, the person has been exposed to that disease. In many cases, once the body makes antibodies to a disease, the person becomes immune to the disease and will not get it in the future.

Infections can range from a mild cold or flu-like illness to life-threatening disease. Certain infections can harm the fetus if the mother is exposed to them during pregnancy. Although a cold or flu often is not harmful to the mother or fetus, over-the-counter medications to treat it may cause harm.

Sometimes an infection may not cause any symptoms or the symptoms may not occur right away. The earlier an infection is found and treated, the less likely it is for long-term health problems to develop.

Some infections can be prevented with vaccines. However, certain types of vaccines are not safe during pregnancy. A vaccine contains either a small amount of the same organism that causes the infection or a small amount of an organism like it. The amount is just enough to cause antibodies to form, but not enough to cause illness.

The best way to protect against infections is to be vaccinated or to avoid being exposed to them before and during pregnancy. If you think you have

Vaccines

Vaccines help prevent diseases caused by infection. Like all medicines, a vaccine should be used during pregnancy only when it is needed and safe. It is best for you to have all your vaccinations before you become pregnant. If a vaccination is needed during pregnancy, waiting until the fourth month is best.

Avoid being exposed to measles, rubella, mumps, and chickenpox during pregnancy. You should be vaccinated against measles, rubella, and mumps at least 1 month before you become pregnant. You also should be vaccinated against chickenpox at least 1 month before becoming pregnant. If you are pregnant but not yet vaccinated, you should ask your doctor when you should be. Vaccination is safe for both you and your baby while you are breastfeeding. Pregnant women also should be vaccinated for influenza if they will be pregnant during the flu season (November–March).

The following vaccines usually are not given to pregnant women as a rule, but the benefits may outweigh the risks if you are likely to come in contact with the infections:

➤ Hepatitis A
➤ Hepatitis B
➤ Pneumonia caused by *pneumococcus*
➤ Rabies
➤ Polio
➤ Diphtheria
➤ Tetanus

The following vaccines contain a live virus and should be avoided during pregnancy:

➤ Lyme disease
➤ Measles
➤ Mumps
➤ Rubella
➤ Varicella (chickenpox)

been exposed to an infection, tell your doctor or nurse right away. Sometimes steps can be taken to avoid problems and decrease any risk to your baby.

Sexually Transmitted Diseases

Sexually transmitted diseases (STDs) are infections that are passed from one person to another during sex. Some STDs can be harmful during pregnancy. For instance, if you have an STD, you are more likely to have preterm labor and an inflammation of the lining of the uterus.

If you think you might have an STD, get tested and treated right away. Your partner also should be treated. Neither of you should have sex until you have finished treatment.

Chlamydia and Gonorrhea

Chlamydia and *gonorrhea* are the most common STDs in the United States. They are caused by bacteria that are passed from person to person during sex. The infections are alike in many ways and often occur at the same time. They infect the same sites in a woman's reproductive tract. In many cases, the cervix, rectum, and urethra (the opening through which urine is passed) are infected.

The most common symptoms in men with chlamydia or gonorrhea are a discharge from the penis and painful urination. Often a woman has no symptoms and learns she has one of these STDs when her sexual partner tells her or she is tested. Screening for these STDs is part of regular prenatal care. They can be treated with antibiotics, even during pregnancy.

Pregnant women who are infected have an increased chance of having premature rupture of membranes and preterm birth. Some women may even have a miscarriage.

Chlamydia and gonorrhea can infect newborns during vaginal birth. A newborn's eyes are an easy target for chlamydia. To prevent damage, the eyes of all newborns are treated at birth whether or not the mother has chlamydia. Chlamydia also can cause pneumonia in a newborn.

Chlamydia and gonorrhea can cause pelvic inflammatory disease. This is a severe infection that spreads from the vagina and cervix through the pelvic area. It may attack the uterus, fallopian tubes, and ovaries.

Herpes Simplex Virus

Genital herpes is an infection caused by herpes simplex virus. Symptoms are painful sores and blisters on or around the sex organs. Herpes also can affect the mouth, eyes, fingers, and other parts of the body. Other symptoms include swollen glands, fever, chills, muscle aches, fatigue, and nausea. Sometimes there are no symptoms.

The infection is spread by direct contact with a person who has active sores.

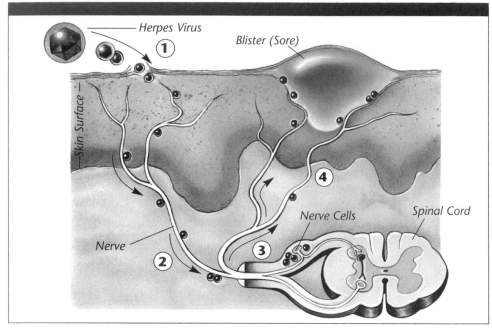

The herpes virus passes through your skin (1). It travels through your body (2) and settles at nerve cells near your spine (3). When something triggers a new bout of herpes, the virus leaves its resting place and travels along the nerve, back to the surface of the skin (4).

In some cases, the virus can be passed to others even when the sores have healed.

There is no cure for genital herpes. However, there are some medications available to treat the symptoms. Herpes sores will heal, but the virus stays in nerve cells near your spine. It stays there until some event triggers a new bout. Then the sores will appear again.

In rare cases, newborns can become infected with the herpes virus during birth. This can cause damage to the nervous system, blindness, mental retardation, or death. The risk is increased when a woman gets herpes for the first time late in pregnancy. Although it is very rare, genital herpes during pregnancy can cause miscarriage.

If you have ever had genital herpes or have had sex with someone who has, tell your doctor or nurse. He or she will want to see if you have open lesions. If you have had herpes in the past but have no herpes sores, the baby can be born vaginally. If there are signs of active infection when you are in labor, you may need to have your baby by cesarean birth. Cesarean birth lessens the chance that the baby will come in contact with the virus. However, a baby can become infected without passing through the vagina. This can occur if the amniotic sac has broken a few hours before birth.

Human Papillomavirus

Human papillomavirus (HPV) is a very common virus that can cause **genital warts.** You can have HPV even without having genital warts. In women, the warts are in clusters on the vulva, inside the vagina, on the cervix, or around the anus. Sometimes the warts cause itching and bleeding. Warts in the genital area are easily passed from person to person during sex. This includes oral and anal sex.

There is a very slight risk that babies born to mothers with HPV can get the infection. In rare cases, a newborn may have warts in his or her throat. This is not a reason for cesarean delivery.

Genital warts may go away on their own. Certain medications that are prescribed to treat the warts should not be used during pregnancy. They are absorbed in the skin and may cause birth defects.

Warts can grow in number and size during pregnancy. Rarely, warts in the vagina or on the cervix can cause problems during birth. They can make the birth canal less elastic or cause a blockage. If this occurs, cesarean birth is needed.

If there are a lot of warts or they are large, minor surgery can be done to remove them. This treatment often is safe during pregnancy. In some cases, it may be best to wait until after the baby is born to begin treatment.

Syphilis

Syphilis can be a severe STD. It is caused by organisms called spirochetes. Syphilis occurs in stages. It is more easily spread in some stages than in others. If not treated, syphilis can cause heart and brain damage, blindness, paralysis, insanity, and death. If syphilis is found and treated early, it may cause less damage.

Syphilis can be passed from a pregnant woman's bloodstream to her baby. This may cause miscarriage, stillbirth, or premature rupture of membranes. Infants born with syphilis may have birth defects. Treating an infected infant after birth will prevent more damage in many cases.

Syphilis can be hard to detect in women. The sore that marks the site of infection—called a *chancre*—is painless. It may be in the vagina where it cannot be seen. A chancre appears only in the early stage of syphilis. Later symptoms are a rash, sluggishness, or slight fever.

In the very early stages of syphilis, a blood test may or may not find the disease. If a chancre is present, syphilis can be diagnosed by scraping tissue from the chancre. The chancre will go away even without treatment, but the infection remains. After the chancre goes away, the only sure way to diagnose syphilis is by a blood test.

Treatment with antibiotics can halt damage to the baby, but it will not reverse any harm already done. Treatment during the first 3–4 months of pregnancy most likely will prevent any long-term damage.

Trichomoniasis

Trichomoniasis is an STD that affects the vagina. There may be no symptoms or, if symptoms occur, there may be a vaginal discharge, burning, and irritation. Infected women have increased risks for premature rupture of membranes and preterm delivery.

It is safe to be treated for trichomoniasis with an antibiotic during pregnancy. This will relieve symptoms, increase the chances of curing it, and make it less likely that the infection will be passed to others.

Human Immunodeficiency Virus Infection

Human immunodeficiency virus (HIV) is spread through contact with body fluids—mainly blood or semen—from an infected person. The most common ways that HIV is passed to others are by sexual contact and by sharing needles used to inject drugs. In rare cases, blood transfusions can transmit the disease. Since 1985, the blood supply in the United States has been tested for HIV. Infected blood is not used. Breast milk

from a woman with HIV also can pass the virus to her baby.

Once in the body, HIV destroys cells that are part of the immune system—the body's natural defense against disease. This leaves the body open to infections that can cause death. When a person with HIV gets one of these infections or has a very low level of these immune-system cells, he or she is said to have *acquired immuno-deficiency syndrome (AIDS)*.

Once infected with HIV, there is no cure. An infected person will have the virus for the rest of his or her life. In most cases, a person who has been infected with HIV doesn't get sick right away. It may take more than 5 years for symptoms to appear. Sometimes people infected with HIV have a brief illness like the flu. Later symptoms can include weight loss, fatigue, swollen lymph nodes, night sweats, fever, diarrhea, and cough.

Following are ways to reduce the risk of HIV infection:

➤ Use latex condoms during sex.

➤ Do not inject drugs.

➤ Avoid having sex with more than one partner.

➤ Avoid having sex with someone who may use drugs or have other sexual partners.

HIV can be passed from mother to baby during pregnancy or at the time of delivery. The baby also can be infected during vaginal delivery. Some women may benefit from a cesarean delivery.

Testing for HIV

In the United States, about 2 out of every 1,000 pregnant women are infected with HIV. A woman may be infected with HIV but not realize it.

Treating an infected mother for HIV greatly reduces the chances that HIV will be passed on to the baby. For this reason, all pregnant women should be tested for HIV as part of routine prenatal testing. If a pregnant woman finds out she is infected, she can start treatment and avoid passing the infection to the baby. If you have questions about the test or the possible results, talk to your doctor.

One test to detect HIV is called the enzyme-linked immunosorbent assay (ELISA). It will show if HIV antibodies are in the blood, which is a sign of infection. If the result is positive, a second ELISA and another test, the Western blot, will be done to double check. If both tests are positive, HIV infection is diagnosed. This means that infection is present and can be passed to others, including a fetus.

Very rarely, the tests will give a false-positive or an unclear result. A false-positive result means the test shows a person is infected when he or she isn't. This occurs in 1–2% of cases.

Other factors can cause test results that are not correct. After a person is exposed to HIV, weeks or months must

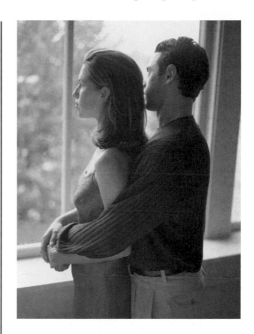

pass before enough antibodies show up in your blood to produce a positive test result. This means that if a person was exposed to the virus only a week before being tested, the test would show a negative result. This is called a false-negative result.

Treatment for HIV

There is no cure for HIV or AIDS, but treatment can prolong life. Women who become pregnant while taking drugs to treat HIV should continue treatment. Being treated for HIV infection greatly reduces the chance that the virus will be transmitted to the fetus.

If a pregnant woman infected with HIV starts treatment during weeks 14–34 of pregnancy, the chance of the fetus getting infected is greatly reduced. Without treatment, about 25% of babies (1 out of 4) born to women infected with HIV will get the virus. With treatment, that number decreases to less than 8%, or about 1 out of 12. For best results, the medication for HIV should be taken during pregnancy, labor, and delivery. Some women may benefit from cesarean delivery. The newborn also should be given the drug during the first 6 weeks of life.

After birth, special care is needed to avoid passing the infection to the baby in other ways. The woman should be careful not to let her body fluids come in contact with the baby's mucus membranes (in the mouth, eyes, nose, and rectum). She should not breastfeed her baby. It is important to continue treatment.

Tuberculosis

Tuberculosis, often referred to as TB, is a disease caused by bacteria that are carried through the air. They are passed on when an infected person coughs or sneezes. Usually, infection occurs in the lungs. But TB infection also can occur in other parts of the body, including the genitals, brain, kidneys, or bones.

A woman should have a TB skin test during pregnancy if she has been exposed to TB, emigrated from a country that has a high rate of TB infection, or has certain medical conditions. If the skin test result is positive, a chest X-ray will be given.

TB can be active or latent. People with active TB have symptoms that can include fever, weight loss, night sweats, a cough, chest pain, and fatigue. Active TB usually shows up on a chest X-ray.

People with latent TB usually have no symptoms and a normal chest X-ray. Most people who are infected with TB have latent TB. Their bodies are able to stop the bacteria from growing. The bacteria become inactive but remain alive in the body and can become active later.

In most pregnant women, treatment of latent TB infection should be delayed until 2 or 3 months after delivery. If TB is latent but threatens to become active, treatment should start right away. Risk factors include being recently infected with TB (in the past 2 years), testing positive for HIV, and injecting drugs.

There are many drugs used to treat latent TB. Treatment lasts from 2–9 months. It is important to finish the treatment. Vitamin B_6 also is given as a part of treatment. It is safe to breastfeed if a woman is still being treated after the baby is born.

Active TB is treated with several drugs for at least 9 months. Most of the drugs used to treat TB are safe to be used during pregnancy. After birth, the baby may need to be kept apart from the mother for a while. Usually, people aren't contagious after 2 weeks of the treatment. After that time, it usually is safe to breastfeed.

With either latent or active TB, the fetus can get infected through blood or breathing in the bacteria at birth. For this reason, the baby may be given treatment for TB after birth.

Hepatitis

Hepatitis is a viral infection that affects the liver. The four common kinds of hepatitis infection are types A, B, C, and D. Type A cannot be passed and type D is rare. Hepatitis B is of the greatest concern during pregnancy because it is most likely to be passed to the baby.

Hepatitis B can be passed between people through infected body fluids. These include blood, semen, vaginal fluids, and saliva. The following factors increase the risk for hepatitis B infection:

➤ Injecting drugs and sharing needles

➤ Having multiple sexual partners

➤ Working in a health-related job that exposes you to blood or blood products

➤ Living with someone infected with hepatitis B

➤ Receiving blood products (for example, for a clotting disorder)

Some people infected with hepatitis B have chronic hepatitis. Symptoms include fatigue, loss of appetite, nausea, and muscle aches. Chronic hepatitis can be life threatening. Some people with hepatitis have liver problems, such as

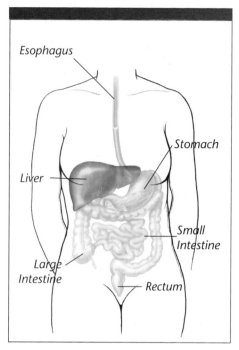

Hepatitis B damages the liver and can cause harm to the fetus during pregnancy. All pregnant women should be tested for this infection.

cirrhosis (hardening) of the liver and liver cancer. Most people who get hepatitis can't pass it on to anyone else after hepatitis has run its course.

Some people with hepatitis B may not feel sick or show any signs of the disease. They are carriers of the infection. They keep the virus in their bodies all their lives and can pass it to other people.

A blood test can show whether someone has been infected with hepatitis B. All pregnant women should be tested for the hepatitis B virus. The infection can be hard to find without testing because its symptoms—nausea and vomiting—often occur in pregnancy anyway. If you might be infected, your doctor may give you **hepatitis B immune globulin**. It contains antibodies to the virus. It can make the illness less severe. Rest, diet, and liquids also may be prescribed.

A woman who is a carrier can pass the hepatitis B virus to her baby at birth. Whether the baby will get the virus depends on when the mother was infected. If it was early in pregnancy, the chances are less than 10% that the baby will get the virus. If it was late in pregnancy, there is up to a 90% chance the baby will be infected. Hepatitis may be severe in babies. It can threaten their lives. Even babies who appear well may be at risk for serious health problems.

Infected newborns have a high risk (up to 90%) of becoming chronic hepatitis B carriers. If they become carriers, as adults they have a 25% risk of dying of cirrhosis or liver cancer.

There is a vaccine to prevent hepatitis B infection. Any teen or adult with a high risk of getting the hepatitis B virus should be vaccinated. All infants too should get the vaccine. The vaccine is given in three doses. The first two doses are given 1 month apart, and the third is given 6 months later.

In infected mothers, the baby also will receive hepatitis B immune globulin soon after birth. With this treatment, the chance of the baby getting the infection is only 1 in 20. If the baby is given the vaccine, it is safe to breastfeed.

Hepatitis B Vaccine

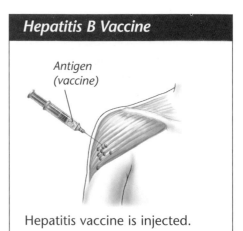

Hepatitis vaccine is injected.

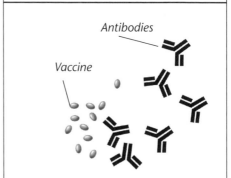

The vaccine triggers antibody production.

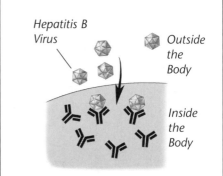

When a person is exposed to hepatitis B virus, the antibodies prevent infection.

Hepatitis C is a disease that occurs more often now than in the past. It is very rare that it is passed to your baby by breastfeeding. There is no vaccine to prevent infection with hepatitis C.

Vaginal Infections

An imbalance of the bacteria growing in the vagina can cause the infection **bacterial vaginosis**. It is the most common cause of a vaginal discharge. The discharge has a fishy odor. Bacterial vaginosis is not an STD. Some women may have a greater risk of having complications, such as preterm birth or premature rupture of membranes if they have this infection.

Bladder and Kidney Infections

Bladder infections (also called urinary tract infections) are common in pregnancy. Severe infections can cause problems for both mother and fetus. Some bladder infections can be found only by tests. Because there may be no symptoms, testing is a part of routine prenatal care. Some symptoms linked with a bladder infection, such as pain with urination, can be caused by other problems such as infection of the vagina or vulva.

Cystitis is a lower-tract (bladder) infection. It is treated with antibiotics. Symptoms may include the following:

➤ Increased need to urinate

➤ Burning and pain when you urinate

➤ Pain in the lower abdomen

➤ Blood in the urine

Pyelonephritis is an upper-tract (kidney) infection. The most common cause is when a bladder infection is not treated or is not cured by treatment. This is why drugs prescribed for a bladder infection should be finished, even if symptoms go away. Symptoms are chills, fever, rapid heart rate, and nausea or vomiting. Kidney infection can lead to premature labor or severe infection. Pyelonephritis is treated with intravenous antibiotics or antibiotic injections. After symptoms clear, the urine is checked for signs of infection that may remain.

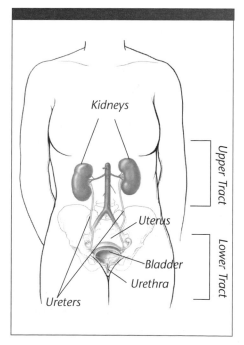

A woman's urinary tract is divided into an upper and lower tract.

Group B Streptococci

Group B streptococci (GBS) bacteria are fairly common in pregnant women. About 10–30% of pregnant women have GBS. The bacteria can be found in the digestive, urinary, and reproductive tract of both men and women. In women, GBS bacteria occur most often in the vagina and rectum. GBS is not a sexually transmitted disease.

The GBS bacteria differ from the streptococcal bacteria that cause strep throat. Group B streptococci can reside in the body without causing symptoms. The bacteria can infect the bladder, kidneys, lungs, or uterus and cause pain and inflammation. These infections often are not serious and can be treated with antibiotics. When GBS bacteria are present but do not cause infection, the person is said to be "*colonized.*"

Although GBS is fairly common in pregnancy, very few babies actually become sick with GBS infection. If GBS bacteria are passed from a woman to her baby, the baby may become infected. This happens to only 1–2% of babies. Babies who do become infected may have early or late infections.

Early infections start when the baby passes through the birth canal colonized with GBS. These infections occur within the first 7 days after birth. Most occur within the first 6 hours. This can cause severe problems. Early infections in some babies may result in death.

Late infections occur after the first 7 days of life. About half of late infections are passed from the mother to the baby during birth. The other half result from other sources of infection, such as contact with people who have GBS.

Testing between 35–37 weeks of pregnancy and treatment greatly decreases the risk, but not all cases can be prevented. Both early and late infections can be serious. They can cause inflammation of the baby's blood, lungs, brain, or spinal cord. Both types lead to death in about 5% of infected babies.

Testing

A culture is the most accurate way to test for GBS. For cultures, a swab is used to take samples from the vagina and rectum. The specimen then is sent to a lab. It may take up to 2 days to get the results.

It is most useful to test for GBS between 35 and 37 weeks of pregnancy. If the test results are positive, showing GBS is present, antibiotics are given during labor to help prevent the baby from being infected.

Women who have already had a baby with GBS infection or had a urinary tract infection caused by GBS during pregnancy do not need to be tested. They will be given antibiotics during labor.

Treatment

All women who test positive for GBS infection must be treated with antibiotics during labor. Women with risk

Risk Factors for Group B Streptococcal Infection

Women with these risk factors are more likely to have babies with GBS infection:

➤ Preterm labor (labor that begins before 37 weeks of pregnancy)

➤ Preterm premature rupture of membranes (breaking of the amniotic sac before 37 weeks of pregnancy)

➤ Prolonged rupture of membranes (18 hours or more before delivery)

➤ Previous birth of baby with GBS infection

➤ Temperature of more than 100.4°

➤ Presence of GBS bacteria in urine

factors for GBS infection also receive antibiotics during labor (see box).

The antibiotic—usually penicillin—is given through a vein. The antibiotics work only if taken during labor. This is because the bacteria grow so fast that, treated earlier, the GBS might grow back before labor.

Group B streptococcal infection in a baby is 20 times more likely if the mother has not been treated with antibiotics. It is not necessary to receive antibiotics during cesarean birth, even if the mother is a GBS carrier.

Other Infections

A number of other infections can cause serious problems in pregnant women or their babies. If you are exposed to these infections during this pregnancy, ask your doctor about their effect during pregnancy. There are vaccines for many of these diseases. If you haven't had these diseases yet, it's a good idea to be vaccinated against them before your next pregnancy. In some cases, vaccination is safe during pregnancy (see box on vaccines).

Cytomegalovirus

Cytomegalovirus (CMV) is the most common virus transmitted during pregnancy. Unlike other viral infections, CMV can come back even if a person has been infected before and has formed antibodies. Those at highest risk for CMV are health care and lab workers, mothers of young children in childcare, and childcare providers.

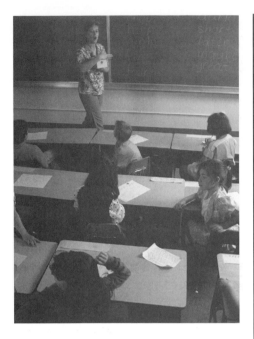

CMV is hard to detect because it rarely causes symptoms. (When it does, the symptoms include fever, swollen lymph glands, sore throat, and fatigue.) Infected women can pass it to their babies during pregnancy, birth, or by breastfeeding. However, healthy full-term babies born to women infected with CMV have protective antibodies, and it is fine for them to be breastfed.

Problems in babies caused by CMV infection include jaundice (yellow skin and eyes caused when the liver doesn't work as it should), microcephaly (having a very small head and being mentally retarded), deafness, and eye problems. The risk of the baby getting infected is greatest if the woman has the infection for the first time during pregnancy. This is rare.

Cytomegalovirus has no treatment. The best way to keep from getting CMV is to avoid contact with infected people and to wash your hands often. Women at high risk may want to be tested to see if they have been exposed to CMV.

Childhood Diseases

Although certain infections are thought of as childhood diseases, they also can occur in adults. Some can cause serious problems in pregnant women. If you have had any of the diseases shown in Table 17–1 (on the following pages) you are not likely to get them again. Also, there are vaccines for many of them. If you are exposed to a child who was recently vaccinated, it does not pose a risk to you or your baby. Because many children have not been vaccinated, these diseases have become widespread. Tell your doctor if you are exposed to these diseases while you are pregnant.

Influenza

Influenza (commonly called the flu) is a contagious infection of the respiratory system. It can be caused by a number of viruses. Major symptoms are fever, headache, fatigue, muscle aches, coughing, congestion, runny nose, and sore throat. Pregnancy can increase the risk for complications from the flu, such as pneumonia.

All women who will be pregnant during flu season (November through March) should be vaccinated for flu.

Protection from the vaccine usually begins 1–2 weeks after getting your flu shot. The protection lasts 6 months or longer. A flu shot is considered safe at any stage of pregnancy. However, the nasal flu mist vaccine is not approved for use in pregnant women.

Lyme Disease

Lyme disease is caused by a bite from an infected deer tick, which often is hard to see. The first sign of Lyme disease is a sore that may look like a bull's-eye. This sore may go away, but the infection remains. Lyme disease also can cause flu-like symptoms, including swollen or painful joints and muscle aches. A few weeks later some people get a rash, meningitis, paralysis of the facial muscles, or heart problems. Antibiotics often will cure the infection.

It is wise to avoid densely wooded areas while you are pregnant. In areas where ticks can be found, wear long-sleeved shirts and long pants tucked into your socks. If you find a tick that has been on you for more than 24 hours, call your doctor. A vaccine is available that may help prevent infection in women who are at high risk for Lyme disease.

West Nile Virus

Infection with the West Nile virus most often is caused by the bite of an infected mosquito. People infected with the West Nile Virus may not have any symptoms. In some cases, the infection can lead to West Nile fever or severe West Nile disease. West Nile fever can cause flu-like symptoms, including a fever, body aches, and headache. There is no certain treatment for the West Nile Virus infection. It is not yet known how or if infection with the West Nile Virus during pregnancy can affect the baby. However, if you are pregnant, it is wise to protect yourself from mosquito bites by wearing long pants and long-sleeved shirts and using insect repellant when outdoors.

Toxoplasmosis

The parasite that causes *toxoplasmosis* can live in any animal that lives outdoors. People can get infected by eating raw or undercooked meat or unwashed vegetables. Infection also can be caused by coming into contact with animal feces. The parasite is not spread from person to person. The most common way infection occurs in the United States is by working in the garden without gloves. Rarely, it occurs from changing a cat's litter box, especially if the cat roams outdoors.

Toxoplasmosis may cause no symptoms or only mild illness in adults. If symptoms do appear, they are flu-like and can last for a few days up to a few weeks. If you were infected before you were pregnant, you won't pass toxoplasmosis on to your baby. You can pass it on to your baby only if you are infected for the first time while you are pregnant. The baby is not likely to become infected if you get toxoplas-

Table 17–1. Childhood Diseases

Illness	Signs	When Signs Appear
Chickenpox (varicella)	➤Rash ➤Fluid–filled, itchy blisters that dry and form scabs ➤Fever ➤Malaise	10–21 days after exposure
Fifth disease (parvovirus B19)	➤Cold-like symptoms followed by rash on the cheeks, arms, legs, and trunk ➤Sometimes joint pain and swelling	Usually 4–14 days after exposure, but sometimes as many as 20 days after exposure
Rubella (German measles)	➤Non–itchy rash ➤Fever ➤Swollen lymph glands ➤Joint pain and swelling	2–3 weeks after exposure
Measles ("red measles")	➤Fever ➤Runny nose and watery eyes ➤Tiny white spots on lining of mouth ➤Skin rash that begins on the forehead and spreads down the body to the feet	7–11 days after exposure
Mumps	➤Fever ➤Swollen glands under the jaw	12–25 days after exposure

When It Can Spread	Risks in Pregnancy
1–2 days before the rash appears and until all blisters have scabs (up to 5 days after the rash appears)	➤ Mother may get pneumonia ➤ Newborn can be seriously ill if mother is infected in last week before birth
Before the rash appears	➤ Miscarriage in first 3–4 months ➤ Anemia in fetus if later in pregnancy
Anytime from 10 days before to 10 days after the signs appear	➤ Miscarriage ➤ Preterm birth ➤ Birth defects, especially if mother has rubella in first month of pregnancy
Anytime from 2 days before to about 4 days after the rash appears	➤ Mother may get pneumonia ➤ Miscarriage ➤ Low birth weight
Anytime from 3 days before to at least 10 days after the signs appear	Miscarriage, preterm labor

mosis in the first 3 months of pregnancy.

If infection does occur, the newborn may have severe eye infections, an enlarged liver and spleen, or pneumonia. Sometimes problems develop months or years later, including hearing loss, vision problems, and mental retardation. Sometimes treatment is available. Infected babies are treated soon after birth to prevent long-term problems.

The best way to protect against toxoplasmosis is to avoid being exposed to it. Be sure meat is well cooked and avoid contact with the cat litter box. Pregnant women should wear waterproof gloves or avoid gardening in areas where there are feces. Always wash your hands with soap and water after touching soil, cats, or uncooked meat or vegetables.

Anthrax

Anthrax is a disease caused by the bacteria *Bacillus anthracis*. There are three ways a person can be infected by anthrax:

1. Cutaneous (through the skin)

2. Inhalation (through the lungs)

3. Gastrointestinal (through the digestive system)

Anthrax infections in the United States are extremely rare. Anthrax is not spread from person to person. A person may become infected with anthrax by handling products or eating under-cooked meat from infected animals. Anthrax also can be used as a weapon. Most people who are exposed to anthrax become ill within 1 week of exposure.

Anthrax usually can be treated with certain antibiotics. In some cases, antibiotics are used to help prevent anthrax infection after a person has been exposed to the bacteria. There are antibiotics available that are safe to use during pregnancy.

Keeping Well

These are the best ways to prevent infections during pregnancy:

➤ Make sure your vaccines are up-to-date before you become pregnant.

➤ Know the symptoms of infections so you can act on them if they occur.

➤ Do not engage in behavior that increases the risk of infections.

➤ Try to avoid being exposed to an infection.

➤ Use good hygiene, including washing your hands often.

If you get an infection during pregnancy, it may be treated to prevent further harm to you or your baby. In some cases, there is no treatment for the disease or it is not safe to have during pregnancy. Your baby may need treatment after birth to treat the illness.

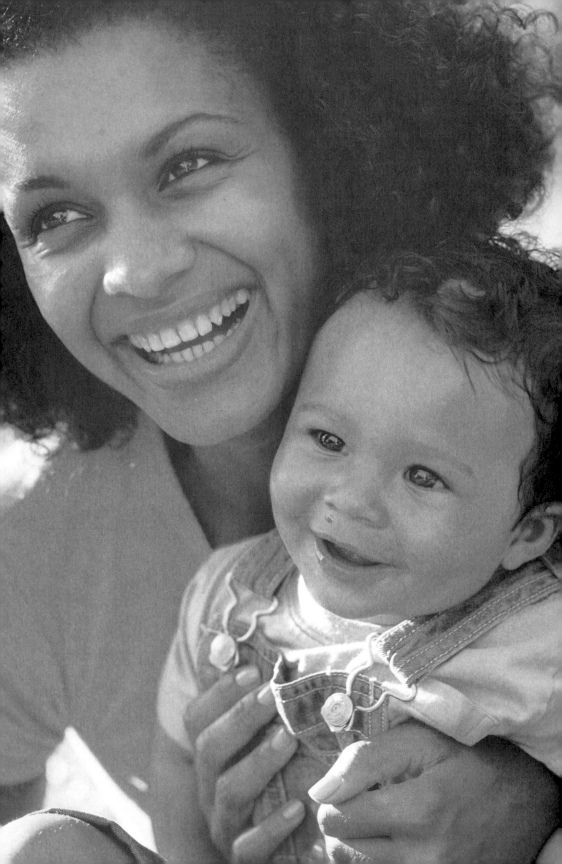

Staying Healthy

Parenting can be one of the hardest and one of the most rewarding jobs you will ever have. Although it may be a challenge to maintain your own health while nurturing a child, it is vital to take care of yourself.

See your doctor regularly for preventive health care. Exams and screening tests can detect problems before you are sick, and immunizations help prevent disease.

Your obstetrician–gynecologist and his or her staff are an important part of a health care team that can advise you on how you can have a healthy lifestyle. Making the right lifestyle choices is the best thing you can do to stay healthy. The choices you make can make you feel better now and prevent health problems later.

CHAPTER 18

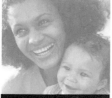

Maintaining Health and Wellness

Now that you've been through pregnancy, you have good reasons to maintain your health. A good diet, a healthy lifestyle, and regular checkups will help ensure your health as well as that of your family. It also will help you prepare for any future children.

A Healthy Diet

Eating well is one of the best things you can do to stay healthy. A good diet increases your energy, improves your sense of well-being, and lowers your risk of disease. What you eat is linked to your risk of serious health problems, such as heart disease, cancer, diabetes, and osteoporosis.

Daily Food Choices

The first step toward healthy eating is to evaluate the foods in your daily diet. Eating a variety of foods each day helps ensure a balanced diet.

The Food Guide Pyramid (see Chapter 6) can help you choose the foods to plan a balanced diet. It shows the number of servings you should have each day from each of these six food groups:

1. Bread, cereal, rice, and pasta
2. Fruit
3. Vegetable
4. Meat, poultry, fish, dry beans, eggs, and nuts
5. Milk, yogurt, and cheese
6. Fats, oils, and sweets

Make it a point to choose most of your foods from the bread, cereal, rice, and pasta group. This group has the largest number (6–11) of recommended servings. Although this may seem like a lot, it really isn't. For instance, one slice of bread is equal to one serving, and so is 1/2 cup of rice or pasta or 1 ounce of

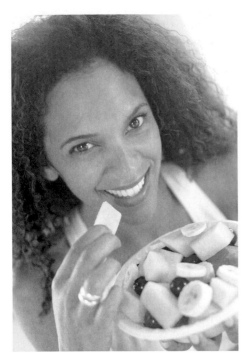

cereal. So, if you eat a bowl of cereal for breakfast, two slices of bread for lunch, and 1 cup of rice or pasta and a roll for dinner, you will get all you need of that food group.

For weight loss purposes, a variety of foods, such as those with more protein and fewer carbohydrates, may be a better option. Talk to your doctor or dietician for more information.

Weight Control

To stay healthy, you should keep your weight at the level best for your height. You may have seen height and weight tables that suggest weights for men and women based on body frame size— small, medium, and large. Today, many doctors use the body mass index (BMI)

table (see Chapter 6) to see if your weight is normal.

The BMI compares a person's height to their weight to see if they are overweight. Having a BMI of 20–24 is normal, and 25–29 is overweight. A woman with a score of 30 or higher is obese.

It is a good idea to lose any weight you gained during your last pregnancy before you become pregnant again. This can help avoid the excessive weight gain that some women experience after multiple pregnancies. It also may help you to avoid diabetes in pregnancy (gestational diabetes) and hypertension in pregnancy. You can lose weight by eating healthy foods and exercising. Talk to your doctor about a weight loss plan that is right for you.

Dietary Supplements

It may be hard to get all the nutrients you need from your diet. Some women may need to take extra vitamins or minerals. It is a good idea to take a daily multivitamin, but talk to your doctor if you think you would benefit from additional vitamin supplements. Do not take more vitamins than your doctor suggests. Iron, calcium, and folic acid are key supplements women should think about taking (see Table 18–1).

Things to Avoid
Too Much Fat

When your body digests food, it breaks the food down into carbohydrates, pro-

Table 18–1. Basic Vitamin Supplements for Women Aged 19–50 Years

Supplement	Use	RDA	Natural sources
Iron	Iron is needed to make new blood cells. Low levels of iron may cause anemia—low blood count. Anemic women feel tired, weak, and look pale.	8 mg	Liver, meat, dried beans and peas, prunes, prune juice
Calcium	Calcium helps keep bones strong and prevent osteoporosis.	1,000 mg	Yogurt, cottage cheese, spinach, tofu, enriched orange juice
Folic Acid	All women who can become pregnant should take folic acid to lower the risk of having a baby with certain birth defects of the spine and skull, especially before pregnancy and during the first months of pregnancy.	400 μg	Spinach, collard greens, oranges, lemons, enriched bread, pasta, flour, crackers, cereal, and rice

teins, and fats and then converts them into energy. You need some fat in your diet for your body to function (for example, to absorb certain vitamins). However, too much fat can add to your weight.

There are two kinds of fat found in food—saturated and unsaturated. Saturated fat is solid at room temperature. Unsaturated fat is liquid at room temperature. Unsaturated fats are better choices than saturated fats—they don't increase your cholesterol level as much. The best choice, though, is to limit all fats.

It is easy to reduce the amount of fat in your diet. Start by eating more fruits, vegetables, and whole grains. Switch from foods high in fat to foods low in fat. For instance, choose skim milk instead of whole milk. Be aware that most "fast food" and prepared foods like snacks and microwave meals have high amounts of fat in them. Chapter 6 has tips on how to reduce the amount of fat in your diet.

Bad Cholesterol

Too much fat in your diet also may lead to high levels of bad cholesterol in your body. The food you eat is broken down in your liver. The liver uses the fat in your food to change it into lipoproteins. Lipoproteins carry the fat through your blood vessels for use or storage in other parts of the body. One type of lipoprotein, called LDL or "bad cholesterol," can stick to the sides of blood vessels.

Over the years, deposits of bad cholesterol may clog your blood vessels, narrow and harden arteries, or even block the arteries in vital organs such as the heart and brain. This may eventually cause a heart attack or a stroke. You can lower your cholesterol levels by eating foods low in fat (especially saturated fat) and cholesterol, and by avoiding excess starches and sweets, which can be converted to fat and cholesterol. You also should keep your BMI between 20 and 24 and exercise.

Smoking, Alcohol, and Illicit Drugs

Smoking lowers your body's ability to reduce the levels of bad cholesterol. It is a leading cause of heart disease, and has even been linked to reproductive problems such as infertility and early menopause. Also, some people (especially children) who live around smokers have health problems from being exposed to second-hand smoke.

Alcohol slows down your body's response to your brain. This affects thinking, talking, walking, driving, and doing day-to-day tasks. Heavy drinking may damage the liver, the heart muscle, and other organs, and it may even increase the risk of osteoporosis, early menopause, irregular periods, infertility, and some cancers. Heavy drinking may also damage your family life, friendships, and lead to criminal activity or suicide.

Like alcohol, drugs can impair your daily life, damage your body, and even cause death. Furthermore, drugs may have long-term harmful effects on your baby's health and future life, as well as the life of your entire family.

It takes patience and plenty of support to end a habit, especially if it's long-standing. Don't be afraid or ashamed to ask for help. Your doctor can suggest ways to get through the early stages and refer you to a support group.

It is up to you to make healthy choices in your life. Healthy eating and avoiding harmful substances in your diet and lifestyle will not only help you maintain your health for years to come, but also set a good example for your family.

Exercise

Another important factor in helping you become and keep fit is regular physical activity. After having a baby, you may start wondering how you can get back in shape. Keeping fit will give you strength and flexibility. It also is a good way to relax and control your weight. An exercise program can help you cope with the rigors of being a new mother and stay healthy for years to come.

When your doctor thinks you are well enough to start exercising, he or she may give you some tips for specific postpartum exercises (or you can refer to Chapter 12 for the postpartum exercise routine). As your body heals after pregnancy and you feel comfortable with your postpartum routine, you may gradually move to more vigorous types of exercise.

Benefits of Exercise

One of the most important benefits of regular physical activity is that it promotes cardiovascular fitness—that is, it strengthens your heart and circulatory system. Having a strong, healthy heart helps lower cholesterol and blood pressure levels—factors that can reduce your risk of heart disease. Regular physical activity also:

➤ Strengthens your muscles

➤ Increases your flexibility

➤ Gives you more energy

➤ Helps control weight

➤ Improves mood

➤ Improves sleep

Physical activity helps build and maintain strong bones. Active women have stronger bones than women who do not exercise. This is important as women age and become prone to weakening of bones known as osteoporosis. Regular physical activity also may reduce the risk of colon cancer and breast cancer.

Physical benefits are not all you get with regular exercise. Staying active promotes mental well-being, relieves stress, and reduces feelings of depression and anxiety. You feel good about your body

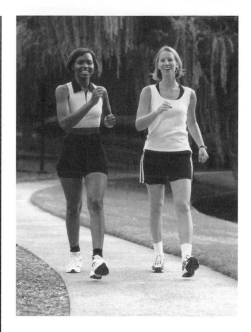

when you exercise regularly, and therefore have a healthier body image.

You do not have to follow an intense exercise routine to benefit. In fact, even moderate daily physical activity totalling 30 minutes, which may be spread throughout the day, can offer health benefits.

Types of Exercise

Three types of exercises—aerobic, flexibility, and resistance training—can help your body in a variety of ways. A combination of all three is the most effective.

Aerobic exercise causes your heart and lungs to work harder and builds fitness. Improving the fitness of your heart and lungs increases your body's ability to use oxygen. It also burns more calories, which helps if you're trying to lose or maintain weight. Aerobic exercise includes walking, jogging, skiing, bicycling, swimming, water aerobics, and dancing.

Flexibility exercise uses stretching movements to increase the length of muscles and your range of motion. This type of exercise may include stretching certain muscles or a yoga or dance class. Stretching exercises will help your body maintain its mobility as you age.

Resistance training builds muscle and slows bone loss. It helps strengthen muscles and bones by exerting force on them. As you build muscle, your body will become more toned. The more muscle you have, the better your body burns calories. Resistance training includes lifting weights and doing leg lifts or squats. Try to avoid exercising the same muscles two days in a row so they have time to recover. You can do resistance exercises for 30 minutes just 2–3 days per week to see results.

Getting Started

Before starting an exercise program, you should be in good health. If you have just had a baby, have a heart condition, or are overweight, talk with your doctor first before beginning an exercise plan (see Chapter 4).

If it has been some time since you've exercised regularly, it's best to start slowly. Begin with as little as 5 minutes per day and add 5 more minutes per week until you can stay active for 30 minutes per day. The box has additional

healthy tips to help you avoid getting hurt during exercise.

Plan your exercise program to suit your interests and lifestyle. If you choose activities that you like, you're more likely to stick to it, which is most important. For example, gardening and dancing are great forms of exercise. Don't forget to count everyday chores and activities, such as climbing stairs, carrying bags, and washing the car. The box "Burning Calories" lists activities that you can select to fit into your daily life. The harder you exercise, the more calories you burn.

Exercising With Baby

Exercising with your baby is a good way to help you get back in shape. It also will give you and your baby a chance to bond and inspire lifelong love of physical activity for you and your family.

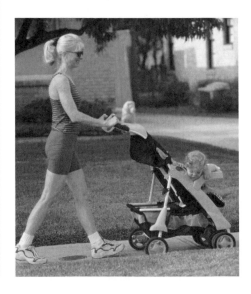

Things to Remember About Exercise

Warming Up—Start each exercise session with a warm-up period of slow walking or stationary cycling and stretching for 5–10 minutes.

Cooling Down—After exercising, cool down by slowly reducing your activity and stretching your muscles for 5–10 minutes.

Frequency of Exercise—Physical activity should be a part of every day. A form of aerobic exercise should be done three times per week. You should maintain your routine throughout the year. If you stop for more than 2 weeks, you may need to work at a lower level when you start exercising again. Then increase your level of exercise as you feel able.

Injuries—Exercise and sports activities can increase your risk of injury to muscle, bones, and joints. It is important not to overdo it when you begin an exercise program. You should alternate between light and heavy activity and even include days of rest into your exercise routine. It also helps to alternate the types of exercise as you get more fit to avoid overworking a particular body part.

Menstrual Changes—Vigorous exercise over a long time span may cause changes in your menstrual cycle. Rarely, a woman's periods stop completely. If you notice changes in your periods or if they stop altogether, see your doctor. Never assume that menstrual changes are related to exercise. A thorough checkup is needed to find the cause.

Walking is probably the best choice for exercising with your baby. It is free, relatively safe, and you can do it almost any place and time soon after your baby is born. Furthermore, seeing other people and being outside can help relieve the stress and depression of the first few weeks as a new mother. You can either put your baby in a baby carrier and take a walk, or push the baby in a stroller. For a more challenging workout, you can choose a neighborhood with hills for your walk.

When you feel up to it and you receive the go ahead from your doctor and your baby's doctor, you can move on to more vigorous exercise. At home you can carry your baby while you walk up and down the stairs or put on your baby's favorite music and move around the room gently bouncing or rocking your baby. You can even try a mother-and-baby exercise video.

When the weather allows, you can take your baby to a park or a school track and let him or her play on a blanket while you exercise nearby.

Burning Calories

Keep track of the number of calories you burn while exercising or performing everyday activities:

Activity	Calories burned per 30 minutes
Dancing	300
Jogging (5mph)	230
Gardening	60–200
Shoveling snow	200
Climbing stairs	200
Low-impact aerobics	200
Mopping floors	100
Walking (3mph)	100
Grocery shopping	100
Raking leaves	100

As your baby gets older (typically by about 6 months), you may consider joining a local health club or a recreation department for a baby-and-mom yoga, aquatics, movement, or play class.

Making exercise a part of your life can pay off in many ways. It can make you look and feel better. Map out a plan that is best for you and your family. Consider which exercises or sports you enjoy—choosing something you like can help you to stick with your routine. Make time for these activities most days of the week.

Routine Health Care

Women of all ages can help to stay healthy by getting regular health care. Women in certain age groups have special health care needs. Some women may have risk factors that require further care. Being aware of things that cause illness in your age group is a good idea. It lets you play an active role in trying to prevent problems.

Age-Specific Assessments

Some health problems are more likely to occur at certain ages. Having regular checkups will help you learn what these common problems are. Your doctor also can show you ways to help prevent them. The goal of preventive care is to prevent or manage problems early.

At routine visits, you will have a physical exam. Your doctor also will ask you about your health history. This is a good chance to talk to your doctor about your health concerns and any problems you may be having. Table 18–2 lists the test needed for women aged 19–39 years. Older women may need additional tests and immunizations. Fill in the blanks on the table to help you keep track of when you last had the test and when you need your next one. If you don't remember when you were last tested or immunized, your doctor may be able to test you to see if you are immune to the disease.

Table 18–2. Test and Immunization for Women Aged 19–39 Years

Test/ Immunization	What and Why	When	Last Done	Next Needed
Pap test	A sample of cells taken from the cervix during a pelvic exam to look for changes that could lead to cancer	Yearly when sexually active or beginning no later than age 21 years, (doctor and patient may decide to have it every 2–3 years after three normal test results in a row)		
Tetanus–diphtheria booster	A shot to immunize against the diseases tetanus and diphtheria	Once every 10 years		

High-Risk Considerations

Women with risk factors may require further screening tests (see Table 18–3). Some people are more likely than others to have certain health problems. Also, where you live, your lifestyle, and your personal and family medical history play a role in the type of health care you may need. For example, if you or a first-degree relative have had breast cancer, you should have mammography done, even if you are younger than 40 years.

Immunizations

Immunizations are injections (shots) that help prevent infections. When your body is invaded by a germ, your immune system—one of your body's natural defenses against disease—produces antibodies to fight the infection. However, it is better to immunize yourself against these diseases rather than fight off the infection or treat them.

Immunizations, or vaccines, offer such protection. Many vaccines are given to children, but adults benefit from some of them as well. Some vaccines last a lifetime, but others need to be renewed from time to time. Some are given to everyone, and others are given only to certain persons. Table 18–2 outlines the standard immunization for women aged 19–39 years. If you have certain risks factors, you may need other immunizations (see Table 18–4).

The vaccines for measles, mumps, rubella, and varicella generally are not recommended for use during pregnancy, but there is no evidence that these vaccines harm the baby you are carrying. So, if you are planning another pregnancy, you should get vaccinated for these diseases at least 1 month before you become pregnant.

Getting the recommended routine health care is one of the easiest and

Table 18–3. Tests and Immunizations for High-Risk Women

You should have this test	If you
Bacteriuria testing	Have diabetes mellitus
Blood count (anemia)	Are of Caribbean, Latin American, Asian, Mediterranean, or African descent; have a history of heavy menstrual flow
Bone density screening	Are a postmenopausal women younger than age 65 years and have a personal history of fracture as an adult or have a history of fracture in a first-degree relative or are Caucasian or have dementia or are in poor health or smoke cigarettes or weigh less than 127 pounds or have low levels of estrogen or have low lifelong calcium intake or alcoholism or have impaired eyesight despite adequate correction or have recurrent falls or are not physically active. All women with certain diseases or medical conditions and those who take certain drugs that increase a woman's risk of osteoporosis
Colorectal cancer screening	Have colorectal cancer or adenomatous polyps in first-degree relative younger than 60 years or in two or more first-degree relatives of any ages; have a family history of familial adenomatous polyposis or hereditary nonpolyposis colon cancer; have a history of colorectal cancer, adenomatous polyps, or inflammatory bowel disease, chronic ulcerative colitis, or Crohn's disease
Fasting glucose testing	Are overweight; have a family history of diabetes; are not physically active; are a member of a high-risk ethnic group (African American, Hispanic, Native American, Asian, or Pacific Islander); have given birth to a baby weighing more than 9 pounds or have had gestational diabetes; have high blood pressure; have a high-density lipoprotein cholesterol level of at least 35 mg/dL; have a triglyceride level of no more than 250 mg/dL; have a history of impaired glucose tolerance or impaired fasting glucose
Flouride supplementation	Live in an area with low amounts of flouride in the water (less than 0.7 ppm)
Genetic testing or counseling	Are planning a pregnancy and are age 35 years or older; have someone in your family (including you) who has a history of a genetic disorder or birth defect; have a partner with a history of a genetic disorder or birth defect; have been exposed to agents known to harm a fetus; are of African, Acadian, Eastern Caucasian, Eastern European (Ashkenazi) Jewish, Mediterranean, or Southeast Asian descent

(continued)

Table 18–3. Tests and Immunizations for High-Risk Women

You should have this test	If you
Hepatitis C virus (HCV) testing	Have injected illegal drugs, received treatment (clotting factor concentrate) for a blood disorder before 1987, are on long-term hemodialysis, received blood from a donor who later tested positive for HCV infection, have persistently abnormal alanine aminotransferase levels, received a blood transfusion or organ transplant before July 1992, are exposed to HCV-positive blood at work
Human immunodeficiency virus (HIV) testing	Are seeking treatment for other STDs, inject drugs, have a history of prostitution, have a past or present sexual partner who is HIV positive or bisexual or injects drugs, have lived for a long time or were born in an area with a high number of HIV infection cases, had a blood transfusion between 1978 and 1985, have invasive cervical cancer, are pregnant (women may think about having this test if planning to become pregnant)
Lipid profile assessment	Have family history of hyperlipidemia, have a first-degree female relative with coronary artery disease before age 60 years or a first-degree male relative with coronary artery disease before age 50 years, have diabetes, smoke
Mammography	Have had breast cancer, have a first-degree relative (mother, sister, or daughter) or multiple other relatives who have a history of premenopausal breast or breast and ovarian cancer
Rubella titer assessment	Are childbearing age and have no proof of immunity
Sexually transmitted disease (STD) testing	Have had more than one sexual partner or a partner who has had more than one sexual partner, have had sexual contact with someone with an STD, have a history of repeated episodes of STDs, have attended a clinic for STDs (sexually active teens and other high-risk women may be tested for gonorrhea and chlamydia as part of routine care)
Skin exam	Work or play in the sunlight often, have a family or personal history of skin cancer, have precancerous lesions
Thyroid stimulating hormone testing	Have a strong family history of thyroid disease, have an autoimmune disease
Tuberculosis skin testing	Have HIV infection, have close contact with persons known or thought to have tuberculosis, have medical risk factors known to increase risk of disease if infected, were born in a country with high rates of tuberculosis, abuse alcohol, inject drugs, live in a long-term care facility (including a nursing home, prison or jail, or mental health institution), are a health professional working in a high-risk care facility, are medically underserved or low income

most important things you can do to increase your chances of staying healthy. Work with your doctor on a regular basis to ensure you have all the tests and immunizations for your age group and risk factors. Practice preventive care to keep yourself healthy for years to come.

Table 18–4. Immunizations for High-Risk Women

You should have this immunization	If you
Chickenpox (varicella) vaccine	Are susceptible to chickenpox, are a health care worker, have household contact with people who are immuno-compromised, are a teacher or daycare worker, live or work in a long-term care facility or institution (including college, the military, or prison), travel outside of the United States, live with children, are a nonpregnant woman of childbearing age
Flu vaccine	Want to reduce the chance of catching the flu, live in a long-term care facility, have chronic cardiopulmonary disorders, have a metabolic disease (such as diabetes or renal problems), are a health care or daycare worker, are pregnant during flu season (pregnant women with medical problems may want to be vaccinated before flu season), live or work with people who are at high risk for health problems if they become infected
Hepatitis A virus (HAV) vaccine	Travel to or work in countries where the population has an increased rate of infection with HAV; use illegal drugs; work with HAV-infected nonhuman primates or HAV in a research lab; have chronic liver disease; have a blood disorder
Hepatitis B virus (HBV) vaccine	Use IV drugs, receive clotting factor concentrates, are a healthcare or public safety worker who is exposed to blood or blood products at work, a training in a school for a health profession, are a patient in a dialysis unit, have household or sexual contact with a carrier of HBV, have had sex with more than one person in the past 6 months, travel for longer than 6 months to countries that have had an increased rate of HBV infection, live or work in an institution for the developmentally disabled or are in a prison or jail, have recently been infected with a sexually transmitted disease (STD), are a patient at an STD clinic
Measles–mumps–rubella vaccine	Were born in 1957 or later and have no proof of being immune or being vaccinated, were vaccinated in 1963–1967, are a health care worker, are starting college, travel overseas, have recently given birth and are rubella negative
Pneumococcal vaccine	Have a chronic illness, are exposed to pneumonia outbreaks, are immunocompromised

Preconceptional Care

If you're planning to have another baby, schedule a pre-pregnancy checkup with your doctor. As a part of this visit, your doctor will ask about your diet and lifestyle. The doctor also will ask you questions about your health and that of your family. For example:

➤ *Your medical history.* Some medical conditions—such as diabetes, high blood pressure, obesity, heart disease, and seizure disorders—can cause problems during pregnancy (see Chapter 14). It's important to be sure these conditions are under control before you try to get pregnant. Keep in mind that the treatment for your medical condition between pregnancies that you worked out with your

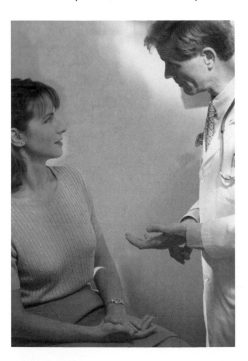

primary care doctor or specialist may need to change during pregnancy.

➤ *Medications you take.* Let your doctor know if you take any medications, herbs, or supplements. You may need to stop using them or switch to others before you try to get pregnant again.

➤ *Past pregnancies.* Your doctor will ask about any previous pregnancies and any problems you may have had during them. If you had a problem in a past pregnancy, that doesn't mean it will happen again or that you should not try to get pregnant. Most women who have had a miscarriage or chose to end their previous pregnancy can go on to have normal future pregnancies and healthy babies. However, it is important to be honest with your doctor. Good preconceptional care often can prevent future problems.

➤ *Your family history.* Your family history or test results may show that you are at risk for having a baby with a birth defect. In that case, it's wise to seek genetic counseling before trying to become pregnant. Genetic counselors have been specially trained to check for the risks of birth defects. They can help you understand your chances of having a baby with such a problem. (For further information about birth defects, see Chapter 13.)

➤ *Immunizations.* Certain infections during pregnancy can cause severe birth defects or illness in a fetus. Some of these can be prevented with proper immunization. Your doctor will determine which diseases you are not immune to and those for which you need immunizations. (For more information on immunizations, see "Routine Health Care" in this chapter as well as "Vaccines" in Chapter 17.)

Be open and honest when you respond to these questions. Your answers will help your doctor decide whether you need special care during pregnancy. This also is a time for you to ask questions. If you have questions about any issues or complications that occurred in your previous pregnancy, talk to your doctor.

Later Childbearing

Older moms often worry that their age will affect their fertility and the health of their babies. There's no set age that is unsafe for women to become pregnant. For women older than 35 years, the chances of having a normal pregnancy and healthy baby are still high—especially if they have good pre-pregnancy and prenatal care. Even so, more mature

---

Are Your Immunizations Up-to-Date?

Although some vaccines are safe to receive during pregnancy, it's best to have all needed immunizations before you become pregnant. Women should have the following immunizations:

One month before pregnancy

___   Measles–mumps–rubella vaccine (if not immune)

___   Varicella vaccine*

Safe during pregnancy

___   Tetanus–diphtheria booster (every 10 years)

___   Hepatitis A vaccine*

___   Hepatitis B vaccine*

___   Influenza vaccine

___   Pneumococcal vaccine*

See Chapter 17 for more information about infections during pregnancy.

*These immunizations are given as needed based on risk factors.

mothers often have to deal with issues in pregnancy that don't apply to younger mothers. Among them:

➤ Infertility. A woman's fertility slowly declines starting in her early 30s. After that time, it may take longer to get pregnant. This is mostly related to problems with ovulation. If you are older than 35 years and you try to become pregnant for more than 6–10 months without success, you may want to talk to your doctor.

➤ Miscarriage. The risk of miscarriage increases as a woman's age increases.

➤ Birth defects. The risk of some birth defects increases with age. In some cases, women aged 35 years and older are offered testing for genetic disorders and other medical problems before and during pregnancy. If there's a problem, it often can be spotted early enough to allow time to decide whether to become pregnant or continue a pregnancy. (For more information on birth defects and testing for them, see Chapter 13.)

Today, more and more couples are starting families later in life. Advances in medicine, along with good care during pregnancy, can help them assess their situation and get the best care they can. Many older women show no greater signs of problems than do younger women. Age need not be a barrier to a safe, healthy pregnancy.

A Healthy Environment: Protecting Current and Future Children

Some substances found in the home or the workplace may make it harder for a woman to conceive and could harm her fetus. These agents also can be dangerous for children. Radiation, toxic substances, and chemicals are just a few of these harmful agents. Discuss your level of exposure and that of your children with your doctor and a pediatrician.

Find out from your employer whether you might be exposed at work to toxic substances such as lead or mercury, chemicals such as pesticides or solvents, or radiation. Then discuss your level of exposure with your doctor as well as your employee health division, personnel office, or union representative. If you do come into regular contact with a substance that may be harmful, take steps to avoid it.

If you have not already, you may want to take some steps to create a healthy and safe environment in your home. Some of the things to consider are:

➤ Replacing batteries in your smoke detectors regularly

➤ Keeping your pets clean and healthy

➤ Banning smoking from your house

➤ Frequently washing your hands and encouraging your children to do the same

➤ Keeping the cosmetic supplies, cleaning detergents, and medications clearly labelled and out of the reach of children

➤ Covering the electric outlets with babyproof caps

You also should try to create a happy home. Raising a child can be stressful. You will have less time for yourself and may need to make changes to your lifestyle. The demands of being a mother may make it harder to reach goals that you have set for yourself. For example, you may need to change the amount of time you spend at your job or at school. You will have less time for other things. If you decide to get pregnant again, one of the greatest challenges will be how to handle your job or school, your family, and your pregnancy while caring for a small child. There may be less time to rest if you have children at home to care for. You may want to consider asking for help. You may need to make more adjustments to your lifestyle to protect yourself and your family from unnecessary stress. For example, you can share chores with other members of your family; even a toddler can do simple tasks such as pick up toys, help you take the laundry out of the dryer, or wipe spilled water. Turn off the TV and spend more quality time with your family walking to the library or a playground or doing an art project. You may even offer to watch a friend's children one night a week if, in turn, he or she watches yours the next time, so that you have more time to rest.

A Healthy Future

It is up to you to make healthy choices in your life. Make changes now: keep fit, eat wisely, avoid things that could be harmful, and visit your doctor regularly. Looking after your own needs and getting support from those around you will help you enjoy your new baby and your family.

Pregnancy Diary

My Health Care Team

Doctors' names:_____

_____

Doctors' address: _____

_____

Telephone/answering service:

Day: _____ Night: _____

Fax: _____ E-mail _____

Pediatricians' names: _____

_____

Pediatricians' address: _____

_____

Telephone/answering service:

Day: _____ Night: _____

Fax: _____ E-mail _____

Hospital: _____

Hospital address: _____

_____

Fax: _____ E-mail _____

Nursing staff: _____ Receptionist: _____

My Childbirth Education

Educator: _____

Address of classes: _____

_____

Telephone: _____

E-mail: _____

First class date: _____ Last class date: _____

First Signs

I first heard my baby's heartbeat: _____

I first felt my baby move: _____

Medications

Medications Taken	Dose	Date Started	Date Ended

Vital Statistics

Date of first day of my last menstrual period: _____

Date I think I ovulated: _____

Date I had a positive pregnancy test result at home: _____

The type of test I used: _____

My pre-pregnancy weight: _____ lb.

Date of my first prenatal check-up: _____

My symptoms: _____

_____

_____

Questions for my doctor: _____

_____

_____

_____

My blood type: _____ Rh factor: _____

Rubella status: _____

Special Tests

Date	Procedure	Findings

Prenatal Visits

Visit	Date	Weeks	Weight	Blood Pressure	Uterus Height (cm)	Questions/ comments
1st						
2nd						
3rd						
4th						
5th						
6th						
7th						
8th						
9th						
10th						
11th						
12th						
13th						

Labor and Delivery

My due date: _____ My labor began: _____

The date my baby was born: _____Time of delivery: _____

Delivered by: _____

My baby's weight: _____ My baby's length: _____

Hospital where my baby was born: _____

Medical Record

Mother: _____   Baby: _____
            (no.)   (no.)

Postpartum Visits

Mother:

Date: _____ Weight: _____ Blood pressure: _____

Family planning: _____

Comments: _____

_____

_____

_____

_____

_____

Baby:

Date: _____ Weight: _____ Length: _____

Special care: _____

Baby's feeding: _____

Comments: _____

_____

_____

_____

_____

_____

My Baby's Growth Charts

Developed by the National Center for Health Statistics in collaboration with the National Center for Chronic Disease Prevention and Health Promotion (2000).

Length-for-Age Percentiles—Boys

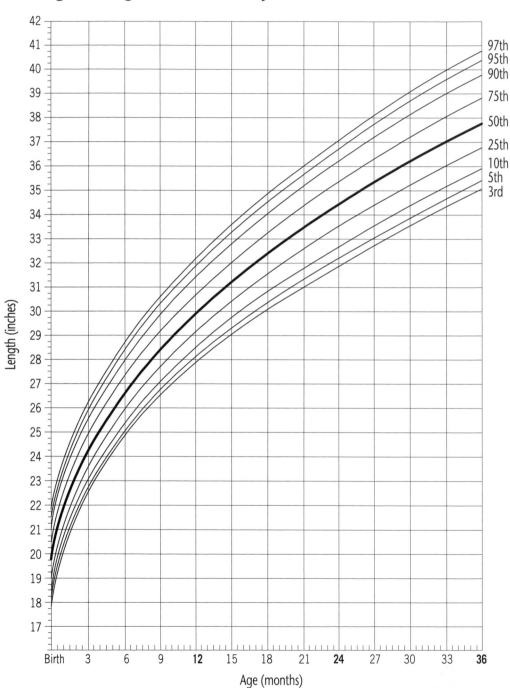

Length-for-Age Percentiles—Girls

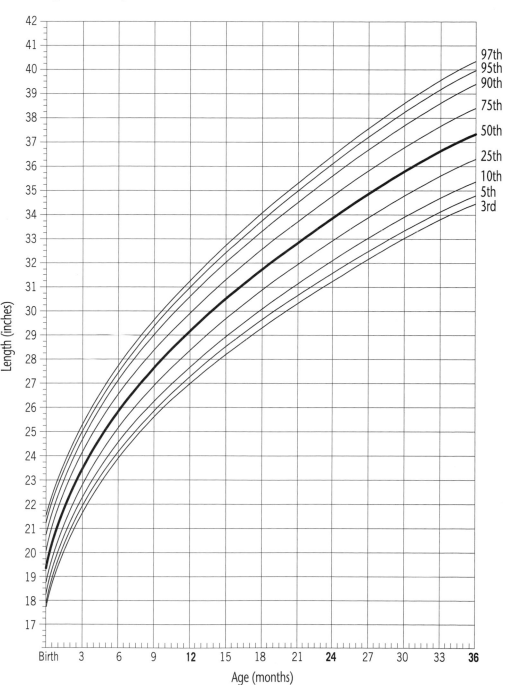

Weight-for-Age Percentiles—Boys

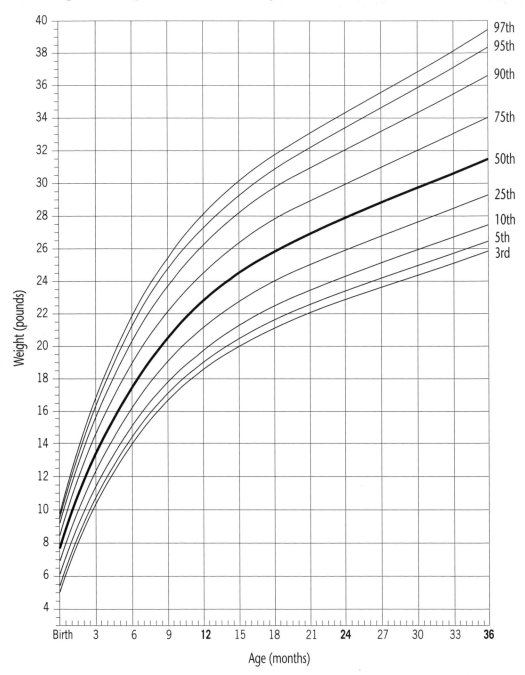

Weight-for-Age Percentile—Girls

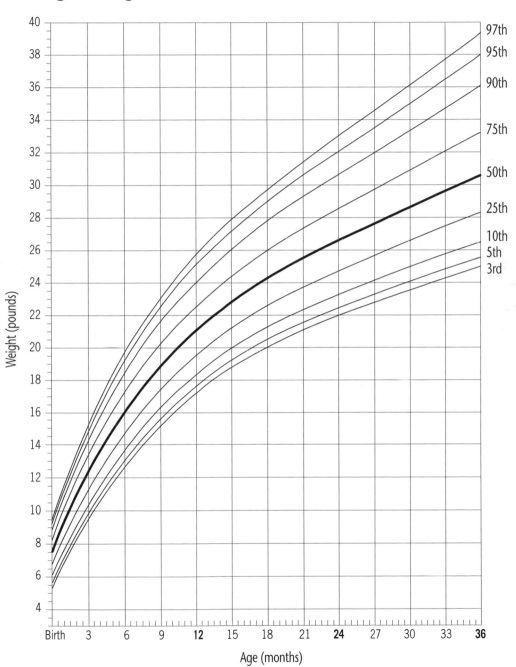

Resources

Pregnancy and Childbirth

The American College of Obstetricians and Gynecologists (ACOG)
409 12th Street, SW
Washington, DC 20024-2188
202-863-2518
E-mail: resources@acog.org
www.acog.org
Offers information and materials on pregnancy, childbirth, breastfeeding, fertility, and women's health.

American Institute of Ultrasound in Medicine (AIUM)
14750 Sweitzer Lane, Suite 100
Laurel, MD 20707-5906
800-638-5352 or 301-498-4100
Fax: 301-498-4450
E-mail: admin@aium.org
www.aium.org
Provides information about ultrasound exams.

American Society for Reproductive Medicine (ASRM)
1209 Montgomery Highway
Birmingham, AL 35216-2809
205-978-5000
Fax: 205-978-5005
E-mail: asrm@asrm.org
www.asrm.org
Offers information on fertility, multiple pregnancy, and assisted reproductive technology.

Maternal and Child Health Library National Center for Education in Maternal and Child Health
2115 Wisconsin Avenue, NW, Suite 601
Washington, DC 20007-2292
202-784-9770
Fax 202-784-9777
E-mail: mchlibrary@ncemch.org
www.ncemch.org
Provides research and information resources on maternal and child health.

National Healthy Mothers, Healthy Babies Coalition
121 North Washington Street, Suite 300
Alexandria, VA 22314-3022
703-836-6110
Fax: 703-836-3470
E-mail: info@hmhb.org
www.hmhb.org
Provides resources and education about healthy pregnancy and prenatal care.

National Institute of Child Health and Human Development (NICHD)
Building 31, 2A32, MSC 2425
31 Center Drive
Bethesda, MD 20892-0001
800-370-2943 or 301-496-5133
Fax: 301-496-7101
E-mail:
NICHDClearinghouse@mail.nih.gov
www.nichd.nih.gov
Provides information and education on pregnancy, infertility, preterm birth, birth defects, contraception, and sexually transmitted diseases.

National Women's Health Information Center
Office on Women's Health
Department of Health and Human Services
200 Independence Avenue, SW, Room 730B
Washington, DC 20201-0004
800-994- 9662
Fax: 888-220-5446 or 202-205-2631
www.4woman.gov
Offers information and resources in Spanish and English about pregnancy, contraception, and diseases affecting women.

Smoking and Substance Abuse

National Clearinghouse for Alcohol and Drug Information
U.S. Center for Substance Abuse Prevention
Parklawn Building
Rockwall Two, Ninth Floor
5600 Fishers Lane
Rockville, MD 20857-0001
800-729-6686 or 800-662-4357
Fax: 301-443-5447
www.ncadi.samhsa.gov
Offers materials for prevention and intervention in alcohol and drug abuse and provides a directory of alcoholism and drug abuse treatment and prevention services nationwide.

National Organization on Fetal Alcohol Syndrome
216 G Street, NE
Washington, DC 20002-4328
800-666-6327 or 202-785-4585
Fax: 202-466-6456
E-mail: info@nofas.org
www.nofas.org
Offers education and information about fetal alcohol syndrome and provides a directory to drug and alcohol abuse treatment programs nationwide.

National Partnership to Help Pregnant Smokers Quit
University of North Carolina, Chapel Hill
Cecil G. Sheps Center for Health Services
Research
725 Airport Road, CB 7590
Chapel Hill, NC 27599-7590
919-843-7663
Fax: 919-966-5764
E-mail:
info@helppregnantsmokersquit.org
www.helppregnantsmokersquit.org
Offers fact sheets and cessation tips and
techniques on quitting smoking.

Environmental Exposure to Toxins

Motherisk
c/o Hospital for Sick Children
555 University Avenue
Toronto, Ontario, Canada M5G 1X8
416-813-6780
Fax: 416-813-7562
E-mail: momrisk@sickkids.ca
www.motherisk.org
Answers questions about potential reproductive risks from exposure to drugs,
chemicals, radiation, and infections during
pregnancy and breastfeeding; will answer
inquiries from Canada or the United
States.

National Institute for Occupational Safety and Health (NIOSH)
4676 Columbia Parkway
Cincinnati, OH 45226
800-356-4674 or 513-533-8326
Fax: 513-533-8588
E-mail: eidtechinfo@cdc.gov
www.cdc.gov/niosh/homepage.html
Identifies workplace hazards and suggests
ways to limit the dangers; will inspect
workplace for hazards on request.

Occupational Safety and Health Administration (OSHA)
Office of Information and Consumer
Affairs
200 Constitution Avenue, NW
Room N-3647
Washington, DC 20210-0001
800-321-6742 or 202-523-1452 (voice)
877-889-5627 (TTY)
www.osha.gov
Provides information about and enforces
federal standards for workplace exposure
to substances and toxins during pregnancy.

Teratology Society
1767 Business Center Drive, Suite 302
Reston, VA 20190-0001
703-438-3104
Fax: 703-438-3113
E-mail: tshq@teratology.org
www.teratology.org
Supports research and provides information on substances affecting birth defects.

High-Risk Pregnancy

Coalition for Positive Outcomes in Pregnancy (CPOP)
507 Capitol Court, NE, Suite 200
Washington, DC 20002-4937
202-544-7499
Fax: 202-546-7105
E-mail: info@positivepregnancy.org
www.positivepregnancy.org
Provides information and responds to inquiries about the risk of preterm delivery.

Confinement Line
c/o Childbirth Education Association
PO Box 1609
Springfield, VA 22151-0609
703-941-7183
Provides telephone support and a newsletter for women confined to bed during pregnancy.

Sidelines National Support Network
PO Box 1808
Laguna Beach, CA 92652-1808
888-447-4754 or 949-497-2265
Fax: 949-497-5598
E-mail: sidelines@sidelines.org
www.sidelines.org
Offers emotional support and resources for women with high-risk pregnancies.

Nutrition

American Dietetic Association
120 South Riverside Plaza, Suite 2000
Chicago, IL 60606-6995
800-877-1600 or 312-899-0040
Fax: 312-899-4739
E-mail: hotline@eatright.org
www.eatright.org
Offers documents and information about nutrition during pregnancy and breast-feeding and provides referrals to nutrition professionals.

Special Supplemental Nutrition Program for Women, Infants, and Children (WIC Program)
Supplemental Food Programs Division
U.S. Department of Agriculture
3101 Park Center Drive, Room 520
Alexandria, VA 22302-1500
703-305-2746
Fax: 703-305-2196
E-mail: wichq-web@fns.usda.gov
www.fns.usda.gov/wic
Provides supplemental foods, nutrition education, and health care referrals for low-income pregnant, postpartum, and breastfeeding women and for infants and children up to 5 years of age.

Childbirth Education and Assistance

American Academy of Husband-Coached Childbirth (The Bradley Method)
PO Box 5224
Sherman Oaks, CA 91413-5224
800-422-4784 or 818-788-6662
www.bradleybirth.com
Provides information on natural childbirth and referrals to childbirth educators.

American College of Nurse–Midwives
818 Connecticut Avenue, Suite 900
Washington, DC 20006-2703
888-643-9433 or 202-728-9860
Fax: 202-728-9897
www.midwife.org
Offers a midwife locator service and information on emergency preparedness for birth.

Association of Labor Assistants & Childbirth Educators (ALACE)
PO Box 390436
Cambridge, MA 02139-0005
888-222-5223 or 617-441-2500
Fax: 617-441-3167
E-mail: info@alace.org
www.alace.org
Provides referrals to childbirth educators and doulas.

Cesarean Sections: Education and Concern (CSEC)
22 Forest Road
Framingham, MA 01701-4230
508-877-8266 (recorded message)
Offers support and information regarding cesarean birth, cesarean prevention, and vaginal delivery after cesarean.

Doulas of North America (DONA)
PO Box 626
Jasper, IN 47547-0626
888-788-3662
Fax: 812-634-1491
E-mail: doula@dona.org
www.dona.org
Provides referrals to birth doulas and postpartum doulas.

International Cesarean Awareness Network (ICAN)
1304 Kingsdale Avenue
Redondo Beach, CA 90278-3926
800-686-4226 or 310-542-6400;
Fax: 310-542-5368
E-mail: info@ican-online.org
www.ican-online.org
Provides information about cesarean delivery and recovery.

International Childbirth Education Association (ICEA)
PO Box 20048
Minneapolis, MN 55420-0048
800-624-4934 or 952-854-8660
Fax: 952-854-8772
E-mail: info@icea.org
www.icea.org
Offers lists of certified childbirth educators and doulas.

Lamaze International
2025 M Street, NW, Suite 800
Washington, DC 20036-3309
800-368-4404 or 202-367-1128
Fax: 202-267-2128
E-mail: info@lamaze.org
www.lamaze.org
Provides information about pregnancy and childbirth and referrals to Lamaze-trained childbirth educators.

Breastfeeding

American Academy of Pediatrics (AAP)
141 Northwest Point Boulevard
Elk Grove Village, IL 60007-1098
847-434-4000
Fax: 847-434-8000
E-mail: lactation@aap.org
Provides written materials about breastfeeding.

International Lactation Consultant Association (ILCA)
1500 Sunday Drive, Suite 102
Raleigh, NC 27607-5151
919-861-5577
Fax: 919-787-4916
E-mail: info@ilca.org
www.ilca.org
Provides a directory of lactation consultants.

La Leche League International (LLLI)
1400 North Meacham Road
Schaumburg, IL 60173-4808
800-525-3243 or 847-519-7730
Fax: 847-519-0035
E-mail: LLLI@LLLI.org
Provides information and support on breastfeeding and referrals to local support groups.

National Women's Health Information Center Breastfeeding Helpline
800-994-9662
Provides telephone support from breastfeeding information specialists and written materials in English, Spanish, and Chinese.

Loss and Grieving

CLIMB: Center for Loss in Multiple Birth, Inc.
PO Box 91377
Anchorage AK 99509-1377
907-222-5321
E-mail: climb@pobox.alaska.net
www.climb-support.org
Offers support for families that have lost twins or high-order multiples during pregnancy and through infancy and childhood.

The Compassionate Friends
PO Box 3696
Oak Brook, IL 60522-3696
877-969-0010 or 630-990-0010
Fax: 630-990-0246
E-mail: nationaloffice@compassionate
    friends.org
www.compassionatefriends.org
Offers support for families experiencing grief following the death of a child of any age.

First Candle/ SIDS Alliance
1314 Bedford Avenue, Suite 210
Baltimore, MD 21208-6605
Phone: 800-221-7437 or 410-653-8226
Fax: 410-653-8709
E-mail: info@firstcandle.org
www.sidsalliance.org
Supports research and education about sudden infant death syndrome; counseling service available at all times.

International Stillbirth Alliance
1427 Potter Road
Park Ridge, IL 60068
E-mail: info@stillbirthalliance.org
www.stillbirthalliance.org
Supports stillbirth research, education, and awareness.

SHARE: Pregnancy and Infant Loss Support, Inc.
St. Joseph's Health Center
300 First Capitol Drive
St. Charles, MO 63301-2893
800-821-6819 or 636-947-6164
Fax: 636-947-7486
E-mail: share@nationalshareoffice.com
www.nationalshareoffice.com
Offers support for families who have lost a baby through miscarriage, stillbirth, or newborn death.

Multiple Pregnancies

Mothers of Supertwins (MOST)
PO Box 951
Brentwood, NY 11717-0627
877-434-6678 or 631-859-1110
Fax: 631-859-3580
E-mail: info@mostonline.org
www.mostonline.org
Provides education, resources, and support during pregnancy, infancy, and childhood for families with triplets or higher numbers of babies.

National Organization of Mothers of Twins Clubs
PO Box 438
Thompsons Station, TN 37179-0438
877-540-2200 or 615-595-0936
E-mail: info@nomotc.org
www.nomotc.org
Provides support and practical advice for women expecting or rearing multiples.

Triplet Connection
PO Box 99571
Stockton, CA 95209-0571
209-474-0885
Fax: 209-474-9243
E-mail: tc@tripletconnection.org
www.tripletconnection.org
Provides information and support for families preparing for or rearing multiples.

Birth Defects

March of Dimes
1275 Mamaroneck Avenue
White Plains, NY 10605-5201
914-428-7100
Fax: 914-997-4537
www.marchofdimes.com
Provides materials in English and Spanish on genetic conditions, birth defects, recommended newborn screening tests, and bereavement materials for pregnancy loss.

National Center on Birth Defects and Developmental Disabilities
4770 Buford Highway, NE
Atlanta, GA 30341-3717
770-488-7150
Fax: 770-488-7156
E-mail: bddi@cdc.gov
www.cdc.gov/ncbddd
Provides information on birth defects, developmental disabilities, and hereditary blood disorders.

Specific Concerns

Motherisk Hotline
c/o Hospital for Sick Children
555 University Avenue
Toronto, Ontario, Canada M5G 1X8
800-436-8477
Provides a hotline for questions about nausea and vomiting in pregnancy.

National Domestic Violence Hotline
800-799-7233 (voice) or 800-787-3224 (TTY)
www.ndvh.org
Offers materials about abuse and domestic violence and referrals to shelters and other community resources.

International Travelers Hotline
(Operated by Centers for Disease Control
and Prevention)
888-232-3228
www.cdc.gov
Provides safety tips about travel in and
up-to-date vaccination facts for many
countries.

DES Action
610 16th Street, Suite 301
Oakland, CA 94612-1284
800-337-9288 or 510-465-4011
Fax: 510-465-4815
E-mail: desaction@earthlink.net
www.desaction.org
Provides materials in English and Spanish
and support for people exposed to diethylstilbestrol (DES) in utero.

Depression After Delivery, Inc.
91 East Somerset Street
Raritan, NJ 08869-2129
800-944-4773
Provides support, information, and referrals for women and families coping with
mental health issues associated with childbearing, both during pregnancy and postpartum.

Group B Strep Association
PO Box 16515
Chapel Hill, NC 27516-6515
919-932-5344
Fax: 919-932-3657
www.groupbstrep.org
Provides information in Spanish and
English and referrals to promote testing
and treatment of GBS.

Glossary

Acquired Immunodeficiency Syndrome (AIDS): A group of signs and symptoms, usually of severe infections, occurring in a person whose immune system has been damaged by infection with human immunodeficiency virus (HIV).

Alpha-fetoprotein (AFP): A protein produced by a growing fetus; it is present in amniotic fluid and, in smaller amounts, in the mother's blood.

Amniocentesis: A procedure in which a small amount of amniotic fluid and cells are taken from the sac surrounding the fetus and tested.

Amniotic Fluid: Water in the sac surrounding the fetus in the mother's uterus.

Amniotic Sac: Fluid-filled sac in the mother's uterus in which the fetus develops.

Analgesics: A type of drug that relieves pain without loss of muscle function.

Anemia: Abnormally low levels of blood or red blood cells in the bloodstream.

Most cases are caused by iron deficiency, or lack of iron.

Anencephaly: A type of neural tube defect that occurs when the fetus's head and brain do not develop normally.

Anesthetics: A type of drug that relieves pain by causing a loss of sensation.

Anesthesiologist: A doctor who is specially trained to give anesthesia.

Anorexia: An eating disorder in which distorted body image leads a person to diet excessively.

Antibiotic: A drug that treats infections.

Antibodies: Proteins in the blood produced in reaction to foreign substances, an antigen.

Anticonvulsant: A drug that controls or prevents seizures (as in epilepsy).

Antigen: A substance, such as an organism causing infection or a protein found on the surface of blood cells, that can induce an immune response and cause the production of an antibody.

Apgar Score: A measurement of a baby's response to birth and life on its own, taken 1 and 5 minutes after birth.

Areola: The darker skin around the nipple.

Auscultation: A method of listening to internal organs, such as the fetal heartbeat during labor.

Autopsy: An exam performed on a deceased person in an attempt to find the cause of death.

Bacterial Vaginosis: A type of vaginal infection caused by the overgrowth of a number of organisms that are normally found in the vagina.

Barrier Methods: Contraception that prevents sperm from entering the female reproductive system.

Bilirubin: A reddish-yellow pigment that occurs especially in bile and blood and may cause jaundice.

Biophysical Profile: An assessment by ultrasound of fetal breathing, fetal body movement, fetal muscle tone, and the amount of amniotic fluid. May include fetal heart rate.

Blastocyst: The ball of cells created when the sperm and egg join and start dividing. The blastocyst travels into the uterus and is embedded in the lining of the uterus.

Braxton Hicks Contractions: False labor pains.

Breast Implants: Sacs filled with saline or silicone gel that are placed in the area of the breast.

Breech: A situation in which a fetus's buttocks or feet would be born first.

Bulimia: An eating disorder in which a person binges on food and then forces vomiting or abuses laxatives.

Calories: Units of heat used to express the fuel or energy value of food.

Carpal Tunnel Syndrome: A condition caused by compression of a nerve where it passes through the wrist into the hand and characterized especially by weakness, pain, and disturbances of sensation in the hand.

Carrier: A person who shows no signs of a particular trait or disorder but has the gene and could pass the gene on to his or her children.

Catheter: A tube used to drain fluid or urine from the body.

Cephalopelvic Disproportion: A condition in which a baby is too large to pass safely through the mother's pelvis during delivery.

Cerclage: A procedure to sew the cervix shut.

Cervix: The lower, narrow end of the uterus, which protrudes into the vagina.

Cesarean Delivery: Birth of a baby through an incision made in the mother's abdomen and uterus.

Chancre: An sore appearing at the place of infection.

Chlamydia: A sexually transmitted disease that can lead to pelvic inflammatory disease, infertility, and problems during pregnancy.

Chloasma: The darkening of areas of skin on the face during pregnancy.

Cholesterol: A natural substance that serves as a building block for cells and hormones and helps to carry fat through the blood vessels for use or storage in other parts of the body.

Chorioamnionitis: Inflammation or infection of the membrane surrounding the fetus.

Chorionic Villus Sampling (CVS): A procedure in which a small sample of cells is taken from the placenta and tested.

Chromosomes: Structures that are located inside each cell in the body and contain the genes that determine a person's physical makeup.

Cleft Palate: A congenital defect in which a gap or space occurs in the roof of the mouth.

Clubfoot: A misshaped foot twisted out of position from birth.

Colonized: Having bacteria in your body that could cause illness, but having no symptoms of the disease.

Colostrum: A fluid secreted from the breasts at the beginning of milk production.

Congenital Disorder: A condition that is present in a baby when it is born.

Contraction Stress Test: A test in which mild contractions of the mother's uterus are induced and the fetus's heart rate in response to the contractions is recorded using an electronic fetal monitor.

Corticosteroids: Hormones given to mature fetal lungs, for arthritis, or other medical conditions.

Crowning: The appearance of the baby's head at the vaginal opening during labor.

Cystic Fibrosis: A life-long illness in infants, children, and young adults that causes problems with digestion and breathing.

Cystitis: An infection of the bladder.

Cytomegalovirus (CMV): A virus in the herpes virus family that can be passed on to a baby during pregnancy, birth, or breastfeeding and can cause problems with the liver, hearing, vision, and mental functioning.

Diabetes: A condition in which the levels of sugar in the blood are too high.

Diastolic Blood Pressure: The force of the blood in the arteries when the heart is relaxed; the lower blood pressure reading.

Doppler: A form of ultrasound that reflects motion—such as the fetal heartbeat—in the form of audible signals.

Down Syndrome: A genetic disorder in which mental retardation, abnormal features of the face, and medical problems such as heart defects occur.

Ectopic Pregnancy: A pregnancy in which the fertilized egg begins to grow in a place other than inside the uterus, usually in the fallopian tubes.

Edema: Swelling caused by fluid retention.

Effacement: Thinning of the cervix during the beginning stages of labor.

Egg: The female reproductive cell produced in and released from the ovaries; also called the ovum.

Electrode: A small wire that is attached to the scalp of the fetus to monitor the heart rate.

Electronic Fetal Monitor: An electronic instrument used to record the heartbeat of the fetus and contractions of the mother's uterus.

Embryo: The developing fertilized egg of early pregnancy.

Epidural Block: Anesthesia that numbs the lower half of the body.

Episiotomy: A surgical incision made into the perineum (the region between the vagina and the anus) to widen the vaginal opening for delivery.

Estrogen: A female hormone produced in the ovaries.

External Version: A technique, performed late in pregnancy, in which the doctor manually attempts to move a breech baby into the head-down position.

Fallopian Tube: A tube through which an egg travels from the ovary to the uterus.

Fertilization: Joining of the egg and sperm.

Fetal Alcohol Syndrome: A pattern of physical, mental, and behavioral problems in the baby that are thought to be due to alcohol abuse by the mother during pregnancy.

Fetal Monitoring: A procedure in which instruments are used to record the heartbeat of the fetus and contractions of the mother's uterus during labor.

Fetoscope: A stethoscope designed for listening to the fetal heartbeat.

Fetus: A baby growing in the woman's uterus.

Fibroids: Benign growths that form in the muscle of the uterus.

Fibronectin: A type of protein made by the fetus that can be measured in secretions from the cervix.

Follicle-Stimulating Hormone (FSH): A hormone produced by the pituitary gland that helps an egg to mature.

Forceps: Special instruments placed around the baby's head to help guide it out of the birth canal during delivery.

Foreskin: A layer of skin covering the end of the penis.

Fragile X Syndrome: A genetic disease, inherited through the X chromosome, that is the most common inherited cause of mental retardation.

Fraternal Twins: Twins, developed from two fertilized eggs, who are not genetically identical.

Fundus: The top part of the uterus.

Genes: DNA "blueprints" that code for specific traits, such as hair and eye color.

General Anesthesia: The use of drugs that produce a sleep-like state to prevent pain during surgery.

Genital Herpes: A sexually transmitted disease caused by a virus that produces painful, highly infectious sores on or around the sex organs.

Genital Warts: A sexually transmitted disease that is linked to cervical changes and cervical cancer.

Gestational Diabetes: Diabetes that arises during pregnancy.

Gestational Hypertension: High blood pressure that occurs during the second half of pregnancy and disappears soon after the baby is born.

Glans: The head of the penis.

Glucose: A sugar that is present in the blood and is the body's main source of fuel.

Gonadotropin-releasing Hormone (GnRH): Medical therapy used to block the effects of certain hormones.

Gonorrhea: A sexually transmitted disease that can lead to pelvic inflammatory disease, infertility, and arthritis.

Hepatitis B Immune Globulin: A substance given to provide temporary protection against infection with hepatitis B virus.

Hepatitis B Virus: A virus that attacks and damages the liver, causing inflammation.

Human Chorionic Gonadotropin (hCG): A hormone produced during pregnancy; its detection is the basis for most pregnancy tests.

Human Immunodeficiency Virus (HIV): A virus that attacks certain cells of the body's immune system and causes acquired immunodeficiency syndrome (AIDS).

Human Papillomavirus (HPV): The common name for a group of related viruses, some of which cause genital warts and are linked to cervical changes and cervical cancer.

Hydramnios: A condition in which there is an excess amount of amniotic fluid in the sac surrounding the fetus.

Hyperemesis Gravidarum: Severe nausea and vomiting during pregnancy that can lead to loss of weight and body fluids.

Identical Twins: Twins, developed from a single fertilized egg, who usually are genetically identical.

Immune System: The body's natural defense system against foreign substances and invading organisms, such as bacteria that cause disease.

Incontinence: Inability to control bodily functions such as urination.

Intrauterine Device (IUD): A small device that is inserted and left inside the uterus to prevent pregnancy.

Inverted Nipples: Nipples that have pulled inward.

Ischial Spines: Bony parts that stick out on each side of the pelvis.

Jaundice: A buildup of bilirubin that causes a yellowish appearance.

Kegel Exercises: Pelvic muscle exercises that assist in bladder and bowel control.

Kick Counts: Records kept during late pregnancy of the number of times a fetus moves over a certain period.

Labor Induction: Using medical or surgical methods to stimulate contractions of the uterus.

Lactation Specialist: A doctor, nurse, or other health professional specially trained to help with breastfeeding.

Lactose Intolerance: Being unable to digest dairy products.

Lanugo: Fine hair that sometimes grows on a baby's back and shoulders at birth; it goes away in 1 or 2 weeks.

Let-Down Reflex: A bodily process, triggered when a baby starts to nurse, that signals ducts in the breasts to contract and release milk from the nipples.

Lightening: When the fetus's head moves down into the uterus and presses against the mother's uterus a few weeks before birth.

Linea Nigra: A line running from the navel to pubic hair that darkens during pregnancy.

Local Anesthesia: The use of drugs that prevent pain in a part of the body.

Lochia: Vaginal discharge that occurs after delivery.

Luteinizing Hormone (LH): A hormone produced by the pituitary gland that helps an egg to mature and be released.

Macrosomia: A condition in which a fetus grows very large.

Maternal Serum Screening: A group of blood tests that check for substances linked with certain birth defects.

Meconium: A greenish substance that builds up in the bowels of a growing fetus.

Miscarriage: Early pregnancy loss.

Multiple Pregnancy: A pregnancy in which there are two or more fetuses.

Neural Tube Defects: Birth defects that result from incomplete development of the brain, spinal cord, or their coverings.

Nonstress Test: A test in which changes in the fetal heart rate are recorded, using an electronic fetal monitor.

Nuchal Translucency Screening: A special ultrasound test of the fetus to screen for the risk of Down syndrome and other birth defects.

Oral Contraceptives: Birth control pills containing hormones that prevent ovulation and thus pregnancy.

Osteoporosis: A condition in which the bones become so fragile that they break more easily.

Ovaries: Two glands, located on either side of the uterus, that contain the eggs released at ovulation and that produce hormones.

Ovulate: To release an egg from one of the ovaries.

Oxytocin: A hormone used to help bring on contractions of the uterus.

Pap Test: A test in which cells are taken from the cervix and vagina and examined under a microscope.

Pelvic Exam: A manual examination of a woman's reproductive organs.

Perineum: The area between the vagina and the rectum.

Pica: The urge to eat nonfood items.

Pituitary Gland: A gland located near the brain that controls growth and other changes in the body.

Placenta: Tissue that provides nourishment to and takes away waste from the fetus.

Placenta Previa: A condition in which the placenta lies very low in the uterus, so that the opening of the uterus is partially or completely covered.

Placental Abruption: A condition in which the placenta has begun to separate from the inner wall of the uterus before the baby is born.

Polydactyly: The condition of having more than the normal number of fingers or toes.

Postpartum Blues: Feelings of sadness, fear, anger, or anxiety occurring about 3 days after childbirth and usually going away (ending) within 1–2 weeks.

Postpartum Depression: Intense feelings of sadness, anxiety, or despair after childbirth that interfere with a new mother's ability to function and that do not go away after 2 weeks.

Preeclampsia: A condition of pregnancy in which there is high blood pressure and protein in the urine.

Premature Rupture of Membranes: A condition in which the membranes that hold the amniotic fluid rupture before labor.

Preterm: Born before 37 weeks of pregnancy.

Progesterone: A female hormone that is produced in the ovaries and that prepares the lining of the uterus for pregnancy.

Progestin: A synthetic form of progesterone that is similar to the hormone produced naturally by the body.

Prostaglandins: Chemicals that are made by the body that have many effects, including causing the muscle of the uterus to contract, usually causing cramps.

Pyelonephritis: An infection of the kidney.

Quickening: The mother's first feeling of movement of the fetus.

Respiratory Distress Syndrome: A condition causing breathing difficulties in some babies in whom the lungs are not mature.

Rh Factor: A kind of protein in some types of blood that causes responses in the immune system.

Rh Immunoglobulin (RhIg): A substance given to prevent an Rh-negative person's antibody response to Rh-positive blood cells.

Ripening: The softening of the cervix that occurs before the onset of labor.

Rupture of Membranes: The breaking of the amniotic sac that surrounds the fetus.

Screening Tests: Tests that look for possible signs of disease in people who do not have symptoms.

Sexually Transmitted Diseases (STDs): Diseases that are spread by sexual contact.

Show: The discharge, often mucus and some blood, that occurs as labor approaches. It also refers to the mucus plug that pushes out when the cervix begins to efface or dilate.

Speculum: An instrument used to spread the walls of the vagina.

Sperm: A male cell that is produced in the testes and can fertilize a female egg cell.

Spina Bifida: A neural tube defect that results from incomplete closure of the fetal spine.

Spinal Block: A form of anesthesia that numbs the lower half of the body.

Station: The relationship of the baby's head to a bony landmark in the pelvis.

Stillbirth: Delivery of a baby that shows no sign of life.

Sudden Infant Death Syndrome (SIDS): The unexpected death of an infant and in which the cause is unknown.

Surfactant: A substance, coating the air sacs in the lungs, that helps the lungs expand.

Syphilis: A sexually transmitted disease that is caused by an organism called *Treponema pallidum*; it may cause major health problems or death in its later stages.

Systemic Analgesics: Drugs that provide pain relief over the entire body without causing loss of consciousness.

Systolic Blood Pressure: The force of the blood in the arteries when the heart is contracting; the higher blood pressure reading.

Teratogens: Agents that can cause birth defects when a woman is exposed to them during pregnancy.

Tocolytics: Medications used to delay preterm labor.

Toxoplasmosis: An infection caused by *Toxoplasma gondii*, an organism that may be found in raw and rare meat, garden soil, and cat feces and that can be harmful to the fetus.

Transducer: A device that emits sound waves and translates the echoes into electrical signals.

Trichomoniasis: A type of vaginal infection caused by a one-celled organism that usually is transmitted through sex.

Trimesters: The three 3-month periods into which pregnancy is divided.

Ultrasound: A test in which sound waves are used to examine internal structures; during pregnancy, it can be used to examine the fetus.

Umbilical Cord: A cord-like structure containing blood vessels that connects the fetus to the placenta.

Uterus: A muscular organ located in the female pelvis that contains and nourishes the developing fetus during pregnancy.

Vaccination: Inoculation with a virus to produce immunity.

Vacuum Extraction: The use of a special instrument attached to the baby's head to help guide it out of the birth canal during delivery.

Vagina: A tube-like structure surrounded by muscles leading from the uterus to the outside of the body.

Varicose Veins: Abnormally swollen or dilated veins.

Vasectomy: A method of male sterilization in which a portion of the vas deferens is removed or blocked.

Vernix: The greasy, whitish coating of a newborn.

Vertex Presentation: A normal position of a fetus in which the head is positioned down, ready to come through the vagina first.

Vibroacoustic Stimulation: The use of sound and vibration to wake the fetus during a nonstress test.

Index

Note: Page numbers followed by letters *f* and *t* indicate figures and tables, respectively.